Endocrine Pathophysiology:

A Patient-Oriented Approach

WAYNE PRATT
1-88

Endocrine Pathop

A Patient-Oriented Approac

JEROME M. HERSHMAN, M.D.

Professor of Medicine,
UCLA School of Medicine,
Chief, Endocrinology Section,
Medical Service,
Veterans Administration Wadsworth Medical Center
Los Angeles, California

Third Edition

Lea & Febiger   *Philadelphia   1988*

Reprinted,

Library of Congress Cataloging-in-Publication Data

Endocrine pathophysiology.

Includes bibliographies and index.
1. Endocrine glands—Diseases. 2. Physiology,
Pathological. I. Hershman, Jerome M., 1932–
[DNLM: 1. Endocrine Diseases—physiopathology.
WK 100 E5155]
RC649.E52   1987   616.4'07   87-3931
ISBN 0-8121-1093-5

PRINTED IN THE UNITED STATES OF AMERICA

Print number: 5   4   3   2   1

Preface

The purpose of this book is to give medical students an understanding of the pathophysiology of endocrine diseases. Although the authors assume that the student has taken introductory courses in biochemistry and physiology that pertain to endocrinology, each chapter begins with a succinct review of the aspects of basic endocrinology that are most relevant to clinical medicine.

Endocrine disorders mainly involve either excessive or decreased secretion of specific hormones. The text presents the modern methods of testing specific glandular function for these disorders, and provides the basic understanding of each test.

Systematic discussions of endocrine pathophysiology explain the symptoms and signs of endocrine diseases. The chapters also present the principles of therapy for each disorder and relevant clinical pharmacology. Descriptions and illustrations of endocrine pathology are brief, so that the student desiring more complete discussions of pathology must consult a standard textbook of pathology.

Chapters 2 through 11 present patients with endocrine disorders to illustrate the clinical findings and the use of diagnostic tests. Questions pertaining to these patients test the reader's understanding of the material, emphasizing clinical concepts and thought processes. The answers to questions appear at the end of the chapter. Students at the UCLA School of Medicine have found that this patient-oriented approach more actively involves them and aids in comprehension.

The third edition of "Endocrine Pathophysiology: A Patient-Oriented Approach" has been completely rewritten and revised to include the many significant advances in understanding endocrine disease that have occurred in the decade since the first edition appeared. Obsolete material has been deleted to maintain a concise text.

Although this book is aimed primarily at medical students, residents in medicine, internists, and family physicians will find it useful as a succinct review of current concepts in clinical endocrinology.

Los Angeles, California   Jerome M. Hershman

Contributors

Shalender Bhasin, M.D.
Assistant Professor of Medicine
UCLA School of Medicine
Division of Endocrinology
Harbor—UCLA Medical Center
Torrance, CA 90509

Glenn D. Braunstein, M.D.
Professor of Medicine
UCLA School of Medicine
Director, Department of Medicine
Cedars-Sinai Medical Center
Los Angeles, California 90048

Harold E. Carlson, M.D.
Chief, Endocrinology Section
Professor of Medicine
State University of New York at Stony Brook
Northport VA Medical Center
Northport, NY 11768

Mayer B. Davidson, M.D.
Professor of Medicine
UCLA School of Medicine
Director, Diabetes Program,
Cedars-Sinai Medical Center
Los Angeles, California 90048

Theodore H. Hahn, M.D.
Professor of Medicine
UCLA School of Medicine
Endocrinology Section
Wadsworth V.A. Medical Center
Wilshire and Sawtelle Blvd.
Los Angeles, CA 90073

Robert A. Kreisberg, M.D.
Professor of Medicine
University of Alabama at Birmingham
Chief, Medical Service
Birmingham VA Hospital
Birmingham, AL

Myron Miller, M.D.
Professor and Vice Chairman
Department of Geriatrics
Mount Sinai University School of Medicine
One Gustave L. Levy Place
New York, NY 10029

Barbara Lippe, M.D.
Professor of Pediatrics
UCLA School of Medicine
Los Angeles, California 90024

Naftali Stern, M.D.
Assistant Professor of Medicine
UCLA School of Medicine
Section of Endocrinology
V.A. Medical Center
Sepulveda, CA 91343

Ronald S. Swerdloff, M.D.
Professor of Medicine
UCLA School of Medicine
Chief, Division of Endocrinology
Harbor-UCLA Medical Center
Torrance, California 90509

Michael Tuck, M.D.
Professor of Medicine
UCLA School of Medicine
Los Angeles, California 90024
Chief, Endocrinology Section
VA Medical Center
Sepulveda, California 91343

Contents

1

Principles of Clinical Endocrinology

Jerome M. Hershman

ABBREVIATIONS

ACTH	adrenocorticotropic hormone
T_4	thyroxine
T_3	triiodothyronine
TSH	thyroid-stimulating hormone

Clinical disorders of endocrine glands are mainly of two types: hyperfunction and hypofunction. Hyperfunction denotes excessive secretion of the hormone. The clinical findings or the signs and symptoms of the disorder reflect the effects of excessive amounts of the hormone on sensitive target tissues. Hypofunction denotes deficient secretion of the hormone: the resulting signs and symptoms occur because the amount of the hormone is insufficient to achieve its normal effect on target tissues.

The concept of hyperfunction and hypofunction of endocrine glands implies that these states differ from normal hormone secretion. Unfortunately, the normal range of many hormone measurements overlaps both deficiency and excess of hormonal blood levels and hormonal production. Single baseline values rarely can be used to establish a definitive diagnosis. The physiologic concept of feedback control also serves as a basis for diagnosing hyperfunction and hypofunction of endocrine glands and allows each hormone system to be considered dynamically.

NEGATIVE FEEDBACK

Pituitary tropic hormones, such as thyroid-stimulating hormone (TSH) or adrenocorticotropic hormone (ACTH), stimulate the target organs (thyroid or adrenal in these cases) to release the target gland hormones (thyroxine, T_4, and triiodothyronine, T_3, or cortisol). In turn, elevated levels of the target gland hormone feed back on the pituitary to inhibit secretion of the tropic hormone. The corollary is that the pituitary detects low levels of the target gland hormone and thus increases its tropic hormone secretion, which causes increased secretion of the target gland hormone. Consider the examples of TSH-T_4 (or TSH-T_3) and ACTH-cortisol in terms of a need to increase the output of the target gland hormone. Application of this concept to all hormones which are controlled by feedback inhibition aids understanding of clinical diagnostic tests.

An x-y plot of tropic verus target gland hormone levels in the blood (Fig. 1–1) illustrates useful dynamic concepts and aids understanding of clinical terminology. Consider the possible levels of ACTH-cortisol or TSH-T_4 based on Figure 1–1.

Hypothalamic hormones, secreted into a portal venous system that reaches the pituitary directly, regulate secretion of the pituitary hormones. For each pituitary hormone, a hypothalamic releasing hormone exists, and for some pituitary hormones, hypothalamic factors inhibit release of the pituitary hormones. The hypothalamic hormones are useful diagnostic tools for testing the response of the pituitary gland and, in turn, the target glands. Several chapters describe the clinical applications of the hypothalamic hormones and the stimuli that alter their secretion.

CATEGORIES OF ENDOCRINE FUNCTION TESTS

Measurement of the basal level of hormone in blood or urine may be satisfactory for making a diagnosis of hyperfunction or hypofunction when

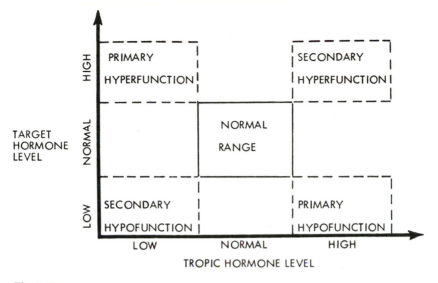

Fig. 1–1.

the disorder is severe, especially when the tests illustrate normal feedback relationships; for example, low T_4 in serum and high TSH in serum indicate primary hypothyroidism.

Stimulation Test. Evaluation of secretory reserve by a stimulation is useful for diagnosing hypofunction and for detecting impaired secretory reserve.

Suppression Test. These tests are useful for diagnosis of hyperfunction because the hyperfunctioning gland is not operating under normal control mechanisms; suppression may be abnormal quantitatively or qualitatively. By negative feedback control, the pituitary gland may be "reset" to respond to high levels of the suppressing hormone; for example, pituitary ACTH secretion in Cushing's disease, which is discussed later. The tropic hormone may be produced in an uncontrolled manner by a cancer, as occurs in the ectopic ACTH syndrome. An abnormal stimulator may be the cause of hyperfunction. A thyroid-stimulating immunoglobulin is responsible for the hyperthyroidism of Graves' disease. On the other hand, the gland may be autonomous and secreting without any control, such as an adrenal adenoma causing hyper-cortisolism or a thyroid adenoma causing hyperthyroidism.

Table 1–1 shows the general scheme of interpretation of suppression and stimulation tests.

TYPES OF HORMONE MEASUREMENTS

These techniques are usually applied to blood serum (or plasma) and urine.

Bioassay. This method is usually not sufficiently sensitive for detection of physiologic levels of hormones and is relatively expensive.

Table 1–1.   General Scheme for Interpretation of Suppression
and Stimulation Tests

Evaluation of Hyperfunction

Baseline Hormone Level or Secretion Rate	Suppression Test	Interpretation of Function
Normal	Normal	Normal
Elevated	Normal	Normal
Elevated	Nonsuppressible	Hyperfunction*

Evaluation of Hypofunction

Baseline Hormone Level or Secretion Rate	Stimulation Test	Interpretation of Function
Normal	Normal	Normal
Low	Normal	Normal
Low	Nonstimulable	Hypofunction
"Low normal"	Nonstimulable	Impaired reserve function†

*Degree of hyperfunction varies from mild to severe.
†Patient may be asymptomatic or have symptoms and signs of hypofunction.

Chemical Measurement. This method measures the hormone, for example, plasma cortisol by fluorimetry, or a hormone metabolite, such as metanephrine in urine as an index of secretion of norepinephrine and epinephrine. Chemical methods are also used to measure a physiologic consequence, such as plasma glucose as an index of insulin secretion.

Radioimmunoassay. A specific antibody is used to recognize the hormone, but the antibody may also detect a biologically inactive portion of the molecule, such as the carboxy-terminal fragment of parathyroid hormone. Because these assays are so sensitive, they are used extensively to measure blood levels of hormones. Usually, the hormone as antigen is labeled with radioactivity as a tracer, but enzymes which yield colorimetric endpoints are also attached as tracers (enzyme immunoassay). The recent use of monoclonal antibodies which are labeled with tracers has led to development of new assays (immunometric) with greatly improved sensitivity.

Radioreceptor Assays. These biologically specific tests may be highly sensitive. An example is the use of plasma membranes of target organs as receptors for peptide hormones, for example, the thyroid plasma membrane for detection of TSH-displacing activity as a marker for Graves' disease.

Metabolic Effects. These tests measure the hormone's effects on a target tissue, for example, systolic time interval to assess the action of thyroid hormone on the heart.

Clinical Assessment Only. In some cases, there is no readily available bioassay, or the clinical situation may provide all of the bioassay data needed; for example, normal menstrual cycles indicate integrity of the hypothalamic-pituitary-gonadal axis in women.

TERMS

The following terms are used in clinical endocrinology.

Primary Hyperfunction. Hypersecretion of a hormone usually due to tumor or disease of an endocrine gland itself.

Secondary Hyperfunction. Hypersecretion of a hormone produced by excessive stimulation from its tropic hormone or its physiologic stimulators; no disease of the gland per se.

Primary Hypofunction. Hyposecretion of a hormone due to disease of the gland of secretion.

Secondary Hypofunction. Hyposecretion of a hormone due to lack of a tropic hormone or lack of the physiologic stimulators.

Suppression Test. Administration of the suppressor to test autonomy of hormonal secretion.

Stimulation Test. Administration of the specific stimulator to test hormonal secretory reserve of the gland.

Secretion Rate. Amount of hormone secreted per unit of time.

Production Rate. Amount of hormone produced outside the gland plus that amount secreted by the gland per unit of time.

Half-Life in Blood. Time for blood level of hormone to fall to half of its original value.

Protein-Bound Fraction of Hormone. That fraction of hormone bound to its specific plasma binding protein and therefore considered to be physiologically inactive.

Free or Unbound Fraction. That fraction of the plasma hormone not protein bound—presumably, the physiologically active fraction.

2

Pituitary Disease

Harold E. Carlson

ABBREVIATIONS

ACTH	adrenocorticotropic hormone
CRH	corticotropin-releasing hormone
Compound S	11-deoxycortisol
FSH	follicle-stimulating hormone
GH	growth hormone
GRF	growth hormone releasing factor
GnRH=	gonadotropin-releasing hormone =
LH-RH	luteinizing hormone releasing hormone
hCG	human chorionic gonadotropin
LH	luteinizing hormone
MSH	melanocyte-stimulating hormone
PRL	prolactin
T_4	thyroxine
T_3	triiodothyronine
TSH	thyroid-stimulating hormone (thyrotropin)
TRH	thyrotropin-releasing hormone

PITUITARY ANATOMY

The anterior pituitary gland or adenohypophysis is derived from an ecto-dermal outpouching of the oropharynx (Rathke's pouch), while the posterior pituitary lobe or neurohypophysis develops as a downward outpouching of the third ventricle. The arterial blood supply of the anterior lobe first enters a capillary network in the median eminence of the hypothalamus where re-leasing and inhibiting factors enter the circulation; these factors are then carried in the long portal veins to the adenohypophysis where they regulate the secretion of the anterior pituitary hormones.

EVALUATION OF ANTERIOR PITUITARY FUNCTION

As described in Chapter 1, the function of an endocrine gland is usually assessed by means of specific stimulation and suppression tests, which make use of known normal responses to perturbation in homeostatic regulatory mechanisms. For the pituitary gland, such tests are commonly used to evaluate the secretory status of most of the individual hormones. The following sections briefly cover the structures and functions of the pituitary hormones, along with the factors (both physiologic and pharmacologic) that alter and regulate their secretion. Table 2–1 summarizes clinically useful pituitary stimulation and suppression tests.

Adrenocorticotropic Hormone (ACTH)

ACTH is a single-chain polypeptide of 39 amino acids whose principal function is the stimulation of cortisol production by the adrenal cortex. ACTH is synthesized in the corticotroph cells of the anterior pituitary as part of a large glycopeptide (mw = 31,000 daltons) called pro-opiomelanocortin. This precursor molecule is cleaved intracellularly into smaller fragments with bio-

Table 2–1.   Clinically Useful Tests of Pituitary Function

Hormone	Stimulation Test	Suppression Tests
ACTH	Insulin hypoglycemia Metyrapone CRH	Dexamethasone administration
TSH	TRH	T_3 or T_4 administration (not standardized)
LH/FSH	GnRH (LH-RH) Clomiphene	Testosterone or estrogen administration (not standardized)
GH	Insulin hypoglycemia Arginine infusion L-dopa GRF	Glucose tolerance
PRL	TRH Chlorpromazine Metoclopramide	None

logic activity, including ACTH and β-lipotropin. Like most polypeptide hormones, ACTH appears to act by binding to a specific cell membrane receptor and activating adenylate cyclase, which raises intracellular levels of cyclic adenosine monophosphate (cAMP). This action initiates a series of biochemical events culminating in cortisol synthesis and release.

Normally, ACTH secretion (and, hence, cortisol secretion) is episodic, with many secretory pulses occurring throughout the day and night; these pulses presumably reflect the episodic secretion of corticotropin-releasing hormone (CRH), the hypothalamic substance which stimulates ACTH secretion. The ACTH pulses appear to be larger and more frequent during the early morning hours resulting, on an average, in a peak of both ACTH and cortisol blood levels at about 6:00 to 8:00 A.M. and a low point in the late afternoon or evening. This 24-hour neural rhythm is basically determined by the sleep-wake cycle and adjusts over a period of 2 to 3 weeks to changes in the pattern of sleep and activity.

When pathologic hypersecretion of ACTH is present, blood levels of ACTH and cortisol (if the adrenal glands are intact) are often elevated in the basal state, and the elevation persists in the face of large doses of exogenous glucocorticoid. Such suppression tests, generally using the administration of dexamethasone, are discussed in detail in later sections dealing with the adrenal cortex (Chap. 4). Normal feedback mechanisms lead to secondary hypersecretion of ACTH in patients with primary adrenal failure; in this instance, the elevation of plasma ACTH is readily suppressed by replacement of the missing glucocorticoid (see Fig. 4–1).

Several factors stimulate ACTH release:
1. Corticotropin-releasing hormone (CRH), the final common pathway for most stimuli to ACTH secretion, is a 41-amino acid polypeptide.
2. Low plasma levels of glucocorticoid.
3. A variety of stresses, such as exercise, anxiety, pain, and anesthesia.
4. Hypoglycemia.
5. Bacterial pyrogens.
6. Vasopressin.

Since most stimuli probably act by increasing hypothalamic secretion of CRH, they depend on an intact hypothalamus and pituitary for a normal response. Vasopressin may act directly on the pituitary corticotrophs, according to some studies.

Procedures commonly used to stimulate ACTH secretion in the clinical evaluation of pituitary function include:
1. Hypoglycemia. Regular insulin, 0.1 or 0.15 U/kg body weight, is injected as an intravenous bolus. The blood sugar drops by at least 50% of its initial level 30 to 45 minutes after injection, provoking ACTH and cortisol secretion, which peaks 60 to 90 minutes after insulin administration. A normal plasma cortisol response consists of a rise of at least 7 µg/dl, reaching peak levels of at least 20 µg/dl (Fig. 2–1).
2. Metyrapone. Oral or intravenous administration of metyrapone, an

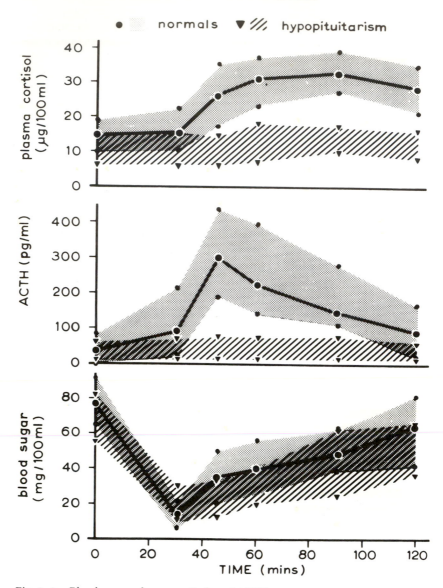

Fig. 2–1. Blood sugar, plasma cortisol, and ACTH responses to intravenous insulin in normal subjects and patients with hypopituitarism; the insulin was given at 0 min. The mean responses in normal subjects are shown by the continuous solid lines, while the shaded areas give the range of the observed responses. (From Donald, R.A.: J Clin Endocrinol Metab, *32*:225, 1971.)

adrenal inhibitor that blocks the 11-hydroxylase reaction (the final step in cortisol synthesis), lowers plasma cortisol and consequently increases ACTH secretion. This increase in ACTH stimulates the adrenal gland and results in an accumulation of cortisol precursors behind the 11-hydroxylase block. In normal subjects, the immediate precursor of cortisol, 11-deoxycortisol (also known as compound S) is secreted in increased amounts and can be easily measured in blood or urine. In one commonly used procedure, 3 g metyrapone are given orally at bedtime; serum compound S and cortisol are measured at 8:00 A.M. the next morning. A fall in serum cortisol to less than 5 μg/dl indicates a valid test, and a serum compound S level of at least 8 μg/dl is a normal response (Fig. 2–2).

3. Corticotropin-releasing hormone. CRH is currently available for investigational use; an intravenous bolus of 1 μg/kg produces a rapid rise of plasma ACTH and cortisol in normal individuals. Patients with pituitary destruction (e.g., from a tumor) will show blunted responses to CRH, as will subjects receiving large pharmacologic doses of glucocorticoids which act on the pituitary to suppress ACTH secretion.

With both hypoglycemia and metyrapone tests, adrenal end products are generally used as an index of ACTH secretion because the direct measurement of ACTH in plasma is difficult and expensive. Therefore, if the cortisol response to either hypoglycemia or metyrapone testing is deficient, it is also

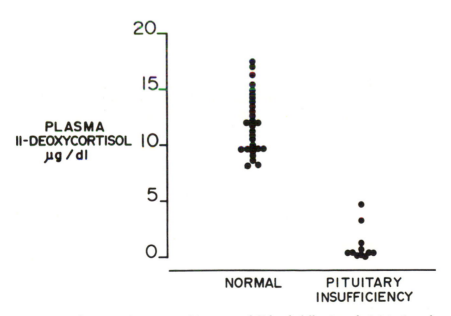

Fig. 2–2. Plasma 11-deoxycortisol (compound S) levels following administration of metyrapone to normal subjects and to patients with hypopituitarism. In this test, 2 or 3 g metyrapone were given at bedtime, with measurement of plasma 11-deoxycortisol the next morning.

necessary to demonstrate that the adrenal glands themselves are capable of responding to ACTH; for this purpose, exogenous ACTH (natural or synthetic) is administered, and plasma or urine steroid responses are measured.

Recent improvements in the methods of ACTH radioimmunoassay have resulted in the availability of reliable plasma ACTH measurements, which have simplified the etiologic diagnosis of adrenal insufficiency: patients with primary adrenal insufficiency have low plasma cortisol levels and elevated plasma ACTH, whereas those with adrenal failure secondary to hypothalamic-pituitary disease have low or low-normal plasma ACTH levels despite low circulating cortisol concentrations. Provocative tests are still needed to document a more modest loss of ACTH reserve.

Melanocyte-Stimulating Hormone (MSH) and β-lipotropin

Besides serving as an ACTH precursor, pro-opiomelanocortin also contains amino acid sequences for several other hormones. Beta-lipotropin, a 91-amino acid peptide, may have lipolytic actions; beta-endorphin, the C-terminal 31 amino acids of β-lipotropin, has opiate activity and may modulate pain perception and stress. Sequences with skin-darkening (melanocyte-stimulating) activity are also found in pro-opiomelanocortin, but are probably not naturally-occurring cleavage products in humans. The intact ACTH molecule, which contains within it the α-MSH sequence (residues 1 to 13), probably accounts for most of the circulating MSH activity in man. Although β-lipotropin and β-endorphin are released from the corticotroph by CRH and plasma levels of these hormones parallel circulating ACTH concentrations in most instances, the functions of these peptides in man are still largely unknown.

Thyrotropin

Thyroid-stimulating hormone (TSH) or thyrotropin, with a molecular weight of about 28,000, is one of the three glycoprotein hormones produced by the pituitary; the others are luteinizing hormone (LH) and follicle-stimulating hormone (FSH). TSH consists of a specific single-chain peptide beta subunit combined with a single-chain peptide alpha subunit; the TSH alpha subunit is virtually identical to the alpha subunit found in the other pituitary glycoprotein hormones, LH and FSH, and also in the placental glycoprotein hormone, human chorionic gonadotropin (hCG). Thyrotropin acts via cyclic AMP to stimulate production of thyroxine (T_4) and triiodothyronine (T_3) by the thyroid gland. Serum levels of TSH, measured by radioimmunoassay, are stable throughout the day with a modest increase in the late evening hours.

Primary hypersecretion of TSH is rare; most of the cases described appear to result from TSH-secreting pituitary tumors. In normal individuals or in those with TSH hypersecretion secondary to thyroid failure (i.e., primary hypothyroidism), TSH secretion may be suppressed by administering T_3 or T_4, which act directly on the pituitary. Somatostatin, dopamine, and large amounts of glucocorticoid also decrease serum TSH levels. Since low serum levels of T_3 and T_4 normally activate feedback mechanisms to increase TSH secretion, secondary hypersecretion of TSH occurs in primary hypothyroidism. Thus, pituitary or hypothalamic disease should be suspected if the serum TSH is not elevated in the presence of documented hypothyroidism; the absence of palpable thyroid tissue in the hypothyroid patient should also alert the physician to the possibility of TSH hyposecretion because TSH is necessary for the maintenance of thyroid size. In human infants, serum TSH is strikingly elevated within an hour after birth and gradually falls to normal adult levels over the first week of extrauterine life.

Thyrotropin-releasing hormone (TRH) is a hypothalamic tripeptide, pyroglutamyl-histidyl-prolinamide. When TRH is given intravenously to normal individuals, a prompt rise in serum TSH occurs, usually peaking about 30 minutes after TRH administration (Fig. 2–3). An exaggerated response to TRH occurs in patients with primary hypothyroidism, while blunted or absent responses may be seen in hyperthyroidism and in hypopituitarism. In hypothalamic disease, hypothyroidism may coexist with a low or normal basal serum level of immunoreactive TSH; this TSH shows reduced bioactivity, however. The TSH response to TRH is usually present in hypothalamic hypothyroidism and may be delayed and prolonged. The TRH test is the best test for evaluating the adequacy of TSH secretion.

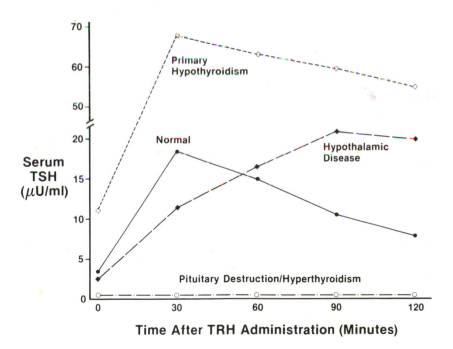

Fig. 2–3. Serum thyrotropin (TSH) response to TRH in normal subjects and patients with disorders of the hypothalamic-pituitary-thyroid axis. Patients with hypopituitarism due to pituitary destruction and those with hyperthyroidism (e.g., due to Graves' disease) both have absent TSH responses following TRH administration.

Gonadotropins

Both LH and FSH are glycoprotein hormones that appear to be secreted by the same pituitary cell. Each consists of the same nonspecific alpha subunit combined with a unique beta subunit that confers hormonal specificity. Each hormone interacts with specific receptors in the gonad, stimulating cyclic AMP production and resulting ultimately in the complex events of gonadal function.

Primary hypersecretion of FSH or LH is rare; when it occurs, it is usually due to secretion of these hormones by a pituitary tumor. Secondary hypersecretion, resulting from gonadal failure, is common and occurs in all normal women after menopause. The secretion of LH and FSH is normally suppressed by elevated serum levels of testosterone or estrogens in both men and women. A poorly characterized product of the testicular germinal epithelium, called inhibin and possibly arising from the Sertoli cells, also appears to suppress FSH secretion and may be important in the normal feedback regulation of this hormone. Inhibin has also been isolated from ovarian follicular fluid and probably arises from the granulosa cells.

Hyposecretion of LH and FSH occurs with many pituitary and hypothalamic diseases. Normally, the secretion of LH and FSH is stimulated by low levels of serum androgens and estrogens, and that of FSH by low levels of inhibin in the male. A hypothalamic factor, designated gonadotropin-releasing hormone (GnRH) or LH-releasing hormone (LH-RH, also abbreviated LRH), is secreted into the hypophyseal portal circulation and causes the release of both LH and FSH from the pituitary (Fig. 2–4). LH-RH, a decapeptide, has been

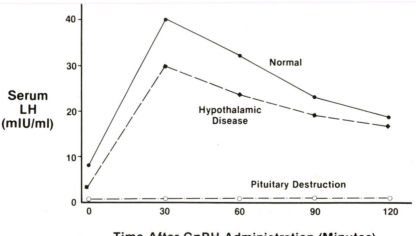

Time After GnRH Administration (Minutes)

Fig. 2–4. Serum LH responses to LH-RH in a normal subject and in patients with hypothalamic and pituitary disorders. Patients with hypothalamic disease but an intact pituitary generally respond to LH-RH, especially after several priming doses of the releasing factor.

isolated, sequenced, and synthesized. Because this single releasing factor is believed to promote the secretion of both LH and FSH, it is likely that other factors (such as circulating androgens and estrogens) play an important role in modifying the response to LH-RH and thus in differentially modulating the secretion of LH and FSH. Intravenous injection of LH-RH, with subsequent measurement of serum LH and FSH, is the most convenient direct test of pituitary gonadotropin secretion.

Clomiphene, a weak synthetic estrogen, is able to bind to hypothalamic receptors for gonadal steroids and block their normal feedback effect; this lack of feedback results in increased secretion of LH and FSH in normal individuals (Fig. 2–5). A combination of both LH-RH and clomiphene testing may be used, in theory, to differentiate hypothalamic from pituitary causes of hypogonadism; with pituitary destruction, responses to both clomiphene and LH-RH are deficient, while normal responses to LH-RH are seen in hypothalamic disease, with absent responses to clomiphene.

Growth Hormone (GH)

GH is a single-chain polypeptide with a molecular weight of about 22,000. Although its principal physiologic effect is stimulation of growth of bone and cartilage (via other peptides, called somatomedins or insulin-like growth factors), GH also generally stimulates protein anabolism, promotes lipolysis, enhances absorption of dietary calcium, and antagonizes the action of insulin.

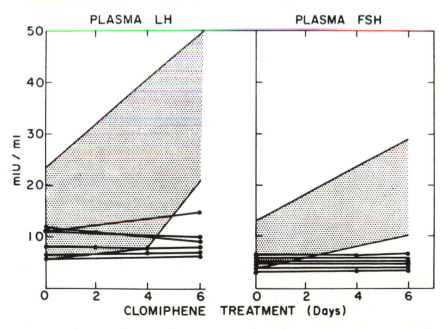

Fig. 2–5. Plasma LH and FSH responses to clomiphene administration in normal men (shaded areas) and patients with isolated gonadotropin deficiency (solid lines). (From Bardin, C.W., et al.: J Clin Invest, *48*:2046, 1969.)

Somatomedins are thought to be synthesized by the liver and perhaps by other organs; the presence of a normal amount of circulating GH is necessary for normal somatomedin production. Somatomedins promote growth of cartilage by stimulating the uptake of amino acids and the synthesis of DNA, RNA, and protein in this tissue; GH itself has little or no stimulating effect on cartilage. The secretion of GH by the pituitary is under both stimulatory and inhibitory control by the hypothalamus. GH-releasing factor (GRF) is a 44-amino acid peptide; somatostatin, a hypothalamic peptide of 14 amino acids, has been shown to inhibit the secretion of GH, as well as TSH.

Sustained hypersecretion of GH produces overgrowth of bone and soft tissue and leads to acromegaly in adults and gigantism in children, in whom the epiphyses of the long bones are still open and capable of further growth. In normal individuals, GH secretion is suppressed by elevations in blood sugar. Thus, the standard glucose tolerance test is widely used to evaluate suppressibility of GH; normally, following a 75 to 100 g glucose load, the serum level of GH falls to less than 5 ng/ml. Other GH suppressants include somatostatin, elevated serum levels of free fatty acids, and glucocorticoid in excess.

GH hyposecretion is often present in hypopituitarism. Many stimuli cause secretion of GH in normal subjects; some of the more common include hypoglycemia, arginine, L-dopa, apomorphine (a dopaminergic agonist), clonidine (an α-adrenergic agonist), GH-releasing factor, vasopressin, glucagon, meals, sleep, exercise, and other stress. Most GH stimuli seem to be potentiated by estrogens; thus, adult women usually respond better than men to any test, and the responses of men and children may be improved by giving pharmacologic amounts of estrogen for a few days. The most commonly used tests for evaluating the adequacy of GH secretion are the insulin hypoglycemia test, the arginine infusion test (0.5 g/kg intravenously over 30 minutes), and the L-dopa test (500 mg orally); the simultaneous administration of propranolol enhances GH responses to L-dopa by blocking β-adrenergic pathways that inhibit GH. All 3 tests give approximately equivalent results in young adults of normal weight (Fig. 2–6). Obesity and hypothyroidism blunt or abolish the GH responses to all tests. A normal GH response to any agent is the achievement, at any time during the test, of a serum GH level of at least 7 ng/ml. Figure 2–7 illustrates the normal mechanisms controlling GH secretion.

Prolactin (PRL)

A single-chain peptide with a molecular weight of about 22,000, PRL appears to exert its main physiologic action on the breast, where it promotes milk production; the role of PRL in males, in children, and in nonlactating females is currently unclear. The primary hypothalamic control of PRL secretion is inhibitory; dopamine probably functions as the major PRL-inhibiting factor, although other unidentified substances may also be involved. Dopamine is produced in the tuberoinfundibular neurons of the arcuate nucleus of the hypothalamus and secreted into the hypothalamohypophysial portal cir-

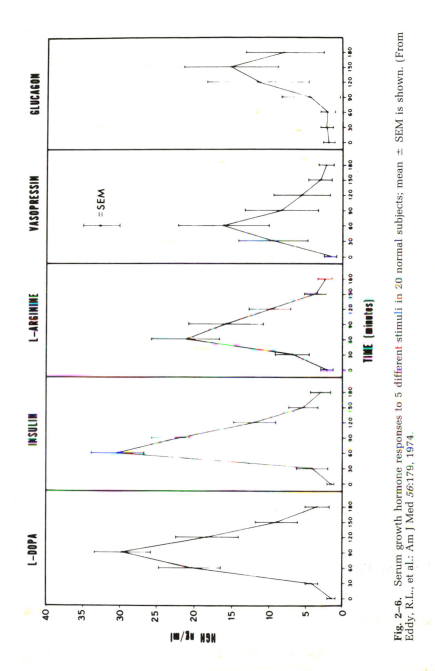

Fig. 2-6. Serum growth hormone responses to 5 different stimuli in 20 normal subjects; mean ± SEM is shown. (From Eddy, R.L., et al.: Am J Med *56*:179, 1974.

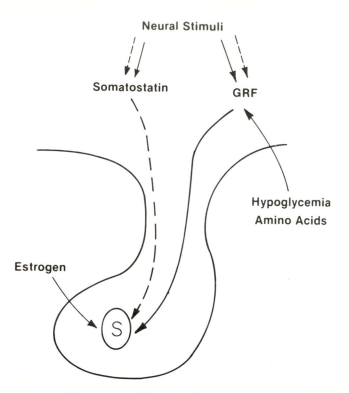

Fig. 2–7. Diagram of factors controlling growth hormone secretion from the pituitary somatotroph (S). Solid arrows indicate stimulatory effects while dashed arrows signify inhibition. GRF indicates growth hormone releasing factor.

culation. Dopamine is then transported to the anterior pituitary where it interacts with specific receptors on the surface of lactotrophs to inhibit PRL secretion. Hypersecretion of PRL may be due to direct production by pituitary tumors, to blockade of dopamine action by drugs such as phenothiazines, or to hypothalamic destruction; it may also be idiopathic. Physiologic hyperprolactinemia normally occurs during pregnancy and lactation; nipple stimulation during suckling stimulates PRL secretion via a neural reflex arc. Hypersecretion of PRL may be asymptomatic or may result in galactorrhea (inappropriate lactation) or hypogonadism. Normally, serum PRL is suppressed by dopaminergic agonists or their precursors, and to some extent, by elevated serum levels of thyroid hormones.

Hyposecretion of PRL may be found with hypopituitarism of varying orgins. In normal individuals, PRL secretion is stimulated by phenothiazines and other dopamine antagonists, tactile breast stimulation, stress, low serum levels of thyroid hormones, and TRH; the role of TRH in the physiologic regulation of PRL is unclear. A modest elevation of serum PRL normally occurs during sleep, especially in the early morning hours. All stimuli to PRL release appear to be potentiated by estrogens. Figure 2–8 illustrates the normal mechanisms

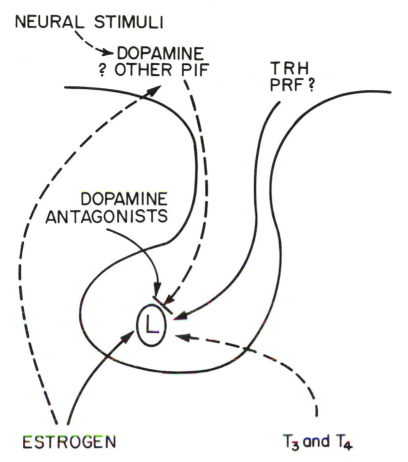

Fig. 2–8. Diagram of factors influencing prolactin secretion from the pituitary lactotroph (L). Solid arrows signify stimulatory effects and dashed arrows denote inhibition. PIF and PRF indicate prolactin inhibiting factor and prolactin releasing factor, respectively.

controlling PRL secretion, while Figure 2–9 demonstrates PRL responses to TRH in a group of normal subjects. As can be seen, serum PRL peaks 10 to 20 minutes after giving intravenous TRH; the peak following intramuscular chlorpromazine (not shown) occurs at about 2 hours.

HYPOPITUITARISM

Causes

Hypopituitarism occurs when the secretion of one or more pituitary hormones is deficient. This state may arise from the effects of disease on the hypothalamic centers that control pituitary hormone release or from processes directly affecting the pituitary gland. Hypothalamic lesions, such as tumors (e.g., craniopharyngioma), trauma, histiocytosis X, or sarcoidosis, may de-

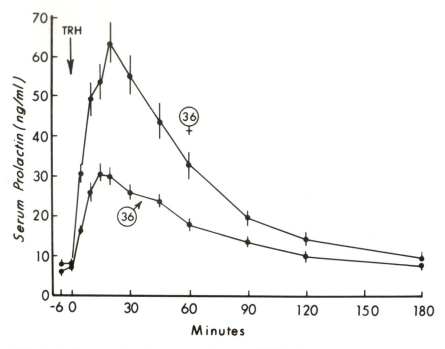

Fig. 2–9. Serum prolactin responses (mean ± SEM) to intravenous TRH in normal subjects. Note that the response in women is larger than that in men. (From Jacobs, L.S., et al.: J Clin Endocrinol Metab, *36*:1069, 1973.

crease secretion of the pituitary hormones that are primarily controlled by releasing factors (e.g., GH, ACTH, TSH, LH, and FSH), while PRL, which is primarily regulated by a hypothalamic inhibitory factor, rises. Some cases of idiopathic or genetic hormonal deficiencies may also be due to deficient or abnormal releasing factors, or to developmental anomalies of midline central nervous system structures.

The pituitary gland itself may commonly be damaged or destroyed by a variety of conditions, including tumors, trauma, infarction (called Sheehan's syndrome when occurring in the postpartum period), surgical procedures, or radiation. Other less common lesions resulting in pituitary destruction include hemochromatosis, granulomas (histiocytosis, sarcoidosis), infections (fungal, tuberculous, luetic, or pyogenic), and aneurysms of the internal carotid artery. The severity of the destructive process causing hypopituitarism varies. Sheehan showed that the classic features of hypopituitarism resulting in death were present when 95% of the pituitary was destroyed. That only 10 to 25% of the pituitary is sufficient for normal hormone secretion implies that the reserve for pituitary hormone secretion in man is substantial.

In addition to destruction of normal pituitary tissue by invasion and compression, pituitary tumors may reduce blood flow in the hypothalamic-hypophysial portal system and interfere with the delivery of releasing factors from the hypothalamus. Thus, pituitary tumors may cause "hypothalamic hypopituitarism."

Pathophysiology

The pathophysiology and clinical expression of hypopituitarism are variable and depend on which hormones are lost. Clinical features result from loss of gonadotropins, causing hypogonadism; deficient growth hormone, causing dwarfism in children but no clinical syndrome in adults; lack of TSH, causing hypothyroidism; prolactin deficiency, resulting in failure of lactation; and lack of ACTH, causing adrenocortical insufficiency. The frequency of hormone loss is usually in this order (most frequent to least frequent): GH, FSH-LH, TSH, ACTH, PRL; however, any combination of hormone loss may be found, even an isolated deficiency of only one hormone. Demonstration of hormonal deficiencies may help to establish the diagnosis of hypopituitarism, to explain the cause of puzzling symptoms, and to determine the need for replacement therapy.

Deficiency of GH is a common result of pituitary lesions that produce functional impairment. In the adult, GH deficiency has no significant consequences, but in the child it causes dwarfism. In congenital dwarfism due to lack of GH, failure to grow is evident within the first year of life. Even though size at birth is normal, subsequent growth rate is retarded. Infants and young children with GH deficiency may have fasting hypoglycemia. Puberty tends to be delayed even though gonadotropin secretion is intact. Children with GH deficiency are chubby and round-faced and may lack normal muscular development. When the diagnosis is established, therapy with GH injections is successful, provided it is started before epiphyseal closure.

Children with hypogonadism fail to enter normal puberty. Females have little or no breast development and primary amenorrhea. Pubic and axillary hair do not develop fully. Males have an infantile phallus and small testes (less than 12 ml in volume or 3.5 cm in length in the long axis). Body hair is sparse. When hypogonadism occurs as an isolated deficiency, growth may be delayed but is continuous and excessive, owing to failure of epiphyseal fusion. The adolescent with isolated hypogonadotropic hypogonadism is taller than one with multiple trophic hormone deficiencies and, if diagnosed late, may have developed eunuchoid proportions with an upper segment/lower segment ratio of less than one (measured as top of head to pubic symphysis/ pubic symphysis to floor), and an arm span greater than height. Familial hypogonadotropic hypogonadism due to absent LH-RH may be associated with anosmia (Kallman's syndrome); some such patients also have midline central nervous system or somatic defects (e.g., cleft palate). In adult women, acquired pituitary hypogonadism causes secondary amenorrhea, some atrophy of the breasts, and thinning of pubic and axillary hair. In men, acquired hypogonadism causes atrophy of the testes, decrease in beard and body hair, decreased libido, and impotence.

Lack of TSH secretion causes involution of the thyroid and features of hypothyroidism; the detailed clinical picture is described in the next chapter. Hypothyroid patients complain of fatigue, weakness, slowness of mental and physical performance, cold intolerance, impaired memory, hoarseness, constipation, muscle cramps, paresthesias, and dry skin. Usually, these patients gain weight despite reduced appetite. The skin is infiltrated by mucopolysaccharide so that the patient with myxedema has a puffy face and coarsening of the features. Speech is slow, body hair is reduced, and scalp hair is dry and coarse. Anemia is common; metabolic rate is reduced and hypothermia may be present. Patients with myxedema may eventually lapse into coma and die unless treated.

Lack of ACTH reduces cortisol production but does not affect aldosterone secretion. Patients are weak and tired; many lose weight because of decreased appetite. They become hypotensive since cortisol is necessary to maintain normal vascular smooth muscle tone. Urinary output is scanty and ability to excrete a water load decreases, resulting in hyponatremia. In contrast with the excessive pigmentation of primary adrenal insufficiency (Addison's disease), patients with secondary (pituitary) adrenal insufficiency have pale skin and fail to tan because of lack of the melanocyte-stimulating effects of ACTH. Response to stress is poor; nausea, vomiting, and diarrhea presage cardiovascular collapse from "adrenal crisis," which leads to death unless glucocorticoid therapy is given. The typical picture of Addison's disease is described in Chapter 4; contrast it with deficiency of ACTH causing a lack of cortisol.

Sheehan's syndrome is postpartum hypopituitarism resulting from ischemic necrosis of the pituitary, which is caused by shock from blood loss sustained at the time of delivery. The pituitary in pregnancy is enlarged and more vulnerable to infarction, which Sheehan believed to be caused by arteriolar spasm from the shock. These women fail to lactate and show rapid mammary involution postpartum; they also do not resume menstruation. Normal strength and vigor are not regained after the delivery; the pubic hair shaved for the delivery does not regrow. Hypothyroidism and adrenal insufficiency usually become manifest eventually, but all variations of hormonal loss may occur. The skin is waxy, and fine wrinkles appear about the eyes and mouth.

Diabetes insipidus results from destruction of hypothalamic nuclei which are the source of vasopressin. Extension of pituitary tumor or other pituitary disease to the hypothalamus may cause diabetes insipidus, so that the symptoms of polyuria, polydipsia, and nocturia must be considered together with manifestations of anterior pituitary insufficiency. Diabetes insipidus is discussed more extensively in Chapter 10.

Pituitary Tumors

Pituitary tumors may not cause any endocrine deficiency, but instead may produce the signs of a space-occupying intracranial neoplasm. Symptoms vary depending on the size and location (local spread) of the tumor. Headache is a common symptom; it is usually frontal or orbital, but location and severity are variable. It is attributed to pressure on the diaphragma sellae or the surrounding dura mater. Compression of the optic chiasm causes defects in the visual fields, usually bitemporal hemianopsia, often starting in the superior quadrants. Optic atrophy and total blindness may ensue; if so, the optic discs become white. The tumors may extend superiorly into the hypothalamus and cause a disturbance of appetite resulting in obesity, alteration of consciousness, and disturbances in temperature regulation. Obstruction of the third ventricle causes internal hydrocephalus. Lateral extension can compress the third (rarely the fourth or sixth) cranial nerves, causing diplopia or ptosis. Anterior or inferior extension may result in invasion of the sphenoid sinus and cerebrospinal fluid rhinorrhea.

With larger pituitary tumors, skull roentgenograms show enlargement of the sella turcica beyond the normal maximum dimension: anteroposterior length of 15 mm and depth of 12 mm on the lateral skull roentgenogram in adults. Erosion of the sella or clinoid processes or a localized bulge in the sellar contour (called a "double floor" when seen on a lateral skull roetgenogram) may also occur. Pituitary tumors, even small "microadenomas" (<1 cm diameter), can usually be visualized by computed tomography (Fig. 2–10). The older invasive technique of pneumoencephalography, in which air is used to fill and outline the brain's ventricular system and subarachnoid cisterns, is now rarely used. Carotid arteriography is also rarely required, but may be useful to demonstrate aneurysms causing sellar enlargement. Nuclear magnetic resonance imaging may also provide detailed resolution of pituitary and parasellar lesions.

It should be emphasized that an enlarged sella turcica does not always mean a pituitary lesion is present. In the primary empty sella syndrome, an incomplete diaphragma sellae allows the arachnoid membrane and cerebrospinal fluid to enter the sella, compressing the normal pituitary gland and, in some cases, enlarging the sella turica. Pituitary function is usually preserved, and

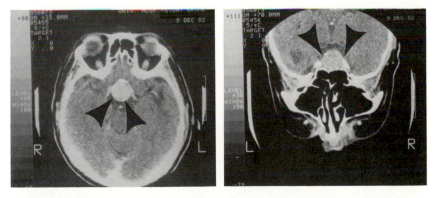

Fig. 2–10. Computed tomography (CT) scan of the sellar region in a patient with a large pituitary tumor; axial (left) and coronal (right) sections are shown. Arrows outline the tumor which fills the sella turcica and extends into the suprasellar area. (Scan courtesy of Dr. A.K. Anand, State University of New York at Stony Brook.)

no treatment is required; the condition must be considered in the differential diagnosis of an enlarged sella. Diagnosis of the empty sella syndrome can usually be made by computed tomography; pneumoencephalography or metrizamide cisternography (in which a water-soluble contrast agent injected into the subarachnoid space can outline the basilar cisterns and the "empty" sella turcica) may also be used. A secondary empty sella may result when sellar contents shrink following infarction, surgery, radiation therapy or medical treatment of a pituitary adenoma; in these cases, it is more likely that abnormal pituitary function will be found.

Hemorrhage into a pituitary tumor (pituitary apoplexy) occurs in about 5% of patients. It causes sudden onset of a severe headache and may progress to unconsciousness; blindness may result from compression of the optic chiasm. Paralysis of the oculomotor nerves, often asymmetric, causes deviation of the eyes and pupillary dilatation. Rapid surgical evacuation of the hematoma is usually required for preservation of vision.

Treatment

Hypopituitarism is treated, rather simply, by replacing the missing hormones or the hormones of the affected end organs.

Cortisol. The usual adult replacement is 15 to 30 mg cortisol given orally in divided doses to mimic normal cortisol secretion (e.g., 15 mg at 8:00 A.M. and 10 mg at noon; or 10 mg at 8:00 A.M., 10 mg at noon, and 5 mg at 6:00 P.M.). Patients should be advised to double the dose for minor stressful illness, and they must carry identification regarding the need to take cortisol. Large amounts of cortisol (such as 300 mg/day), together with glucose and sodium chloride, are given intravenously for adrenal crisis.

Thyroid. The usual daily maintenance dose in adults is 0.1 to 0.2 mg L-thyroxine given orally as a single dose. It must not be given in hypopituitarism unless cortisol is also given or the adequacy of ACTH secretion assured; otherwise, increased metabolic demands may precipitate an adrenal crisis if the patient cannot respond with increased ACTH and cortisol secretion.

Gonadal Steroids. Men may be treated with a depot testosterone preparation, 200 to 300 mg intramuscularly every 2 to 4 weeks, or methyltestosterone 10 to 40 mg orally daily. Methyltestosterone has hepatic toxicity and is not as potent as injected testosterone. Adequate therapy with either preparation restores muscularity, potency, libido, and body hair.

Women may be given a variety of estrogen preparations in a physiologic replacement dosage. In contrast, contraceptive pills are larger than physiologic dosage in order to suppress gonadotropin secretion.

Fertility in men may be achieved by administration of hCG possibly with addition of a human FSH preparation in proper dosage, but this therapy is difficult and expensive. Treatment of women with cyclic administration of human FSH and hCG may result in ovulation so that fertility may be achieved.

Growth Hormone. Children may be treated with human GH by intramuscular injection. Biosynthetic human GH produced by recombinant DNA techniques is now readily available commercially.

In some cases (such as pituitary tumors), the cause of the hypopituitarism can also be treated; these treatments (usually surgical procedures or radiation) are of major value in relieving and preventing the deleterious local effects of the intracranial mass lesion (such as loss of vision or obstruction of the flow of cerebrospinal fluid).

HYPERPITUITARISM

Hyperpituitarism refers to the pathologic overproduction of one or more pituitary hormones not secondary to end-organ failure. (This definition thus excludes the TSH overproduction occurring in primary hypothyroidism, for example.) Most cases of hyperpituitarism are due to hormone production by functioning pituitary tumors. Oddly, some pituitary hormones are much more commonly overproduced than others. PRL and GH overproduction are common, ACTH is occasionally overproduced, whereas primary TSH, FSH, or LH overproduction is rare (Table 2–2).

Acromegaly and Gigantism

These conditions, resulting from the effects of excess GH, differ only in their age of onset. In the child, when long-bone growth is possible, excess GH greatly increases height, resulting in gigantism; in the adult, following closure of the long-bone epiphyses, bones may grow wider and thicker, and soft tissues may proliferate, leading to characteristic changes in the appearance of the face and extremities (acromegaly literally means enlargement of the distal parts of the body).

The cause of GH overproduction in acromegaly is unclear; in most cases, an autonomously functioning pituitary tumor appears to be the cause, since normal GH secretion may be restored by removal of the tumor. On the other hand, several cases of acromegaly due to ectopic production of GRF by distant tumors have been reported. This has raised the possibility that abnormal hypothalamic regulation of GH secretion might be present in ordinary cases of acromegaly and could be responsible for the overproduction of GH (and

Table 2–2.   Relative Incidence of Pituitary Tumors

	Percent Occurrence
GH-secreting	15
PRL-secreting	30
ACTH-secreting	14
TSH-secreting	1
Gonadotropin-secreting	4
Nonfunctional	25
Mixed tumors (mostly GH & PRL)	11

Modified from Asa, S.L., and Kovacs, K., Clin Endocrinol Metab, 12:567, 1983.

possibly for the tumor formation) observed. Against this hypothesis is the observation that a discrete pituitary adenoma rather than somatotroph hyperplasia can be demonstrated in most cases. With routine hematoxylin and eosin staining, the cells of the adenoma may be either eosinophilic or chromophobic; however, electron microscopy usually shows specific GH secretory granules in both varieties and adenoma cells are seen to contain GH when immunohistochemical techniques are applied. Some patients with acromegaly have other endocrine tumors (syndrome of multiple endocrine neoplasia, type I, with tumors of pituitary, parathyroid and pancreatic islets).

The symptoms of acromegaly derive from the effects of both excess GH and a pituitary tumor; in general, they are more pronounced with longer duration of disease. The nose, jaw, tongue, and soft tissues of the hands and feet are often enlarged (Fig. 2–11). Protrusion of the jaw may result in dental malocclusion; the teeth may also become widely separated. Excessive sweating and oily skin are other common complaints, possibly because of hypertrophy of sweat and sebaceous glands. Bony overgrowth and deformity around joints may result in accelerated osteoarthritis, while soft tissue proliferation

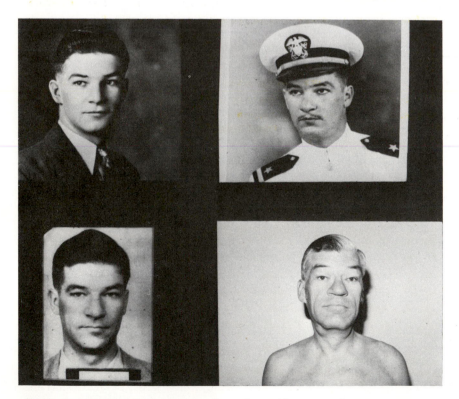

Fig. 2–11. Sequential photographs of a patient with acromegaly. Note progressive coarsening of the facial features with time. Patient is seen at 18 years of age in the upper left photo, 22 years in the upper right, 27 years in the lower left, and 53 years in the lower right.

in the carpal tunnel of the wrist may compress the median nerve, leading to weakness and paresthesias in the hand. Lactation may be due to the intrinsic lactogenic properties of GH or to the presence of a "mixed" adenoma containing both lactotrophs and somatotrophs. Symptoms of hypogonadism, hypothyroidism, or hypoadrenalism may result from compression or destruction of normal pituitary tissue. Headaches and visual changes occur frequently, owing to the pituitary tumor.

Signs of acromegaly include the changes in appearance just mentioned and visual abnormalities, including extraocular palsies and the classic bitemporal hemianopsia; additionally, hypertension is often seen. Deepening of the voice due to vocal cord thickening is characteristic. Generalized visceromegaly, with enlargement of the heart, liver, and kidneys, is frequent; although the enlarged kidneys may have increased glomerular filtration rate (creatinine clearance may be 150 to 300 ml/min), the cardiac enlargement may be associated with congestive heart failure. Cardiac and cerebrovascular diseases are responsible for most of the increased mortality in acromegaly. The relative contributions of elevated GH, hypertension, and glucose intolerance to the heart disease remain to be defined. There also appears to be an increased incidence of colonic polyps and colon cancer in acromegaly.

Routine laboratory studies may show glucose intolerance (45% of patients), hyperphosphatemia and hypercalciuria. Although basal fasting serum GH is usually elevated in acromegaly, stress may produce similar elevations in normal individuals. Since GH secretion is normally suppressed by glucose, the best diagnostic test for acromegaly uses the measurement of GH during a standard oral glucose tolerance test; as previously mentioned, serum GH in normal subjects should be less than 5 ng/ml 1 to 2 hours after glucose ingestion, whereas most subjects with acromegaly fail to show this degree of suppression (Fig. 2–12). Many patients with acromegaly also show transient GH stimulation following administration of TRH or LH-RH and suppression of GH after L-dopa; none of these responses are seen in normal subjects. Serum somatomedin levels are usually moderately increased in acromegaly. X-ray studies in acromegaly may show bony enlargement of the jaw, paranasal sinuses, hands, and feet. Soft tissue enlargement may also be seen; the heel pad thickness is measured in this regard and is greater than 20 mm in acromegaly. Skull x-rays often reveal an enlarged sella turcica. Computed tomography is used to delineate the size and extent of the tumor and is particularly useful in guiding the neurosurgeon or radiotherapist.

The treatment of acromegaly has been reasonably successful in 60 to 80% of patients through the use of pituitary ablative techniques (surgical procedures or radiation). Radiation therapy is associated with a slower fall in GH levels (over 1 to 5 years); both surgery and radiation may result in hypopituitarism. Medical treatments such as somatostatin and bromocriptine administration are being investigated for use when patients are not cured by ablative techniques or when these treatments are unsuitable. A long-acting somatostatin analog has been moderately successful in treating acromegaly. Bromocriptine, a drug

SERUM GH RESPONSE TO ORAL GLUCOSE IN ACROMEGALY

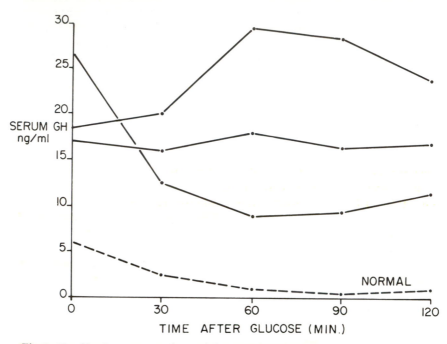

Fig. 2–12. Varying patterns of growth hormone responses to an oral glucose load in three patients with acromegaly (solid lines). Although one patient showed partial suppression of serum growth hormone, this did not reach the low levels seen in normal subjects (dashed line).

that has dopamine-like actions and may be given orally, has longer-lasting effects, but lowers GH to normal in only a small minority of patients.

Hyperprolactinemia

The inappropriate production of breast milk (i.e., not associated with normal postpartum nursing) is known as galactorrhea; although it may occur in both men and women, it is much more common in women, probably because of their greater breast development. Since lactogenic hormones are necessary for normal milk production, it is not surprising that an excess of one such hormone, PRL, would be associated with galactorrhea; indeed, in many cases of galactorrhea, serum PRL levels are elevated. PRL elevations commonly result from various medications (phenothiazines, butyrophenones, metoclopramide and other dopamine antagonists), from diseases affecting the hypothalamus or pituitary stalk (since PRL is primarily under hypothalamic inhibitory control), or from direct overproduction by pituitary tumors. Nonfunctioning pituitary tumors can compress the pituitary stalk, interfere with the delivery of dopamine to the lactotrophs, and thereby raise serum PRL.

In cases of pituitary tumors making PRL, the adenoma may be either eosinophilic or chromophobic on routine staining with hematoxylin and eosin, but electron microscopy usually reveals PRL secretory granules and immunohistochemical techniques show specific staining with anti-PRL antibodies. Small pituitary tumors (called microadenomas) producing PRL are usually located in the lateral wings of the pituitary, where lactotrophs are normally concentrated; somatotrophs (and therefore GH-secreting adenomas) are found in this same region also. The cause of PRL-secreting tumors is unknown. Although some tumors seem to have a reduced sensitivity to the inhibitory effects of dopamine, it is unclear whether this is a cause of the neoplastic transformation or a result of it.

Apart from the symptoms of a pituitary tumor per se (such as headache), excessive PRL secretion may result in galactorrhea, amenorrhea, decreased libido, impotence, and possibly gynecomastia (male breast enlargement); amenorrhea without galactorrhea is probably the most common complaint. Although some of the features of hypogonadism may be due to compression of the normal pituitary by the tumor, in many cases the high serum levels of PRL suppress LH and FSH release, probably by inhibiting LH-RH secretion. Few signs of excessive PRL production exist; careful breast examination may be necessary to demonstrate minimal galactorrhea. The pituitary tumor may produce visual field defects, extraocular palsies, and signs of hypopituitarism.

Unfortunately, no dynamic testing procedures can reliably differentiate functional (i.e., nontumorous) from tumor-produced hyperprolactinemia. Administration of L-DOPA or other dopaminergic agonists often suppresses serum PRL in both tumor and nontumor cases. The PRL response to TRH and other secretagogues is often blunted in cases of PRL-secreting tumors, although this reduced response is not universal. Perhaps the most useful procedure is simply multiple measurements of basal serum PRL; persistent elevation of serum PRL to levels above 100 ng/ml (normal male levels are less than 15 ng/ml; normal female less than 20 ng/ml) usually indicates the presence of a PRL-secreting pituitary tumor. Small tumors, of course, may be associated with less severe hyperprolactinemia.

Although x-ray findings of generalized sellar enlargement provide evidence to support the diagnosis of pituitary tumor, computed tomography provides the best demonstration of both small and large PRL-secreting adenomas.

Surgical removal restores normal pituitary-gonadal function in the majority of patients; however, there is an appreciable incidence of recurrence. Although radiation therapy usually controls tumor growth, the fall in serum PRL is slow and gradual over many years. Medical treatment with bromocriptine, lisuride or other dopaminergic ergot alkaloids suppresses PRL in nearly all patients and shrinks PRL-secreting tumors in many patients.

Other Hormones

Primary overproduction of other pituitary hormones is less common. Inappropriate ACTH overproduction occurs in Cushing's disease, usually due to a small ACTH-secreting pituitary tumor (see Chap. 4). Following bilateral adrenalectomy (an older treatment for Cushing's disease), ACTH secretion increases greatly; the ACTH-secreting pituitary tumor may then enlarge, leading to signs of an expanding sellar mass as well as intense hyperpigmentation due to the intrinsic melanocyte-stimulating action of ACTH or possibly coexistent overproduction of a human MSH. In this situation, known as Nelson's syndrome, serum ACTH levels are often elevated to several thousand picograms per milliliter (normal serum ACTH levels are about 40 to 100 pg/ml). The radiologic findings are similar to those for other pituitary tumors, and either neurosurgical removal or radiation therapy may be effective treatment.

A small number of TSH-producing pituitary tumors have been reported. These tumors result in hyperthyroidism in the presence of elevated serum TSH levels. Nontumorous hyperplasia of the thyrotrophs sufficient to enlarge the sella turcica may occur in primary hypothyroidism and needs to be differentiated from a TSH-secreting tumor; the demonstration of hypothyroidism rather than a hyperthyroid state is usually adequate to make this distinction.

Gonadotropin-secreting tumors are also uncommon; some may arise as a consequence of primary hypogonadism, while others may be associated with normal or increased gonadal function. Gonadotroph hyperplasia may result from primary hypogonadism and may also produce sellar enlargement.

Thyrotroph and gonadotroph tumors may also produce excessive amounts of free glycorotein hormone alpha-subunit. Some tumors which are otherwise non-functional appear to secrete only alpha-subunit as well.

CLINICAL PROBLEMS

Patient 1. A 28-patient-old woman had suffered a severe postpartum hemorrhage 2 years before examination. She had been in shock at least 4 hours and had required transfusion of 2500 ml of blood. Failure of lactation, permanent amenorrhea, some atrophy of the breasts, and excessive fatigue followed the delivery.

PHYSICAL EXAMINATION. This examination revealed a well-nourished woman; temperature was 36.5°C, pulse was 88/min, blood pressure (BP) 90/60, weight was 125 pounds (57 kg) and height was 64 inches (163 cm). Visual fields were normal by the confrontation method. Oral mucous membranes were normal. The thyroid gland was not palpable. Chest, cardiac, and abdominal examination was normal. Pelvic examination showed decreased vaginal secretions, small uterus, and nonpalpable adnexa. Axillary and pubic hair were diminished. The skin and areolar pigment were pale. Neurologic examination was normal.

LABORATORY DATA
Complete blood count—normal. Urinalysis—normal.
Chest roentgenogram: small cardiac silhouette.
Skull roentgenogram: relatively small sella turcica
CT Scan: empty sella
Serum T_4—6.6 μg/dl (normal, 5 to 12 μg/dl). Cortisol—3 μg/dl at 8:00 A.M. (normal, 7 to 18 μg/dl).
Serum LH—<1 mIU/ml (normal, 4 to 30 mIU/ml). FSH—<1 mIU/ml (normal, 4 to 30 mIU/ml).
Serum estradiol—20 pg/ml (normal premenopausal female, greater than 25 pg/ml).

The patient was given 0.1 U/kg regular insulin intravenously at zero time for testing GH and ACTH reserve:

Time (min)	Glucose (mg/dl)	GH (ng/ml)	Cortisol (μg/dl)
0	80	<1	4
30	30	1	5
60	40	2	6
90	60	1	7
120	70	1	5

The patient was next given 500 μg TRH intravenously at zero time:

Time (min)	TSH (μU/ml)	PRL (ng/ml)
0	2	3
30	9	5
45	12	4
60	7	3
90	4	3

QUESTIONS
1. What is the pathogenesis of this disorder?
2. Which hormones are deficient and which appear intact?
3. What would be the hazards of testing her with metyrapone?
4. Predict the likely results of testing her with GRF and LH-RH.

Patient 2. A 49-year-old man came to the emergency room complaining of 3 days of increasing retro-orbital headache and diplopia. Additional history included: 10 years of decreased libido; 5 years of chronic fatigue, cold intolerance, decreased beard growth, and poor tanning of the skin. On questioning, he admitted to a progressive increase in shoe and ring size over the past 20 years, along with increasing enlargement of his nose, lips, tongue, and jaw.

PHYSICAL EXAMINATION. BP was 100/60 lying and 80/50 standing. The right pupil was dilated and did not react to light. The right eye was deviated laterally and could not be adducted past the midline. Visual fields by confrontation demonstrated a bitemporal hemianopsia. Pubic and axillary hair was scanty. The testes were 2.5 cm in length and were softer than normal. The skin was dry and pale, and appeared thickened. Deep tendon reflexes showed a prolonged relaxation phase. The nose, jaw, zygomata, and lips were prominent; the tongue was large. Soft tissues of the hands and feet were increased.

LABORATORY DATA. Skull roentgenograms showed an enlarged sella turcica; chest roentgenogram revealed a normal cardiac silhouette. Laboratory studies included an unremarkable urinalysis; hematocrit was 36 (normal, 42 to 52); white blood count was 7500, with 6% eosinophils on the differential (normal 3% or less); serum sodium was 130 mEq/L (normal, 135 to 145 mEq/L); potassium was 4.8 mEq/L (normal, 3.5 to 5.0 mEq/L); plasma cortisol was 4 μg/dl (normal, 7 to 18 μg/dl); serum calcium was 12.1 mg/dl (normal 9.0 to 10.5 mg/dl).

Over the next 8 hours, the patient was given fluids and hydrocortisone intravenously; although his BP increased to 120/80, his headache worsened, and vision in the nasal field of the left eye deteriorated. An emergency surgical procedure was performed.

Other laboratory studies (specimens drawn on admission, but results returned postoperatively) included: serum thyroxine—1.7 μg/dl (normal, 5 to 12 μg/dl); serum TSH—less than 0.5 μU/ml (normal, less than 5 μU/ml); serum testosterone—170 ng/dl (normal male, 300 to 1100 ng/dl); serum LH—2 mIU/ml (normal, 1 to 15 mIU/ml); serum PRL—6 ng/ml (normal male, less than 15 ng/ml); serum GH—59 ng/ml (normal basal GH, less than 5 ng/ml).

QUESTIONS
1. What chronic processes affected this man's pituitary gland? How long ago did they begin?
2. What acute process was superimposed on this condition?
3. Interpret the history and laboratory findings in relation to these processes.
4. Other similar cases may have elevated serum PRL levels. How would you explain this finding?

5. What kind of operation do you think was performed? Why was a surgical procedure chosen over radiation? What long-term endocrine treatment would you recommend?
6. What other endocrine disorder may exist in this patient? What further diagnostic studies should be done (when the patient can tolerate them)?
7. If surgical intervention had not been necessary, what might have happened to this patient's elevated serum GH over the next few weeks?

Patient 3. This 9-year-old boy had a 4-year history of slow growth, and a 7-month history of intermittent headaches.

PHYSICAL EXAMINATION. The examination revealed a short (3 SD below the mean), mildly obese (sixteenth percentile) prepubertal male with dry skin. The optic fundi showed pale discs, and visual fields revealed bitemporal hemianopsia. A skull roentgenogram showed erosion of the posterior clinoids of the sella turcica and calcification in the suprasellar region. Surgical exploration revealed a large suprasellar cystic tumor, with involvement of the optic chiasm. The cyst was drained and some tumor removed; pathologic diagnosis was craniopharyngioma. Post-operatively, the patient developed polyuria.

LABORATORY DATA. The following postoperative laboratory studies were obtained:
Serum thyroxine—3.1 µg/dl (normal, 5 to 12 µg/dl).
Serum TSH-4 µU/ml (normal, 0.5 to 5 µU/ml).
A TRH stimulation test was performed using 7 µg/kg TRH intravenously:

Time (min)	TSH (µU/ml)	PRL (ng/ml)
0	4	45
15	8	110
30	18	106
45	20	87
60	26	60
75	22	52
90	14	48

Evaluation of GH and ACTH: The patient was pretreated with diethylstilbestrol, 5 mg twice daily for 3 days; regular insulin 0.1 U/kg was given intravenously at zero time, with the following results:

Time (min)	Blood sugar (mg/dl)	Serum GH (ng/ml)	Plasma cortisol (µg/dl)
0	84	2	7
30	31	2.4	
45	46	3.3	
60	59	2	12

QUESTIONS
1. Why was the patient pretreated with diethylstilbestrol prior to GH testing? What effect may the diethylstilbestrol have on the plasma cortisol concentrations?
2. Can you be sure the patient is GH deficient? What would you do before retesting GH secretion?
3. Explain the results of the TRH stimulation test based on the location of the tumor. Since basal serum TSH is normal, why is the patient hypothyroid?

Patient 4. A 31-year-old woman underwent menarche at age 13. After 5 years of normal menses, her menstrual periods became scanty and finally ceased entirely at age 21. Bilateral milky nipple discharge has been present since age 24. She has had frequent occipitofrontal headaches for the past 2 years, but denies visual disturbance.

PHYSICAL EXAMINATION. Vital signs were normal. There was no abnormal pigmentation of the skin, plethora, or acne. The extraocular movements were full, but visual fields showed bilateral superior temporal defects. No masses were noted in the breasts; a milky discharge could be expressed from each nipple.

LABORATORY DATA. CBC, urinalysis and serum electrolytes were normal. CT scan of the sella showed a 3-cm pituitary mass with significant suprasellar extension and erosion into the sphenoid sinus (similar to Fig. 2–10).

Serum FSH—5 mIU/ml (normal 4 to 30 mIU/ml)
Serum LH—3 mIU/ml (normal 4 to 30 mIU/ml)
Serum estradiol—18 pg/ml (normal >25 pg/ml)
Serum thyoxine—5.6 µg/dl (normal 5 to 12 µg/dl)
Serum TSH—2.2 µU/ml (normal 0.5 to 5 µU/ml)
Serum PRL—740 ng/ml (normal <20 ng/ml)
Serum cortisol—9 µg/dl (normal 7 to 18 µg/dl)
Metyrapone test for ACTH reserve (3 g given orally at bedtime: At 8:00 the next morning, serum 11-deoxycortisol was 4 µg/dl.

COURSE. She was begun on bromocriptine therapy; on a dose of 5 mg twice a day, serum PRL was 18 ng/ml. Galactorrhea disappeared and menses resumed after 3 months of treatment. Her headaches and visual fields improved, but she developed a watery nasal discharge. Repeat overnight testing with metyrapone yielded a serum 11-deoxycortisol value of 16 µg/dl.

QUESTIONS
1. What is the pretreatment status of the pituitary hormones?
2. What is the cause of the amenorrhea and low gonadotropins?
3. How did the bromocriptine treatment produce cerebrospinal fluid rhinorrhea? Why did the metyrapone test normalize following bromocriptine therapy?

SUGGESTED READING

Normal Physiology and Testing

Ben-Jonathan, N.: Dopamine: a prolactin-inhibiting hormone. Endocr Rev, 6:564, 1985.
Chrousos, G.P., et al.: Clinical applications of corticotropin-releasing factor. Ann Intern Med, 102:344, 1985.
Guillemin, R., et al.: Somatocrinin, the growth hormone releasing factor. Recent Prog Horm Res, 40:233, 1984.
Hammond, C.B., and Ory, S.J.: Diagnostic and therapeutic uses of gonadotropin-releasing hormone. Arch Intern Med, 145:1690, 1985.
Ho, K.Y., Evans, W.S., and Thorner, M.O.: Disorders of prolactin and growth hormone secretion. Clin Endocrinol Metab, 14:1, 1985.
Jackson, I.M.D.: Thyrotropin-releasing hormone. N Engl J Med, 306:145, 1982.
Lamberton, R.P., and Jackson, I.M.D.: Investigation of hypothalamic-pituitary disease. Clin Endocrinol Metab, 12:509, 1983.
Streeten, D.H.P., et al.: Normal and abnormal function of the hypothalamic-pituitary-adrenocortical system in man. Endocr Rev, 5:371, 1984.

Hypopituitarism

Abboud, C.F.: Laboratory diagnosis of hypopituitarism. Mayo Clin Proc, 61:35, 1986.
Veldhuis, J.D., and Hammond, J.M.: Endocrine function after spontaneous infarction of the human pituitary: Report, review and reappraisal. Endocr Rev, 1:100, 1980.

Pituitary Tumors

Asa, S.L., and Kovacs, K.: Histological classification of pituitary disease. Clin Endocrinol Metab, 12:567, 1983.
Ekblom, M., et al.: Pituitary function in patients with enlarged sella turcica and primary empty sella syndrome. Acta Med Scand, 209:31, 1981.
Kaplan, N., Day, A.L., Quisling, R., and Ballinger, W.: Hemorrhage into pituitary adenomas. Surg Neurol, 20:280, 1983.
Kendall, B.: Current approaches to hypothalamic-pituitary radiology. Clin Endocrinol Metab, 12:535, 1983.
Odell, W.D., and Nelson, D.H. (eds.): Pituitary Tumors. Mount Kisco, Futura Publishing Co., 1984.
Smallridge, R.C., and Smith, C.E.: Hyperthyroidism due to thyrotropin-secreting pituitary tumors. Arch Intern Med, 143:503, 1983.
Snyder, P.J.: Gonadotroph cell adenomas of the pituitary. Endocr Rev, 6:552, 1985.
Wass, J.A.H., and Besser, G.M.: The medical management of hormone-secreting tumors of the pituitary. Ann Rev Med, 34:283, 1983.
Wilson, C.B., and Dempsey, L.C.: Transsphenoidal microsurgical removal of 250 pituitary adenomas. J Neurosurg, 48:13, 1978.

Valenta, L.J., et al.: Diagnosis of pituitary tumors by hormone assays and computerized tomography. Am J Med, 72:861, 1982.

Acromegaly

Ch'ng, J.L.C., et al.: Growth hormone secretion dynamics in a patient with ectopic growth
hormone-releasing factor production. Am J Med, 79:135, 1985.

Jadresic, A., et al.: The acromegaly syndrome. Relation between clinical features, growth
hormone values and radiological characteristics of the pituitary tumours. Q J Med, 51:189,
1982.

Melmed, S., et al.: Pathophysiology of acromegaly. Endocr Rev, 4:271, 1983.

Thomas, J.P.: Treatment of acromegaly. Br Med J, 286:330, 1983.

Whitehead, E.M., et al.: Pituitary gigantism: a disabling condition. Clin Endocrinol, 17:271,
1982.

Wright, A.D., et al.: Mortality in acromegaly. Q J Med, 39:1, 1970.

Hyperprolactinemia

Blackwell, R.E.: Diagnosis and management of prolactinomas. Fertil Steril, 43:5, 1985.

Franks, S., and Jacobs, H.S.: Hyperprolactinemia. Clin Endocrinol Metab, 12:641, 1983.

Koppelman, M.C.S., et al.: Hyperprolactinemia, amenorrhea, and galactorrhea. A retrospective
assessment of twenty-five cases. Ann Intern Med, 100:115, 1984.

Cushing's Disease

Krieger, D.T.: Physiopathology of Cushing's Disease. Endocr Rev, 4:22, 1983.

ANSWERS TO QUESTIONS

Patient 1

1. Pituitary infarction and necrosis due to hypotension and vasoconstriction have led to loss
   of anterior pituitary function. The specific hormonal deficiencies have produced failure
   to lactate, hypotension, and amenorrhea.

2. GH, PRL, ACTH, LH, and FSH are deficient. Neither GH nor ACTH responded to
   insulin hypoglycemia, and prolactin showed only a minimal response to TRH. Although
   no specific stimulation test of gonadotropin release was performed, serum LH and FSH
   were both inappropriately low in the face of a hypogonadal serum estradiol concentration.
   TSH secretion is intact, based on a normal serum thyroxine concentration and a normal
   TSH response to TRH.

3. Metyrapone, by inhibiting the patient's already deficient secretion of cortisol, could
   provoke a severe hypoadrenal crisis with hypotension and cardiovascular collapse.

4. Since this patient's hypopituitarism is due to pituitary destruction, she would probably
   have no hormonal response to the administration of the releasing factors GRF and LH-
   RH. In contrast, patients with hypopituitarism secondary to a hypothalamic disorder
   usually show pituitary responses to the releasing factors, especially after several repetitive
   "priming" doses.

Patient 2

1. This patient has probably had acromegaly for at least 20 years; additionally, several
   clinical features of hypopituitarism have been present for 10 years.

2. Pituitary apoplexy (hemorrhage into his tumor) occurred acutely.

3. Features of acromegaly noted to be present include the increase in shoe and ring size, as
   well as enlargement of the facial features, tongue, and soft tissues of the extremities.
   The elevated serum GH is somewhat supportive of the diagnosis of acromegaly, although
   the stress of the acute illness might raise serum GH to this level in a normal subject.

   The slow growth of the pituitary tumor has enlarged the sella turcica. While some
   visual field abnormalities may have resulted from the tumor alone, the subsequent pituitary
   hemorrhage undoubtedly expanded the sellar contents and further compressed the optic
   chiasm. Lateral expansion accounts for the third cranial nerve palsy.

   Hypogonadism is revealed by the history of decreased libido and beard growth, by the
   physical findings of scanty hair and atrophic testes, and by the low serum testosterone
   and LH. Hypothyroidism is suggested by the history of fatigue and cold intolerance, by
   the dry skin and delayed reflexes on physical examination, and by the low serum thyroxine
   and TSH. Deficient ACTH secretion may have produced poor tanning of the skin, or-

thostatic hypotension, and hyponatremia; the increased number of eosinophils seen on the white cell differential count may also be a result of hypoadrenalism. The low serum cortisol in the face of major stress supports the diagnosis of hypoadrenalism.

4. Elevated serum PRL is a common finding with pituitary tumors. This finding may result either from direct production of PRL by the tumor or by interruption of the hypothalamic-pituitary portal vessels by the expanding tumor, with a resultant decrease in dopamine at the pituitary.

Tumors which produce more than one hormone may be composed of several cell types with each cell type producing one hormone (e.g., a mixed adenoma composed of somatotrophs and lactotrophs) or, alternatively, a single cell type may produce more than one hormone.

5. A transfrontal hypophysectomy was probably done; this approach is traditionally used when significant suprasellar extension accompanies compression of the optic chiasm. The transsphenoidal route is used when there is less need for suprasellar dissection. Although radiation therapy might have been appropriate at any prior time in the patient's course, it would not be useful in the present situation since it would not produce the rapid decompression of the tumor needed to preserve vision. Treatment with glucocorticoid was given before, during, and after the operation. When the patient had recovered from the operation, it would be reasonable to begin replacement therapy with L-thyroxine and testosterone, and to continue hydrocortisone.

6. The elevated serum calcium raises the possibility that this patient may also have hyperparathyroidism; acromegaly and other pituitary tumors may occur with hyperparathyroidism and pancreatic islet-cell tumors in the familial syndrome of multiple endocrine neoplasia, type 1. The patient's parathyroid status should be further investigated with a measurement of serum parathyroid hormone. Serum gastrin and fasting blood sugar should also be measured (gastrin, insulin and glucagon may be produced by islet-cell tumors of the pancreas).

7. In some cases of pituitary apoplexy in acromegaly, enough tumor is destroyed to cure the acromegaly; thus, the serum GH might fall to normal levels over several days or weeks following the acute infarction and hemorrhage. If the serum GH remained elevated, either surgical or radiation therapy could be given.

Patient 3

1. In normal men and prepubertal children, GH responses to provocative testing are sometimes inadequate. Brief pretreatment with large doses of estrogens will enhance GH responses to all stimuli and will thus help separate normal from abnormal responses. Estrogens also increase the production of serum cortisol-binding globulin, the carrier for circulating cortisol. In a normal individual, these extra binding sites are rapidly filled with additional cortisol; thus, this patient's relatively low serum cortisol concentration after estrogen administration and the deficient rise in cortisol after hypoglycemia both suggest that cortisol production is impaired.

2. GH deficiency is not yet established. Since hypothyroidism impairs GH responses to provocative tests, the practical approach is to give replacement thyroid hormone, if necessary, before evaluating GH secretion.

3. Since serum TSH rose adequately following TRH administration, the pituitary's capacity to secrete TSH appears to be intact. Thus, the inappropriately normal basal TSH in the face of hypothyroidism is probably due to TRH deficiency produced by hypothalamic disease. The delayed and prolonged peak of TSH following TRH injection also supports the diagnosis of hypothalamic hypothyroidism.

The elevated basal serum PRL value is also consistent with a hypothalamic lesion leading to impaired delivery of dopamine to the pituitary. Following TRH administration, serum PRL more than doubled, indicating normal pituitary PRL reserve.

Although the immunoreactive basal serum TSH level is normal, the TSH is probably of reduced bioactivity, accounting for his hypothyroidism.

Patient 4

1. TSH secretion is intact; based on the insufficient response to metyrapone, ACTH reserve is impaired. GH was not assessed; PRL hypersecretion is present, reflecting direct secretion by the pituitary tumor. Basal LH and FSH concentrations are low or low-normal in the

face of hypogonadism with low serum estradiol, suggesting that gonadotropin secretion is deficient.

2. Elevated serum PRL probably suppresses hypothalamic production or release of LH-RH, leading to low serum gonadotropins and amenorrhea. Additionally, a pituitary tumor of this size could compress the adjacent normal pituitary tissue and pituitary stalk, further impairing the function of the gonadotrophs.

3. Bromocriptine commonly produces shrinkage of PRL-secreting pituitary tumors. In this patient, tumor had broken through the floor of the sella into the sphenoid sinus; when the tumor shrank in response to bromocriptine therapy, a channel through the sellar floor was opened, allowing cerebrospinal fluid to leak into the sinus. As the tumor shrank, pressure on the normal pituitary and the pituitary stalk was relieved, allowing the delivery of CRH and permitting the corticotrophs to function normally.

3

Thyroid Disease

Jerome M. Hershman

ABBREVIATIONS

DIT	diiodotyrosine
FT_3	free triiodothyronine
FT_4	free thyroxine
FT_4I	free thyroxine index
FT_3I	free triiodothyronine index
MIT	monoiodotyrosine
RAIU	radioiodine uptake of thyroid
T_3	triiodothyronine
rT_3	reverse triiodothyronine
T_3U	T_3 uptake
T_4	thyroxine
TBG	thyronine-binding globulin
Tg	thyroglobulin
THBR	thyroid hormone binding ratio
TRH	thyrotropin-releasing hormone
TSH	thyroid-stimulating hormone

Thyroid diseases are the most common endocrine disorders worldwide. An understanding of their pathophysiology provides a logical guide to their management. Examination of the thyroid gland is simple. The examiner palpates the gland while standing behind the patient using the forefinger and third finger of each hand which is placed over the corresponding lobe just inferior to the larynx. The gland rises while the patient swallows, thus confirming that the tissue being palpated is the thyroid. (Providing a glass of water makes it easier for the patient to swallow.) The normal gland is just palpable in most adults and weighs about 15 to 25 g.

PHYSIOLOGY AND BIOCHEMISTRY

Biosynthesis of Thyroid Hormone

Dietary iodine is essential for synthesis of thyroid hormone. The usual dietary iodine intake is 100 to 500 μg per day. Diets in the United States often contain about 400 μg due to enrichment of food with iodine and the use of iodized salt (76 μg per g salt). Iodine is absorbed in the upper gastrointestinal tract, enters the blood stream, and is *trapped* by an *active transport system* in the thyroid follicular cells. The iodide which is not concentrated by the thyroid is rapidly cleared by the kidneys.

The trapped iodide is oxidized by thyroid peroxidase and hydrogen peroxide to an unstable intermediate which is rapidly incorporated into tyrosine to form monoiodotyrosine (MIT) and diiodotyrosine (DIT) in peptide linkage within the thyroglobulin molecule. This step of *oxidative iodination* of thyroglobulin is called *organic binding of iodine*. The iodotyrosines couple to form thyroxine (3,5,3′,5′-tetraiodothyronine) or triiodothyronine (3,5,3′-triiodothyronine), a reaction that is also catalyzed by thyroid peroxidase. The peroxidase is present mainly in the apical portion of the thyroid epithelial cell. This location of the peroxidase restricts the iodination to the cell-colloid interface and provides the thyroid with a mechanism for minimizing accidental iodination of non-thyroglobulin intracellular protein. Once iodinated, thyroglobulin containing newly formed iodothyronines is stored in the follicular lumen.

The thyroxine (T_4) and triiodothyronine (T_3) are secreted by proteolytic digestion of thyroglobulin in response to activation of the gland by thyrotropin, TSH. *Release of iodothyronines* involves endocytosis of thyroglobulin from the follicular lumen, and enzymatic hydrolysis of thyroglobulin in the follicular cells to liberate free iodoaminoacids (T_4, T_3, MIT, and DIT). Figure 3–1 summarizes the various steps of biosynthesis of thyroid hormone.

Thyroglobulin, Tg, is a large molecule, 660,000 daltons, consisting of two equal subunits. Within the molecule, there are many tyrosines, but only a few tyrosines are in sites favored for iodination and coupling to form T_4 or T_3. On the average, each molecule of Tg contains three molecules of T_4, and only one of every 3 Tg molecules contains a T_3 molecule. The T_4/T_3 ratio within the thyroid is about 10. Thyroglobulin also contains MIT and DIT which are released by the proteolytic digestion. The MIT and DIT are deiod-

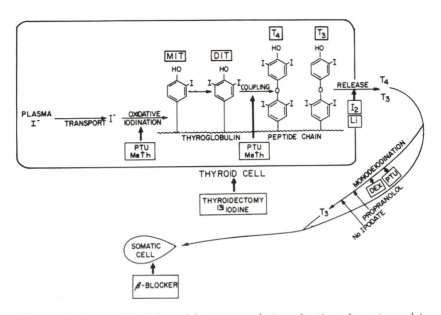

Fig. 3–1. Biosynthesis of thyroid hormone and sites of action of agents used in treatment of hyperthyroidism (PTU: propylthiouracil; Meth: methimazole; I_2: stable iodine; Li: lithium; Dex: dexamethasone).

inated by iodotyrosine deiodinase within the thyroid in order to conserve iodine which then reenters the thyroid iodine pool.

Action of TSH

TSH (described in Chap. 2) binds to specific receptors on the thyroid cell membrane and exerts its stimulatory action by activation of adenylate cyclase and increase of cyclic AMP. TSH causes the release of thyroid hormone and stimulates all of the metabolic processes within the thyroid, including growth and thyroid hormone synthesis.

Extrathyroidal Production of T_3 from T_4

The daily production of T_4 is about 80 μg and that of T_3 is 32 μg. Only 8 μg of T_3 is secreted directly by the thyroid gland. The other 24 mcg arises from outer ring deiodination of T_4 in other tissues, such as the liver and kidney. There are two 5′-deiodinases in peripheral tissues. Table 3–1 summarizes their characteristics. Deiodination of the inner ring of T_4 yields $3,3′,5′$-T_3, called reverse T_3, which is metabolically inactive. Outer ring deiodination of T_4 is a pathway of activation to produce the more active hormone, T_3, while inner ring deiodination is a pathway of inactivation (Fig. 3–2). These processes are carefully regulated. Table 3–2 shows the production rates and serum concentrations of the iodothyronines.

Table 3–1.   Characteristics of Two T_4 5'-Deiodinases

	Type 1	Type 2
Tissues	Liver, kidney, other organs	Brain, pituitary, placenta, brown fat
V_{max}	High	Low
Affinity	Low	High
Inhibition by pro- pylthiouracil	Yes	No
Activity in:		
Hyperthyroidism	Increased	Decreased
Hypothyroidism	Decreased	Increased
Role	Maintenance of circulating T_3 concentration	Maintenance of local T_3 concentration

Table 3–2.   Mean Euthyroid Values of Iodothyronine Serum Concentrations and Kinetics

		T_4	T_3	rT_3
Serum concentration	μg/dl	8	0.12	0.025
	nmol/L	102	1.8	0.37
Distribution volume	L	10	38	98
Metabolic clearance rate	L/day	1	27	100
Production rate	μg/day	80	32	25
	nmol/day	102	49	37
Plasma $t_{1/2}$	days	8	1	0.2

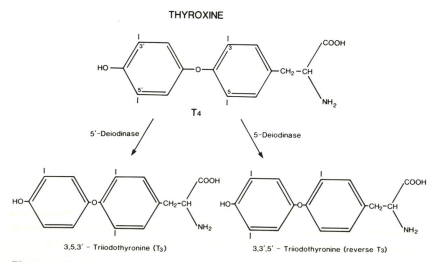

THYROXINE

5'-Deiodinase   5-Deiodinase

T_4

3,5,3' – Triiodothyronine (T_3)   3,3',5' – Triiodothyronine (reverse T_3)

Fig. 3–2.   Structures of T_4, T_3, and rT_3, and the enzymatic pathways for deiodination of T_4 to produce T_3 and rT_3 in peripheral tissues.

Transport and Peripheral Metabolism

In the blood, T_4 and T_3 bind tightly to serum proteins, thyronine-binding globulin (TBG), prealbumin, and albumin. Table 3–3 shows the relative distribution of these hormones among the binding proteins.

The free hormone is that portion that is not bound to serum proteins and is thus able to enter the cells readily. Equation 1 shows the equilibrium between T_4, TBG, and the complex: T_4-TBG.

$$T_4 + TBG \longleftrightarrow T_4\text{-}TBG \qquad\qquad (1)$$
$$K = [T_4\text{-}TBG]/[T_4][TBG] \qquad\qquad (2)$$
$$[T_4] = [T_4\text{-}TBG]/K[TBG] \qquad\qquad (3)$$

where T_4 represents free T_4, TBG is the unoccupied TBG, and T_4-TBG is T_4 bound to TBG. Free T_4 is directly proportional to the bound T_4 and inversely proportional to the unoccupied TBG. Only 0.02% of T_4 in the serum is free and 99.98% is bound to protein; 0.3% of serum T_3 is free and 99.7% is bound to protein. The free fraction of these hormones is a small fraction of the circulating pool.

The free hormone hypothesis assumes that (1) only the free hormone is available to enter body tissues and (2) that only the free hormone is carefully regulated and maintained constant. Assumption (1) is probably incorrect because some of the bound T_4 and T_3 is readily available to tissues. The T_4 bound to prealbumin and albumin is loosely bound; this T_4 diffuses through capillary pores in the liver and brain and enters cells. T_3 bound to TBG and albumin is also loosely bound and may leave the capillary bed to enter cells readily. Only T_4 bound to TBG or to an abnormal variant of albumin (dysalbumin) is so tightly bound that it does not dissociate in the capillary beds of the liver or brain. Thus a much larger fraction of the circulating T_4 and T_3 is available to cells than the free fraction.

Action of Thyroid Hormone

Thyroid hormones (T_3 and T_4) act on many tissues to increase metabolic activity and protein synthesis. In fact no tissue or organ system escapes the adverse effects of an excess or deficiency of thyroid hormone. Thyroid hormone is essential for normal growth and development. T_3 and T_4 bind to nuclear receptors and influence gene transcription. The affinity of T_3 for the nuclear receptor is 10-fold greater than the affinity of T_4. The hormones increase the synthesis of certain hepatic enzymes and the activity of

Table 3–3. Distribution of T_4 and T_3 Among Serum Binding Proteins

	TBG	Prealbumin	Albumin
Capacity	low	high	high
Affinity	high	low	low
T_4 (%)	70	20	10
T_3 (%)	70	0	30

$Na^+K^+ATPase$, which is coupled to Na^+-K^+ transport across cell membranes. T_3 binds to mitochondrial receptors and has direct effects on the mitochondria. It also affects transport of sugars and amino acids across plasma membranes within minutes, an effect unrelated to nuclear binding. Thyroid hormones influence many aspects of carbohydrate and lipid metabolism. They increase the action of epinephrine on glycogenolysis, increase glucose uptake by fat, increase lipolysis, and increase oxidation of free fatty acids.

THYROID FUNCTION TESTS

Thyroid function tests define: (1) the level of thyroid function (euthyroid, hyperthyroid, or hypothyroid), (2) the cause of any departure from euthyroidism, and (3) the nature of abnormalities of thyroid structure.

Serum Thyroxine (T_4)

The test measures the total amount of thyroxine in serum. The normal range is about 4.5 to 11 mcg/dl serum (58 to 140 nmol/L). Serum T_4 is elevated in hyperthyroidism and is low in hypothyroidism. Elevation of TBG increases the serum T_4. This happens during pregnancy or with estrogen therapy because estrogen increases hepatic production of TBG. Serum T_4 is low in euthyroid persons who have a low TBG, which occurs in cirrhosis owing to a low synthesis of TBG and in the nephrotic syndrome because of a loss of TBG in the urine. Only rarely is a low TBG congenital.

Free Thyroxine Concentration (FT_4)

The *percentage* of free T_4 (%FT_4) is measured by determining what proportion of a tracer amount of radioactive T_4 added to the patient's serum will pass through a dialysis or ultrafiltration membrane. Normally this fraction of T_4 is only 0.02% of the total serum T_4 (range 0.014 to 0.029%). Then the free thyroxine concentration may be calculated by:

$$FT_4 = \text{Total } T_4 \times \%FT_4$$

Normally, its approximate range is 1 to 3 ng/dl (13 to 38 pmol/L). FT_4 is high in hyperthyroid and low in hypothyroid patients.

Because of the difficulty of the dialysis and ultrafiltration methods, several new methods have been developed. These techniques, which employ radioactive T_4 derivatives as indicators, use antibodies to T_4 which bind the free T_4. Because of their simplicity and speed, they are now widely used.

Triiodothyronine Uptake (T_3U)

This test indicates the degree of saturation of the thyroid hormone binding proteins. Radioactive T_3 is used as an indicator. The result depends on competition for radioactive T_3 between the unsaturated binding sites on TBG in the patient's serum and a resin which binds T_3 (an antibody to T_3 or another T_3-binder may be used in place of resin). As the test is usually performed, the patient's serum is incubated with the T_3-binder and radioactive T_3; then the radioactive T_3 attached to the T_3-binder is counted. Because the T_3-binder has fixed affinity for the hormone, differences in uptake of the radioactive T_3 by the T_3-binder reflect variations in the hormone binding capacity of the serum proteins. The uptake of radioactive T_3 by the T_3-binder is high in hyperthyroidism because the binding sites on TBG are relatively saturated, so more of the tracer T_3 is available to bind to the T_3-binder. The uptake of radioactive T3 is low in hypothyroidism because the serum binding sites are relatively unsaturated, so less of the tracer is taken up by the T_3-binder. The T_3 uptake is increased in sera with a relative deficiency of binding proteins as occurs in cirrhosis, nephrotic syndrome, or as a hereditary trait. The T_3 uptake is decreased in sera with an increase in TBG which occurs in pregnancy.

The T_3 uptake does not measure the serum concentration of T_3. Because T_3 binds to TBG with one-tenth of the avidity of T_4, changes in serum T_3 have little effect on the T_3 uptake. Radioactive T_4 could be used in place of radioactive T_3 (T_4 uptake). The T_3 uptake is usually expressed as a ratio (T_3U ratio) by comparing the patient's result with that of a normal serum pool run simultaneously. This ratio is also termed thyroid hormone binding ratio, THBR.

Free Thyroxine Index (FT_4I)

The FT_4I is calculated as the product:

$$FT_4I = T_4 \times T_3U \text{ ratio}$$

As an example, one might look at typical results in a euthyroid woman taking birth control pills that contain estrogen.

Results: $T_4 = 15$ mcg/dl, $T_3U = 20\%$ (normal pool $= 30\%$)

T_3U ratio $= 20\%/30\% = 0.67$

Calculation: $FT_4I = 15 \times 0.67 = 10$

The normal range of $FT_4I = 4.5$ to 11, same as for T_4.

Remember that the FT_4I has essentially the same significance as FT_4; only the numbers and units are different. To show that FT_4I is only an index rather than a direct measurement of the free hormone, it does not have units.

Serum Triiodothyronine (T_3)

The serum T_3 measures the total amount of T_3 in serum by radiommunoassay. The normal range is about 80 to 180 ng/dl (1.2 to 2.7 nmol/L). It is a useful test for mild hyperthyroidism since T_3 rises earlier and more markedly than does T_4 in all common forms of hyperthyroidism. "T_3-thyrotoxicosis" is the name given to hyperthyroidism associated with supranormal serum T_3 and normal serum T_4 concentrations.

Measurement of T_3 concentration is less useful in the diagnosis of many forms of hypothyroidism because an insufficient thyroid remnant, driven by TSH, secretes a hormone mixture high in T_3 relative to T_4. Thus, while serum T_4 may be distinctly subnormal, serum T_3 may be within the normal range, and the patient may indeed be hypothyroid.

Serum Free T_3 Concentration (FT_3)

FT_3 is measured and calculated in the same way as FT_4 and has the same significance. The normal range for the percentage of free T_3 is about 0.15 to 0.35%, and the normal range of FT_3 is 1.5 to 3.5 pg/ml (2.2 to 5.2 pmol/L).

A serum free T_3 index (FT_3I) can be calculated by the same manipulation of data for T_3 as was done for T_4. As an example, let us examine typical results in a hyperthyroid patient.

Results: T_3 = 400 ng/dl, T_3U = 40%, control T_3U = 30%,
   T_3U index = 40%/30% = 1.33
Calculation: FT_3I = 400 × 1.33 = 533

Serum Thyrotropin (TSH)

Serum TSH is measured by immunoradiometric methods using monoclonal antibodies, one of which is labeled with radioactivity (or attached to an enzyme in the enzyme immunoassay). With the current sensitive methods for measuring TSH, the normal range is about 0.5 to 5 $\mu U/ml$. The TSH level in hyperthyroidism is low except in the rare TSH-induced hyperthyroidism. Serum TSH is particularly useful in the diagnosis of hypothyroidism and for separation of thyroidal from pituitary-hypothalamic causes of hypothyroidism. In thyroidal hypothyroidism, serum TSH is supranormal. In pituitary-hypo-thalamic hypothyroidism, the serum TSH is low or sometimes normal. The normal level of TSH in this circumstance is attributed to secretion of TSH with reduced biologic activity because, in the absence of TRH, the glyco-sylation of TSH is deficient. Although the poorly glycosylated TSH molecules may be detected by the antibody, they do not have full biologic activity in hypothyroid patients with hypothalamic disease.

TRH Test

Thyrotropin-releasing hormone (TRH) may be administered to test the adequacy of pituitary TSH secretion, as described in Chapter 2. The peak TSH response to TRH is usually proportional to the baseline TSH level. In hyperthyroidism, the low serum TSH does not rise after TRH because the pituitary cannot overcome the negative feedback inhibition of the high circulating levels of T_4 and T_3.

Serum Thyroglobulin (Tg)

The serum Tg concentration can be measured by radioimmunoassay. TSH increases secretion of Tg. Higher serum Tg levels occur in any goitrous process or inflammation of the thyroid. After removal of the thyroid gland, serum Tg levels are undetectable. The test is useful for monitoring therapy of thyroid carcinoma. Endogenous antibodies to Tg interfere with the determination. The normal serum levels are about 2 to 20 ng/ml, but there is considerable methodologic variability.

Thyroid Uptake of Radioiodine (RAIU)

A tracer dose of radioactive iodide, ^{123}I or ^{131}I, is given to the patient by mouth. The radioactivity over the thyroid gland is counted at various intervals of time, usually 4 or 6 hours and 24 hours. The normal 24-hour thyroid uptake is about 10 to 35% of the tracer dose. Figure 3–3 shows examples of the RAIU in different conditions.

The thyroid uptake is increased in hyperthyroidism and reduced in hypothyroidism. It is also reduced (1) in euthyroid patients who take drugs or chemicals containing iodine, since the pool of iodide in the body is expanded and the tracer is diluted in a larger pool; (2) in patients taking thyroid hormone, which suppresses TSH; and (3) in patients taking antithyroid drugs that interfere with trapping of iodide (perchlorate or thiocyanate) or organic binding (propylthiouracil or methimazole, which are used for the treatment of hyperthyroidism). Since the average American diet is high in iodine, normal thyroid uptake overlaps that in hypothyroidism. The RAIU is increased in euthyroid patients on a low iodine diet.

Perchlorate Discharge Test

The monovalent anion, perchlorate, competes with iodide in the thyroid trap. Administration of 1 g potassium perchlorate will cause release of radiodide which is trapped but not organically bound, so that it tests the efficiency of organic binding. The test (see Fig. 3–3) is used to diagnose defects in the peroxidase enzyme system.

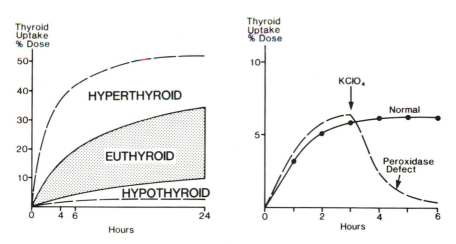

Fig. 3–3. Thyroid uptake of radioiodine. Left panel: the shaded region shows the normal range. The upper dashed line shows a typical hyperthyroid uptake and the lower dashed line a hypothyroid uptake curve. Right panel: Perchlorate discharge test. The solid line shows the plateauing of the thyroid uptake after oral ingestion of potassium perchlorate at 3 hours, and the dashed line shows the discharge of thyroidal radioiodine in a patient with a deficiency of organic binding (peroxidase defect).

Thyroid Scan

A scan is not indicated to determine the *level* of thyroid function. A scan after the administration of ^{123}I, ^{131}I or ^{99m}Tc-pertechnetate shows the distribution of the isotope in the thyroid gland. It shows whether a thyroid nodule concentrates radiodine to the same extent as the other thyroid tissue (isofunctional) or whether it is "cold" (hypofunctional) or "hot" (hyperfunctional). In hyperthyroid patients, a scan may distinguish among Graves' disease, multinodular goiter, and hyperfunctioning adenoma. Figure 3–4 shows typical abnormal thyroid scans.

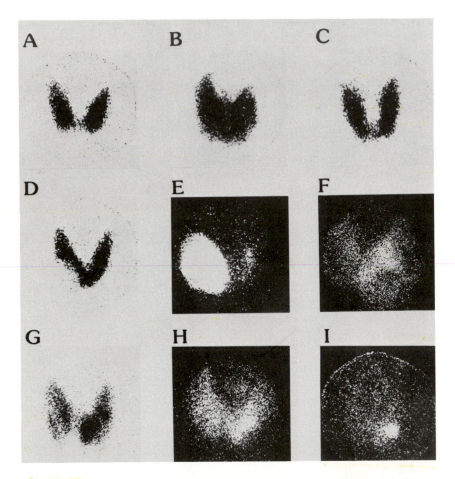

Fig. 3–4. Thyroid radioiodine scans. A-normal, B-hyperthyroidism with a large gland, C-hyperthyroidism with a symmetric gland and prominent isthmus, D-cold nodule in right lower lobe, E-hot nodule in right lobe with faint uptake in left lobe, F-colloid goiter with warm and cool areas, G-colloid goiter with increased uptake in nodules in inferior left lobe and cold nodule in right medial lobe (a bloody cyst on needle aspiration), H-multinodular colloid goiter with warm area in lower left lobe, I-same patient 2 years later with hot nodule in left lobe.

Tests of the Actions of Thyroid Hormone

The serum TSH level is sensitively affected by thyroid hormones. There are no other widely used, sensitive, specific tests of the actions of thyroid hormone. Instead, the assumption is made that the action is proportional to the serum free hormone levels of T_4 and T_3. Thyroid hormones (1) increase oxygen consumption and the basal metabolic rate (BMR, oxygen consumption at rest), (2) increase the speed of tendon reflexes, (3) shorten systolic time intervals and the pre-ejection period of cardiac contractility. Measurements of these effects are not usually performed.

HYPOTHYROIDISM

Hypothyroidism is the syndrome resulting from a deficiency of thyroid hormones, which causes many metabolic processes to slow down. Symptoms include fatigue, slowing of mental and physical performance, cold intolerance, impaired memory, change in personality (apathy or irritability), exertional dyspnea, hoarseness, constipation, muscle cramps, paresthesias, and dry skin. In newborns, hypothyroidism imparts a characteristic picture called cretinism. Cretins show retarded development of the brain, which may be irreversible, and retardation of growth leading to dwarfism. In children, growth retardation, delayed dentition, and delayed bone maturation are characteristic manifestations of thyroid hormone deficiency.

Pathophysiology

The skin is infiltrated by mucopolysaccharide, which retains sodium and water so that the face is puffy, especially around the eyes. The features become coarse and the eyebrows thinned. The tongue may enlarge and the vocal cords become thick, leading to hoarseness. Retarded cerebration slows speech because thyroid hormone affects the brain directly. Muscle contraction and relaxation (tendon reflexes) are slowed. There is mild weight gain, but never severe obesity as a result of hypothyroidism. Myocardial contractility is reduced, and the pulse tends to be slow because of a lack of the chronotropic effect of thyroid hormone. Effusions may occur in serous cavities including the pericardium causing distant heart sounds. Atherosclerosis is accelerated because of high serum levels of cholesterol and triglyceride. The rate of degradation of lipids is even slower than the rate of synthesis. The skin tends to be dry and has a yellow tinge, possibly due to carotene accumulation caused by a reduced rate of conversion of carotene to vitamin A. Body hair may be lost and not replaced, and scalp hair often becomes dry and coarse. Anemia may occur, usually owing to a reduced rate of red cell production. The anemia is normochromic and normocytic, but may be macrocytic or microcytic. Menorrhagia secondary to anovulatory cycles may also contribute to the anemia. In some women with primary hypothyroidism, amenorrhea develops and suggests the incorrect diagnosis of hypopituitarism.

The spectrum of severity ranges from severe hypothyroidism with its classic

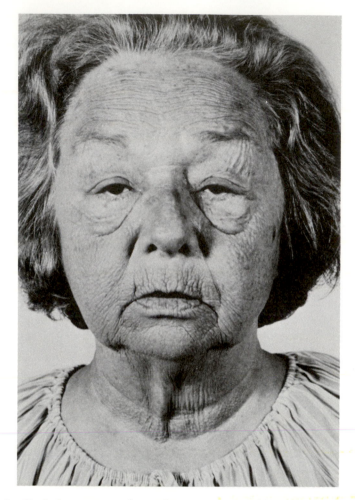

Fig. 3–5. Typical appearance of myxedema in a 60-year-old woman; note the swelling beneath and around the eyes and at the base of her nose, thin lateral eyebrows, droopy eyelids with wrinkling of forehead to keep eyes open, and poorly groomed hair.

features (called myxedema) to a mild, nearly asymptomatic subclinical disorder that requires sensitive thyroid function tests to establish the diagnosis. Figure 3–5 shows a woman with myxedema. Severe hypothyroidism may progress to myxedema coma, which is usually precipitated by another stressful illness. Such patients are hypothermic because of a marked reduction of metabolic rate, and they have typical features of myxedema. Hypoventilation leads to respiratory acidosis and carbon dioxide narcosis. Some patients experience emotional instability, overt psychosis (myxedema madness), or dementia, which is irreversible.

Causes

Hypothyroidism may be either congenital or acquired. The etiologic classification is as follows.

Congenital
1. Thyroid dysgenesis
   a. Thyroid aplasia
   b. Thyroid hypoplasia
   c. Ectopic thyroid (usually hypoplastic)
2. Inborn defects in thyroid hormone synthesis or metabolism
   a. TSH nonresponsiveness
   b. Inability to trap iodide
   c. Inability to organify iodide (peroxidase defect)
   d. Inability to couple iodotyrosines
   e. Iodotyrosine deiodinase defect
   f. Deficient or abnormal thyroglobulin synthesis
   g. Peripheral unresponsiveness to thyroid hormone
3. Pituitary or hypothalamic disorder

Acquired
1. Chronic lymphocytic (Hashimoto's) thyroiditis
2. Idiopathic atrophy
3. Iatrogenic
4. Endemic hypothyroidism
5. Hypopituitarism or hypothalamic disease

Congenital Hypothyroidism

Thyroid Dysgenesis. These infants have a deficiency in the volume of thyroid tissue. Most (80%) have a small amount of glandular tissue, often located ectopically, such as at the base of the tongue (lingual thyroid). Screening of newborns by measuring serum T_4 and TSH shows that this congenital disorder occurs in 1 per 4,000 births.

Inborn Defects in Thyroid Hormone Synthesis. The patients usually have goiter and may be cretinous, hypothyroid, or euthyroid depending on the severity of the defect. These defects are rare and occur in 1 per 40,000 births.

TSH NONRESPONSIVENESS. The patients have a small gland with a low radioiodine uptake, hypothyroid function tests, and lack of response to exogenous TSH.

IODIDE TRANSPORT DEFECT. Features include low thyroid uptake of radioiodine and low thyroid concentration of iodine. The iodide transport system is also missing in the salivary glands and gastric mucosa. Administration of iodine raises plasma iodide, which, by diffusion, increases intrathyroid iodide and thus permits synthesis of normal amounts of hormone.

ORGANIFICATION DEFECT. Failure of oxidative iodination results in rapid and high uptake of radiodine, but the radiodine is not oxidized and organically bound; thus it can be displaced from the gland by perchlorate (see Fig. 3–3). The specific oxidative enzyme system (peroxidase) for organification of iodine is deficient. Some patients with a milder form of this syndrome have nerve deafness. The combination of nerve deafness and familial goiter is called Pendred's syndrome.

DEFECTIVE COUPLING OF IODOTYROSINES. Radioiodine tracer is taken up rapidly and retained (organified), but there is a defect in coupling iodotyrosines to form iodothyronines. Thyroidal iodine is primarily in the form of MIT and DIT with trace amounts of T_4 and T_3. This defect is probably not attributable to a single specific deficiency. It may be enzymatic or may be due to a structural defect in the thyroglobulin molecule that prevents iodotyrosines from coming into close proximity for coupling.

DEFICIENT IODOTYROSINE DEIODINASE. Normally MIT and DIT, released by proteolysis of thyroglobulin, are rapidly deiodinated in the thyroid. Little MIT or DIT is secreted. Iodotyrosine deiodinase is present in many organs. Patients with this defect have high MIT and DIT concentrations in the blood. When they are given labeled MIT or DIT, they excrete the intact molecule in the urine. Synthesis of T_4 and T_3 can occur, but leakage of MIT and DIT depletes iodine stores. This defect is inherited as an autosomal recessive.

DEFICIENT OR ABNORMAL THYROGLOBULIN SYNTHESIS. These patients are goitrous cretins whose thyroid glands transport and oxidize iodide, but most of the iodine in the thyroid is bound to albumin, and thyroglobulin is absent. The thyroglobulin gene is one of the largest eukaryotic genes characterized, and many aberrations in the structure of thyroglobulin probably exist.

PERIPHERAL RESISTANCE TO THYROID HORMONE. Families have been reported with stippled epiphyseal centers and deaf-mutism (indicating congenital hypothyroidism), goiter, and *elevated serum T_4*. The findings indicate peripheral resistance to the effects of thyroid hormone. The defect may be binding to the receptor or a postreceptor defect.

Pituitary or Hypothalamic Disorder. Hypothalamic hypothyroidism with TRH deficiency, isolated TSH deficiency, congenital absence of the pituitary and other causes of hypopituitarism cause hypothyroidism in 1 per 80,000 births.

Acquired Hypothyroidism

Hashimoto's Lymphocytic Thyroiditis. This condition is the most common cause of hypothyroidism in adults and in children after 8 years of age. Most patients with Hashimoto's thyroiditis have mild to moderate enlargement of the thyroid, but they are euthyroid and asymptomatic. About one-fifth of cases are hypothyroid, and a few are hyperthyroid.

Idiopathic Atrophy. This disorder, the second most common cause of adult hypothyroidism, is usually due to lymphocytic thyroiditis. There are small remnants of thyroid tissue with occasional follicles, fibrous tissues, and lymphocytic infiltration. Most patients have antibodies to thyroid tissue, and TSH-blocking antibodies have been found.

Iatrogenic Hypothyroidism. This common disorder occurs after surgical thyroidectomy, after ^{131}I treatment of hyperthyroidism or thyroid cancer, after radiation therapy to the neck for cancer of the larynx or lymphoma, with overdosage of antithyroid drugs (a reversible condition), and with high doses of iodine in susceptible individuals.

Endemic Hypothyroidism Including Cretinism. Patients with this condition and their parents usually have goiter. This syndrome occurs in regions of severe iodine deficiency. Endemic cretins may be hypothyroid or euthyroid in later life, but they retain short stature and the characteristic appearance of cretinism. Mental retardation, deafness, and other neurologic abnormalities may predominate, leading to the term "neurologic cretin."

Hypopituitarism. Lack of TSH may be associated with deficiencies of other pituitary hormones, but unitropic loss of TSH occurs. Most pituitary lesions cause a loss of growth hormone and gonadotropin before loss of TSH and ACTH. This condition is called pituitary or secondary hypothyroidism.

Hypothalamic Disease. Organic suprasellar lesions or biochemical defects may cause a deficiency of TRH, alone or in combination with loss of other hypothalamic hormones. The diagnosis is established in hypothyroid patients by finding a low serum TSH that increases after administration of TRH.

Therapy

Administration of exogenous thyroid hormone will completely reverse the features of hypothyroidism with the exception of cretinism. The following are among the preparations available.

	Average daily adult replacement dose
1. Sodium l-thyroxine (synthetic T_4)	100 to 200 μg
2. Sodium l-triiodothyronine (synthetic T_3)	50 to 75 μg
3. Preparations of mixed synthetic T_4 and T_3 in a ratio of 4:1	50 to 100 μg T_4 + 12.5 to 25 μgT_3
4. Thyroid USP (desiccated thyroid) A dried, powdered preparation of animal (usually pig or cattle) thyroid glands.	90 to 180 mg

L-Thyroxine is the preferred preparation for replacement therapy because it is more uniform than biologic preparations, its absorption is reliable, and it is easily measured in serum. Because the circulating T_3 in T_4-treated patients comes from conversion of T_4 to T_3 in tissue, normal ranges for T_4 and T_3 can be used to monitor therapy.

NONTHYROIDAL ILLNESS AND THYROID FUNCTION

Severe illnesses that do not involve the thyroid directly may cause changes in serum thyroid hormone levels. Reduction of the serum T_3 occurs commonly with many forms of metabolic stress, such as starvation, any serious illness such as pneumonia or septicemia, and after major surgery. The low serum T_3 level results from impairment of 5'-monodeiodination of T_4 in tissues such as the liver, which is the main source of T_3 production. There is a reciprocal increase in the 5-deiodinase, which produces more reverse T_3. With more severe illnesses, serum T_4 concentrations also fall, but free T_4 usually remains normal. This may be due to circulating inhibitors of binding of T_4 to serum proteins. High levels of several unsaturated free fatty acids will inhibit this binding. In some patients, free T_4 is also low. These patients with low T_3 and

CONTINUUM OF THYROID HORMONE AND THYROTROPIN PROFILES IN NONTHYROIDAL ILLNESS AND RECOVERY

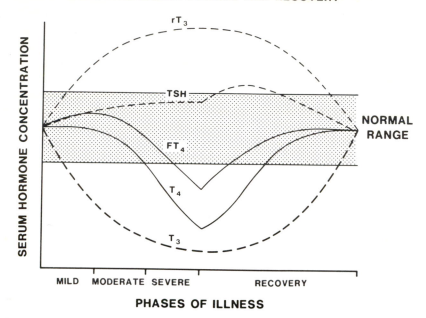

Fig. 3–6. Patterns of serum T_4, T_3, FT_4, TSH, and rT_3 for increasing severity of nonthyroidal illness and for recovery. Serum T_3 is subnormal in mild illness, with serum T_4 and FT_4 falling only with more severe illness. Reverse T_3 rises as T_3 falls. The recovery is generally a reverse of the illness pattern with a slight elevation of serum TSH in many instances. (From Brent, G.A., and Hershman, J.M.: In The Thyroid Gland. Edited by L. Van Middlesworth, Chicago, Year Book Medical Publishers, 1986, with permission.

T_4 levels have normal serum TSH levels, which excludes the diagnosis of primary hypothyroidism. The normal serum TSH in the face of low T_4 and T_3 concentrations suggests that pituitary TSH secretion is inhibited by the effects of the systemic illness. During recovery from the severe illness, serum T_4 and TSH levels rise concomitantly. In this recovery phase, serum TSH may exceed the normal range. With further recovery, serum T_3 normalizes. Figure 3–6 diagrams these events. The reduction of serum T_3 and T_4 may be a homeostatic adaptation to the illness that spares the patient from the catabolic actions of thyroid hormones. Limited trials of therapy with T_4 or T_3 have not been beneficial.

AUTOIMMUNE THYROID DISEASE

There are three forms of autoimmune thyroid disease: Hashimoto's thyroiditis, Graves' disease, and lymphocytic thyroiditis with hyperthyroidism. In a given patient, one disorder may eventually develop into another, and in a single family, siblings may develop different forms of autoimmune thyroid disease. These disorders are about 3 to 6 times more common in women compared with men.

The major histocompatibility complex of chromosome 6 contains genes for three major classes of molecules called HLA, which are glycoprotein antigens expressed on the surface of cells. Patients with autoimmune endocrine disease have an increased prevalence of certain antigens. Class I antigens are involved in cytotoxic T-cell responses. Class II antigens, which are present mainly in the macrophage or B lymphocyte, interact with helper T-cells to promote antibody formation. Graves' disease is associated with an increased prevalence of the class I antigen HLA-B8 and the class II antigen HLA-DR3 in Caucasians. Patients with atrophic Hashimoto's thyroiditis have an increase in HLA-B8 and HLA-DR3 while patients with goitrous Hashimoto's thyroiditis have an increase in HLA-DR5. The precise role of these antigens in the pathogenesis of autoimmune thyroid disease is unclear.

Several antibodies are found in the serum of these patients. These are:

1. Antibody to thyroid microsomes. The major antigen is thyroid peroxidase, an organ-specific antigen.

2. Antibody to thyroglobulin.

3. Antibodies to thyrotropin receptor. These antibodies are detected in several ways and may differ in activity qualitatively in the following ways: (1) displace TSH without activating the receptor, (2) activate the receptor and mimic TSH action, (3) block the action of TSH and cause atrophy of the thyroid, (4) stimulate growth of the thyroid without increasing secretion of thyroid hormone.

The principal theory in regard to pathogenesis of these disorders is that there is a defect in suppressor T-lymphocytes, which permits the expression of antibodies that are not normally produced.

HYPERTHYROIDISM

Hyperthyroidism is a clinical syndrome that occurs when excessive amounts of thyroid hormones in the circulation affect peripheral tissues. The most common cause of hyperthyroidism is Graves' disease, characterized by one or more of three pathognomonic clinical entities: (1) hyperthyroidism associated with a diffusely enlarged thyroid gland, (2) infiltrative ophthalmopathy (exophthalmos), and (3) infiltrative dermopathy (pretibial myxedema). Hyperthyroidism is the most frequent clinical entity in patients with Graves' disease. When infiltrative ophthalmopathy (or dermopathy) occurs in the absence of hyperthyroidism, the condition is referred to as "euthyroid Graves' disease."

The causes of hyperthyroidism other than Graves' disease include:

1. Hyperfunctioning solitary thyroid adenoma ("hot" nodule)

2. "Toxic" multinodular goiter

3. Lymphocytic thyroiditis with low thyroid radioiodine uptake

4. Subacute (granulomatous) thyroiditis (early phase)

5. Ingestion of excessive amount of thyroid hormones (thyrotoxicosis factitia)
6. TSH-producing pituitary adenoma
7. Pituitary resistance to suppression of TSH-secretion by thyroid hormone
8. Trophoblastic tumors (hydatidiform mole, choriocarcinoma) that secrete excessive amounts of chorionic gonadotropin, a weak thyroid stimulator.
9. Thyroid carcinoma (follicular type) with widespread metastases
10. Struma ovarii (ovarian teratoma with thyroid elements)

Pathogenesis of Graves' Hyperthyroidism

The serum IgG of patients with Graves' hyperthyroidism contains a thyroid stimulator that has been detected by several methods. In bioassays, this stimulator has a longer duration of action than TSH, leading to the term long-acting thyroid stimulator. Incubation of cultured thyroid cells with the serum IgG of the patient increases production of cyclic AMP by these cells. This is the best current method to measure the stimulator. With sensitive assays, thyroid-stimulating activity is found in the serum of over 90% of patients with active hyperthyroidism. Another technique measures displacement of radioactive TSH from a thyroid membrane preparation by the IgG of the patient, a test which is positive in about 70% of hyperthyroid patients. However, this TSH-binding inhibition activity does not prove that there is stimulatory activity in the patient's serum.

Pathology of the Thyroid in Graves' Disease

The thyroid gland is diffusely enlarged and has soft-to-normal consistency. Microscopically, the follicles are small and lined with hyperplastic columnar epithelium. Colloid is scanty, and marginal scalloping and vacuolization are evident. The nuclei are vesicular and mitoses are frequently seen. Hyperplastic epithelium shows frequent papillary projections into the lumen of the follicles. Vascularity of the gland is increased, and it is generally infiltrated with lymphocytes and plasma cells that are frequently aggregated in the form of lymphoid follicles. Figure 3–7A shows the typical histopathology.

Symptoms and Signs

The clinical features of hyperthyroidism mainly reflect two effects of excessive circulating thyroid hormone levels: (1) increased metabolic activity in various tissues due to direct effects of thyroid hormones, and (2) increased sensitivity of tissues to catecholamines due to an increased number of receptors for catecholamines rather than increased circulating catecholamines.

Patients complain of nervousness, weight loss despite good appetite, heat intolerance, and increased perspiration. The skin is warm and moist to dissipate the increased heat production. Vitiligo (patchy depigmentation) may occur as an associated autoimmune disorder. There is an abnormally deep separation of the distal end of the fingernail from its base (onycholysis).

Cardiovascular manifestations, directly reflecting the effect of thyroid hor-

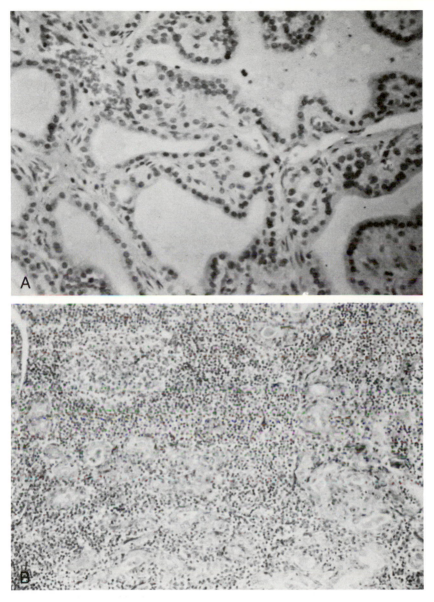

Fig. 3–7. *A.* Graves' thyroid gland. The thyroid follicles have a columnar epithelial lining and there are intraluminal epithelial infoldings; the colloid is water clear. *B.* Hashimoto's lymphocytic thyroiditis. There is diffuse lymphocytic infiltration of the thyroid with a germinal center on the upper left. The thyroid follicles are small and colloid is sparse; follicular cells have abundant cytoplasm characteristic of Askanazy cells.

mone on the heart, are prominent, with tachycardia; tachyarrythmias such as atrial fibrillation and paroxysmal atrial tachycardia; systolic hypertension; and widened pulse pressure. The cardiac impulse is forceful and provides a useful clinical sign for evaluating thyroid hyperfunction. Congestive heart failure is usually related to the tachycardia, increased cardiac work, and sometimes underlying heart disease, and may occur despite a high cardiac output.

Dyspnea is related to intercostal muscle weakness and increased oxygen utilization. Patients often have increased appetite and mild hyperdefecation, but diarrhea is unusual. Nervousness, emotional lability, and hyperkinesia are common since thyroid hormone affects the nervous system.

Muscle weakness is more marked proximally because of catabolism of muscle protein. Patients complain of weakness in walking up stairs and may have difficulty rising from a squatting position. Muscle wasting may be striking. Myasthenia gravis or hypokalemic periodic paralysis may coexist. Mobilization of bone mineral leads to osteoporosis, and hypercalcemia occurs in some patients.

Hematologic manifestations include neutropenia, lymphocytosis, anemia, and increased red cell mass due to the excess demand for oxygen. Oligomenorrhea, amenorrhea, and decreased libido occur. Gynecomastia is found in 10 to 20% of men and may be related to a high serum estradiol/testosterone ratio because of increased conversion of androgen to estrogen.

Ophthalmopathy

Patients with Graves' disease are characterized classically by bilateral proptosis (exophthalmos) that may be asymmetrical; exophthalmos may even be unilateral (Fig. 3–8). The cause of the ophthalmopathy is unclear, but is probably due to antibodies directed against retro-orbital antigens such as extraocular muscle constituents. Proptosis is due to swelling of the retro-orbital muscles with a mixture of mononuclear cell inflammation and edema. Besides proptosis, ophthalmic symptoms may include increased lacrimation, gritty sensation in the eyes, diplopia, and diminution in vision. Clinical findings may include lid lag, lid retraction (causing a ''stare''), conjunctival congestion, conjunctival edema (chemosis), congestion of the lateral rectus muscle insertion (which can be seen on lateral gaze), and limitation of extraocular muscle movement, commonly involving the inferior rectus muscle and leading thereby to diplopia upon upward and lateral gaze.

Figure 3–9 shows a computed tomographic scan of the orbit in a patient with Graves' ophthalmopathy. Approximately 1% of patients develop severe and progressive (malignant) exophthalmos, which may result in exposure keratitis, diminution in visual acuity due to optic nerve involvement, panophthalmitis, and even dislocation of the globe.

Infiltrative Dermopathy

This condition is present in a small percentage of patients. It is frequently associated with ophthalmopathy and usually involves the pretibial region of

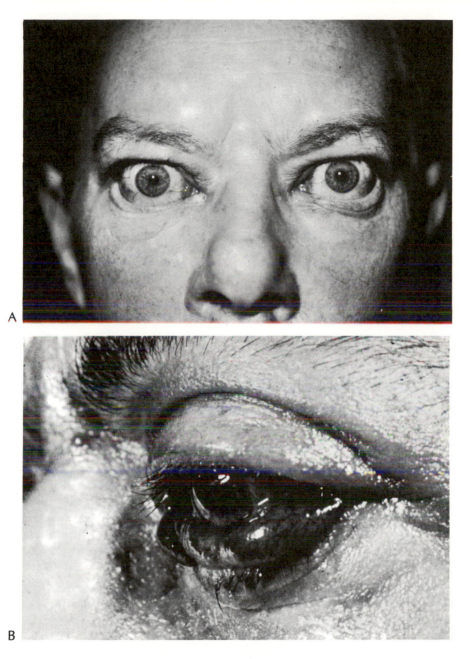

Fig. 3–8. *A*, 45-year-old man with Graves' disease showing typical stare and ex-ophthalmos. *B*, Severe exophthalmos with periorbital swelling and chemosis in a woman.

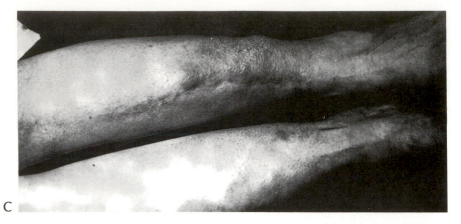

C

Fig. 3–8 (Cont'd).   *C,* Pretibial dermopathy in a 40-year-old woman who has nodular areas of induration and violaceous thickened skin (right).

the legs (see Fig. 3–8). The skin is thickened and shiny, violaceous, difficult to raise into a fold, and may resemble an orange peel. Microscopically, the dermis is thickened and infiltrated with glycosaminoglycans and cells of chronic inflammation.

Laboratory Diagnosis

Elevated serum levels of thyroid hormones are the hallmark of the diagnosis. Ordinarily, serum T_4, T_3, free T_4, and free T_3 are all elevated, and serum TSH is suppressed. The low serum TSH does not rise after administration of TRH. There is increased saturation of thyroid hormone binding proteins, as assessed by the T_3 uptake test.

Some hyperthyroid patients have an elevated serum T_3 concentration and a normal serum T_4 concentration. This entity, T_3-thyrotoxicosis, may occur in patients who have Graves' disease or hyperfunctioning nodular goiter as the cause for their hyperthyroidism.

Although thyroid radioiodine uptake is high in most forms of hyperthyroidism, it is low in patients who are hyperthyroid owing to lymphocytic thyroiditis, subacute thyroiditis, or ingestion of thyroid hormone. The thyroid scan in Graves' disease shows diffuse uptake of radioiodine. The scan is helpful if a solitary hyperfunctioning thyroid adenoma is being considered as the cause of hyperthyroidism (see Fig. 3–4).

Treatment of Hyperthyroidism

Three definitive modes of treatment are available for hyperthyroidism: drugs, ^{131}I, and surgical thyroidectomy.

Drugs. Thionamide drugs, propylthiouracil and methimazole, inhibit the peroxidase enzyme system of the thyroid gland and reduce synthesis of thyroid hormone. In addition, propylthiouracil (but not methimazole) inhibits monodeiodination of T_4 to T_3 in peripheral tissue. Figure 3–1 illustrates these

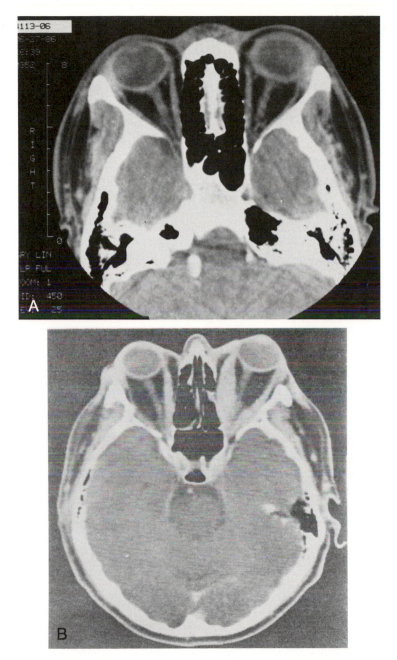

Fig. 3–9. Computed tomographic scan of the orbit of a normal person (A) and of a patient with Graves' ophthalmopathy (B) seen from below. The left medial rectus is massively enlarged, and the left lateral rectus and right medial rectus are moderately enlarged. (Reprinted from Trokel, S.L., and Jakobiec, F.A.: Ophthalmology, *88*:553, 1981, with permission.

mechanisms. After a course of treatment lasting 12 to 18 months, nearly one-half the patients have a lasting remission.

Iodine in a dose of 6 to 2000 mg/day inhibits release of hormone from the gland, probably by interfering with proteolysis of thyroglobulin, resulting in a rapid fall of serum T_4 and T_3 levels. A large amount of iodine may block the peroxidase system also. Unfortunately many patients escape from these effects in several weeks. Lithium also slows the release of hormone from the gland by interfering with proteolysis of the colloid.

Beta-adrenergic receptor blocking drugs produce significant improvement in many features of hyperthyroidism. They reduce tachycardia, tremor, nervousness, and perspiration without affecting the secretion of thyroid hormone. Propranolol, and possibly other beta blockers, also blocks peripheral conversion of T_4 to T_3 and will lower serum T_3 levels to a modest extent.

Radioiodine-131

[131]I destroys thyroid tissue mainly by the beta radiation, which is selectively concentrated in the thyroid follicular cells. The radiation also impairs the ability of residual tissue to replicate and damages the microvasculature. Administration is simple: the patient merely swallows the radioiodine. The usual dose is 3 to 10 millicuries. The only significant undersirable effect is permanent hypothyroidism, which appears in 30 to 70% of patients. Although hypothyroidism often develops in the first year after treatment, it may not become manifest until many years later.

Surgical Procedure

Subtotal thyroidectomy rapidly cures hyperthyroidism. It is carried out when the patient has been made euthyroid with antithyroid drugs to prevent a serious exacerbation of hyperthyroidism ("thyroid storm") in the postoperative period. Stable iodine is given for 10 days preoperatively to control the hyperthyroidism and to reduce the vascularity of the thyroid gland. Unfortunately, a significant incidence of serious complications occurs with surgical thyroidectomy: hypothyroidism, hypoparathyroidism from inadvertent removal or damage of the parathyroid glands, and vocal cord paralysis from cutting the recurrent laryngeal nerves. Other complications include hemorrhage necessitating tracheostomy, cosmetic disfigurement, and recurrent hyperthyroidism.

THYROIDITIS

The various types of thyroiditis are (1) chronic lymphocytic (Hashimoto's) thyroiditis; (2) subacute (acute) granulomatous thyroiditis; and (3) acute suppurative thyroiditis (rare).

Chronic Lymphocytic Thyroiditis

This disease is the most frequently observed thyroid disorder in the United States. It is about three-fold more common in women than in men. Its incidence is about 3 to 4% of the population, 1.4% in euthyroid asymptomatic adolescents, and up to 16% of elderly women. The disease is characterized by infiltration of the thyroid tissue by lymphocytes and plasma cells. Some follicular cells are enlarged with vacuolized cytoplasm containing eosinophilic granules (Askanazy cells). There is a variable degree of fibrosis. Figure 3–7B shows typical histopathology.

In most patients, there is a minimal to moderate-sized firm, nobby, non-tender goiter with sharply defined margins. Signs of an infection are absent. The disease usually is detected incidentally by palpation, but some patients have thyroid dysfunction.

Associated Disorders. Certain families tend to develop Hashimoto's thyroiditis. It occurs with increased incidence in patients with chromosomal disorders (Turner's and Klinefelter's syndromes). It also occurs in association with other endocrine gland deficiencies of autoimmune origin, including Addison's disease, hypoparathyroidism, and diabetes mellitus; pernicious anemia and moniliasis may also be found in these patients. These syndromes occur in various combinations; Schmidt's syndrome is the combination of Hashimoto's thyroiditis and adrenal insufficiency with or without diabetes mellitus.

Clinically, about three-fourths of the patients with Hashimoto's thyroiditis have euthyroid goiter, one-fourth have hypothyroidism with or without goiter, and a small proportion are hyperthyroid. Nearly one-third of patients with lymphocytic thyroiditis have a nodular goiter.

Diagnosis. Several markers for Hashimoto's thyroiditis aid in diagnosis, especially the presence of circulating antibodies. The anti-microsomal antibody is much more frequently detectable than anti-thyroglobulin antibody. The thyroid scan is spotty and uneven because of the lymphoid infiltration and fibrosis of the gland. Iodide organification is abnormal, so that administration of perchlorate discharges a large proportion of the trapped radioiodine (positive perchlorate discharge test, see Fig. 3–3). As the disease progresses and thyroid tissue is damaged, the serum TSH increases. The Hashimoto's gland is unusually sensitive to administered iodine, which will reduce synthesis and secretion of T_4 leading to hypothyroidism that is reversible when the iodine is stopped.

Lymphocytic Thyroiditis with Hyperthyroidism. Hyperthyroidism associated with low thyroid uptake of radioiodine is usually due to lymphocytic thyroiditis. The thyroid is not tender and is only slightly enlarged. Apparently, the inflammatory process causes a leak of thyroid hormone into the circulation, but biosynthesis is reduced. Patients usually go through a hypothyroid phase. Figure 3–10 diagrams the course of the condition. The disease is self-limited, subsides in 1 to 3 months, and usually does not result in permanent hypothyroidism. The pathophysiologic basis for the functional difference between this disorder and Hashimoto's thyroiditis with *hypothyroidism* is unclear.

Pregnancy influences the clinical course of autoimmune thyroid disease. As pregnancy advances, the levels of thyroid autoantibodies decline. Follow-

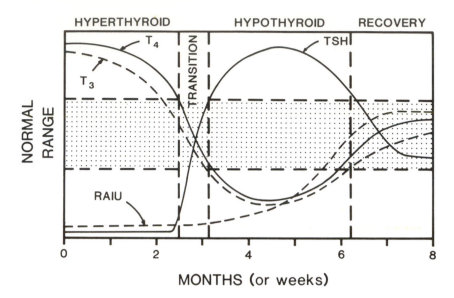

Fig. 3–10. Diagram of the course of lymphocytic thyroiditis with hyperthyroidism. The shaded region shows the normal range. The same general pattern occurs in subacute thyroiditis, but the duration of each phase is weeks rather than months.

ing delivery, the titers rise, reaching a peak 3 to 4 months postpartum. This transient rebound of the autoimmune process causes postpartum thyroiditis in about 5% of mothers. The most common course is transient hyperthyroidism followed by hypothyroidism and then recovery. There may occur only a hypothyroid phase with spontaneous recovery in several months.

Therapy. No specific treatment exists for Hashimoto's thyroiditis. Some evidence suggests that thyroid hormone suppresses the disease and decreases goiter size by inhibiting TSH secretion, but the thyroid antibodies generally persist. Hypothyroidism, once present, is usually permanent and requires treatment with thyroid hormone. Postpartum women undergo spontaneous recovery from hypothyroidism, however, as do a few adolescents.

Subacute Granulomatous Thyroiditis

Acute-subacute nonsuppurative granulomatous thyroiditis is usually referred to as subacute thyroiditis because the course runs from 2 weeks to several months. The etiology is unknown, although a viral origin seems most likely. The onset is characterized by fever, malaise, and a firm, tender goiter. Often an upper respiratory infection or a prodrome of malaise, myalgia, and fatigue precedes this condition. The frequent presence of fever and systemic features suggests an infectious process. The disease often occurs in association with viral epidemics, including mumps, influenza, measles, and the common cold, and antibodies to viral antigens may be detected. The histologic picture varies with the stage of the disease. There is infiltration of the tissue with inflammatory cells, disruption of the follicular architecture, and multinucleated giant cells congregating around masses of colloid.

Antithyroid antibodies occur in many of these patients, but the titers are low, peak several weeks after the onset, and disappear after several months. They probably occur as a result of the disease and are not involved in the pathogenesis. The frequency of the HLA-B8 antigen is increased six-fold compared with normal controls, suggesting a hereditary predisposition to this disorder. The signs and symptoms can be divided into three subgroups: local, systemic, and metabolic.

Local manifestations are due to the inflammation of the gland and include neck pain in the area of the thyroid, sometimes with radiation to the ears; pain on swallowing; sore throat; and often visible swelling in the area of the thyroid gland. Thyroid tenderness is pathognomonic of the disorder.

Malaise and fatigue are present in 80% of patients. Fever, anorexia, myalgia, occasionally chills, and features of an upper respiratory infection also may occur.

Hypermetabolism. In the early phase of the disease, about half the patients complain of nervousness, sweating, heat intolerance, tachycardia, insomnia, and weight loss. These manifestations presumably relate to the release of thyroid hormones from the severe thyroid cell damage caused by the infectious agent. The serum T_4 and thyroglobulin are increased because of release caused by the destructive process. The damaged thyroid cells fail to trap iodine, and the thyroidal radioiodine uptake is reduced early in the disease. The local and systemic symptoms and signs and the elevated T_4 concentration in association with a low thyroid uptake of radioiodine suggest the diagnosis. The hyperthyroidism is self-limited, usually subsiding in 2 to 6 weeks. Figure 3–10 shows the course of the illness; note that the time scale is in weeks rather than months, in contrast with lymphocytic thyroiditis with hyperthyroidism.

Therapy and Course. No specific therapy exists, and antithyroid medication offers little benefit because of the short duration of hyperthyroidism. Symptomatic therapy for the local or systemic discomfort may be helpful. Glucocorticoids have been given with good results.

During recovery, the radioactive iodine uptake increases as the follicular cells resume normal function. The elevated levels of T_4 fall as glandular colloid is depleted and may reach hypothyroid levels if recovery of follicular cell function is delayed. At this point, features of hypothyroidism appear in about one-fourth of the patients. Thyroid function eventually returns to normal; however, an enlarged, hard, nontender thyroid gland may persist for weeks or months after the acute phase. In some patients with protracted or recurrent thyroid tenderness, administration of thyroid hormone appears beneficial.

ENDEMIC GOITER

Endemic goiter is defined as enlargement of the thyroid gland to twice the normal size or larger in at least 10% of the population of an area. Endemic goiter still occurs in all continents, even though its incidence in most areas of the world has decreased because of the prophylactic use of iodine in the form of iodized salt.

Etiology

The principal cause of endemic goiter is deficient dietary iodine intake. The minimal essential dietary requirement is 100 μg/day. Diets containing about 50 to 70 μg/day are associated with a 25% prevalence of goiter and diets containing only 20 to 50 μg/day are associated with a 50% prevalence of goiter (Fig. 3–11). Dietary deficiencies of iodine occur in areas where the soil is poor in iodine, resulting in low iodine content of the food and water

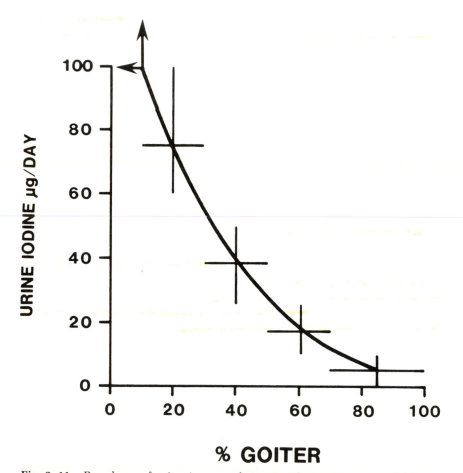

% GOITER vs. URINE IODINE

Fig. 3–11. Prevalence of goiter in a population in relation to mean urine iodine content which reflects dietary iodine intake. The size of the horizontal and vertical lines through each point approximates the range of values in different populations.

of the region. Oceans are the world's chief iodine store. The sea's iodine is continually redistributed in the atmosphere and returns to the land by precipitation with rain. Major areas of natural iodine deficiency include the northwestern and Great Lakes areas of the United States, the mountainous areas of Central and South America, the Alps and the Himalayas, central Africa, and many regions of Asia. Saltwater fish and shellfish are rich in iodine; smaller amounts are found in eggs, meat, milk, and cereals. Dietary iodine deficiency tends to be prevalent in impoverished populations of developing countries. Goitrogenic substances in the food or water have been postulated to cause goiter in some regions by blocking formation of thyroid hormone, but the evidence for this is inconclusive.

The deficiency of iodine prevents adequate production of thyroid hormone. Increased secretion of TSH occurs resulting in compensatory thyroid hyperplasia and increased efficiency of iodine transport and biosynthesis of hormone in an attempt to maintain normal thyroid hormone levels. The iodine deficient thyroid gland is more sensitive to the growth-promoting effect of TSH. Patients with endemic goiter have low urinary iodine excretion which reflects their dietary intake, an elevated thyroid radioiodine uptake, and an elevated serum TSH level. In the compensated state, serum T_4 levels are normal to low and serum T_3 levels are normal to high.

The use of iodized salt in many areas of the world, such as the United States, and intramuscular injection of iodized oil in other areas (New Guinea, central Africa, China) have reduced the development of goiter in these areas and the size of existing goiters. An injection of iodized oil provides an adequate iodine store for 4 years.

Clinical Features

The patients are euthyroid in the compensated state. The thyroid can be moderately to grossly enlarged. Table 3–4 gives the staging classification system of the World Health Organization. In childhood and adolescence, the gland is diffusely enlarged. With the passage of time, nodules form, so that multinodular goiter is found in older adults. Figure 3–12 shows goiter in three generations of a family. Females are twice as likely to develop goiter compared with males for reasons which are still unclear. In the decompensated state,

Table 3–4. Staging of Endemic Goiter, World Health Organization Criteria

Stage	Criteria
0	No goiter
I	Enlargement of each lateral lobe equivalent in size by palpation to patient's distal phalanx of thumb
II	Visible enlargement of thyroid readily apparent on close inspection
III	Large goiter easily visible at distance of 10 m

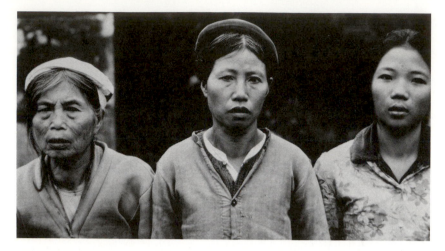

Fig. 3–12. Goiter in three generations of a family in Vietnam. The grandmother has stage 3 multinodular goiter; the mother and granddaughter have stage 2 diffuse goiters.

hypothyroidism develops. Severe iodine deficiency in pregnancy causes cretinism in the offspring. In severe endemic goiter areas where the prevalence of goiter is more than 70%, the incidence of cretinism may be as high as 10%.

THYROID NODULES AND THYROID CARCINOMA

A thyroid nodule (little node) is a common deformity of the thyroid gland found during careful physical examination by inspection and palpation. A thyroid nodule may not be detectable clinically when it is less than 1 cm in diameter even though it may be readily found on pathologic examination of the gland. Figure 3–13 shows a typical thyroid nodule.

Etiology

A thyroid nodule can result from nearly all of the pathologic processes in the thyroid gland. The following pathologic entities frequently cause nodule formation (single or multiple nodules): (1) colloid goiter (may be cystic), (2) adenomas, (3) thyroid carcinoma, (4) chronic lymphocytic thyroiditis, (5) subacute thyroiditis, (6) metastatic cancer, and (7) granulomatous involvement of the thyroid gland (tuberculosis, sarcoidosis).

Adenomas and Carcinomas

In experimental animals, prolonged and increased stimulation of the thyroid gland by TSH, induced by iodine deficiency or antithyroid drugs, can be responsible for thyroid hyperplasia and tumor formation of the follicular cells. In cultured thyroid cells, TSH activates various oncogenes. If the animal thyroid is exposed to x-irradiation during dietary iodine deficiency, tumor formation increases. When these tumors are transplanted to histocompatible

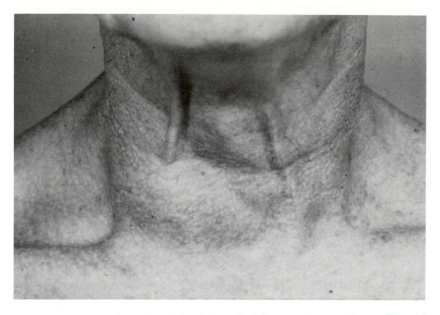

Fig. 3–13. A 5-cm thyroid nodule of the right lobe in a 70-year-old man. Thyroid scan (Fig. 3–4, middle row, 2nd scan) showed that it was hot; he was hyperthyroid.

hosts, the tumors may metastasize. In man, clinical evidence strongly suggests that the incidence of both benign and malignant thyroid tumors increases following exposure to ionizing radiation. Children who were given x-ray therapy for thymic or tonsillar enlargement (in which the thyroid was incidentally irradiated) have a striking increase in the incidence of thyroid tumors (papillary and follicular carcinomas as well as adenomas). Exposure to radiation from fallout of the atomic bomb, which contains ^{131}I, also led to the development of benign and malignant tumors. The latent period between the radiation and the recognition has been 10 to 40 years.

Colloid Goiter

Colloid goiters become nodular in their end stage. The first stage, hyperplasia of the thyroid cells, is followed by colloid accumulation. In the final stage, degenerative changes (infarction hemorrhage, necrosis) occur and lead to nodularity. These nodules can be distinguished clinically from true adenomas because of the multiplicity of nodules in the colloid goiter.

Metastatic Thyroid Cancer

Secondary metastatic lesions to the thyroid are frequent pathologically in patients with disseminated metastatic tumors because of the vascularity of the thyroid, but these lesions are rare clinically. Lymphomas may involve the thyroid gland secondarily or may originate in the thyroid gland.

Clinical Presentation

Symptoms. Benign or malignant nodules of the thyroid gland are symptomless most of the time and are usually found on a routine physical examination. If a nodule is large, it can compress the esophagus leading to dysphagia, it can compress the trachea leading to respiratory difficulties, and it can compress the ipsilateral recurrent laryngeal nerve and cause impairment of the voice, such as hoarseness or even vocal cord paralysis. A malignant lesion is rarely painful. As a rule, benign lesions are not painful except in acute or subacute thyroiditis.

Signs. The nodule is usually discovered by inspection and palpation of the thyroid gland. The consistency of nodules varies from soft to firm. A nodule that is fixed to adjacent tissue and does not move with swallowing is likely to be malignant. Cervical lymphadenopathy suggests that a thyroid nodule is malignant.

Classification of Carcinoma

Table 3–5 lists the classification and frequency of various thyroid cancers. Differentiated thyroid carcinomas (papillary and follicular) make up approximately 85% of all malignant tumors of the thyroid. Differentiated carcinomas are far less malignant than anaplastic carcinomas. If the papillary or follicular carcinoma is confined to the thyroid gland in a patient less than 40-years-old, long-term survival is not reduced. Papillary carcinoma spreads through the lymphatics to the regional lymph nodes. Follicular carcinomas tend to invade blood vessels and metastasize to lung and bone.

Medullary carcinoma of the thyroid, which often has amyloid stroma, originates from the parafollicular C-cells. This tumor is of considerable interest because of its familial incidence in patients with the syndrome of multiple endocrine neoplasia (type 2) consisting of medullary thyroid carcinoma, pheochromocytoma, and hyperparathyroidism. Some of the families have mucosal neuromas and a characteristic appearance with a long thin face, long extremities, and poor musculature. About one-half of the cases of medullary carcinoma are sporadic (nonfamilial). High serum calcitonin level serves as a marker for the medullary carcinoma. Stimulation of calcitonin release by infusion of calcium or pentagastrin gives an excessive calcitonin response in these patients and aids diagnosis of the tumor in a preclinical phase (C-cell

Table 3–5. Histopathologic Classification of Thyroid Cancer

Type	Frequency (%)
Papillary (with or without follicular foci)	60
Follicular	20
Medullary	5
Undifferentiated	10
Lymphoma	5

hyperplasia) in afflicted family members. Although the patients have excessive calcitonin secretion, they are not hypocalcemic; their apparent resistance to the metabolic effect of calcitonin may be explained by a reduction in the number of receptors for calcitonin caused by the high serum levels of the hormone (see Chap. 9).

Separation of Benign from Malignant Lesions

Important factors in the investigation of the patient with a thyroid nodule include a history of radiation therapy to the neck in childhood or a family history of medullary thyroid carcinoma.

The following physical findings suggest malignancy: (1) enlarged lymph nodes in the cervical area, (2) pressure symptoms of hoarseness, and (3) fixation of the nodule to adjacent structures.

Thyroid function is usually normal in the patient with a nodule. If the patient has hypothyroidism or hyperthyroidism, the nodule probably represents lymphocytic or subacute thyroiditis. Serum calcitonin is increased in patients with medullary carcinoma.

X ray of the neck shows small dense calcifications (aggregated psammoma bodies) in papillary carcinoma. Shell-like calcifications usually indicate calcification of a degenerative colloid goiter.

Scanning of the thyroid gland with radioactive iodine has been widely used in an attempt to distinguish benign from malignant lesions. Hyperfunctional ("hot") nodules that concentrate nearly all the radioiodine are rarely malignant. Although "cold" nodules may be malignant, at least 80% of the lesions that do not concentrate radioiodine are benign.

Thyroid ultrasonography is a useful method to distinguish the solid from the cystic lesion. Most malignant lesions are solid by ultrasonography, but not all solid lesions are malignant. Cystic lesions are almost uniformly benign; mixed solid and cystic lesions are sometimes malignant. Ultrasonography has shown that about 20% of thyroid nodules are cystic.

Aspiration of the nodule with a fine needle yields cellular material or fluid that may be diagnostic. This technique of fine-needle aspiration is the most useful method for making a diagnosis without subjecting the patient to surgical operation. Cytologic examination of the aspirate is often successful for making the diagnosis of colloid goiter, lymphocytic thyroiditis, granulomatous thyroiditis, papillary carcinoma, medullary carcinoma, and anaplastic carcinoma. Unfortunately, the cytologic examination usually cannot distinguish the common follicular adenoma from a follicular carcinoma. Figure 3–14 shows examples of the cytology. Cystic contents can be aspirated through the needle to decompress the cyst.

Therapy

Two general forms of therapy have been advocated for the management of thyroid nodules: (1) thyroid hormone to suppress TSH secretion because TSH may be a growth factor for the nodule, (2) surgical removal of the nodule.

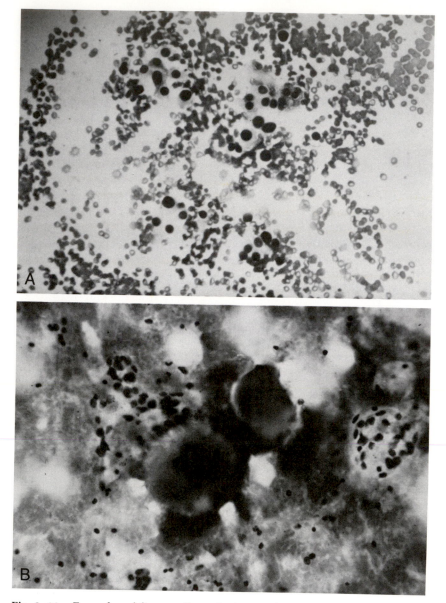

Fig. 3–14. Examples of fine needle aspiration cytology. *A.* Normal thyroid cells, some in follicular arrangement, against a background of red blood cells. *B.* Colloid goiter. There is abundant colloid with scattered normal follicular cells, some in follicular arrangement.

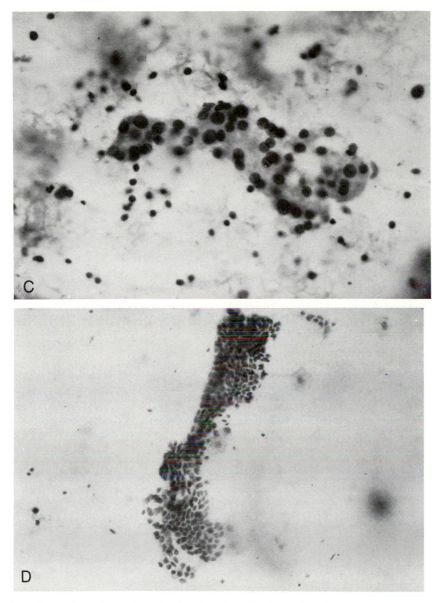

Fig. 3–14 (Cont'd). *C.* Hashimoto's lymphocytic thyroiditis. There are numerous lymphocytes in the background. Thyroid cells have abundant cytoplasm (Askanazy cells). *D.* Papillary carcinoma showing a diagnostic monolayer sheet of cells.

Lesions with definite suspicion of malignancy based on clinical evaluation and needle aspiration cytology are removed surgically. Nodules that are not likely to be malignant, such as colloid nodules, multinodular goiters, cysts, and adenomas, can be treated with doses of thyroid hormone which suppress TSH secretion, such as 100 to 200 mcg thyroxine daily.

After thyroidectomy for differentiated thyroid carcinoma, treatment with ^{131}I is often given to destroy residual malignant tissue, and it is given subsequently when functional metastases become evident. The serum thyroglobulin level is a helpful guide for following the patient; an elevated level indicates persistent or residual functioning tissue.

CLINICAL PROBLEMS

Patient 1. A 36-year-old woman complains of a 15 pound weight gain in 1 year, amenorrhea for 6 months, fatigue, difficulty remembering phone numbers and being "slowed up" mentally, a lower voice and constipation.

PHYSICAL EXAMINATION. She has a puffy face and cool dry skin. Temperature 35°C, pulse 56, BP 120/85. Her thyroid gland is firm, lobular, and nontender. Tendon reflexes are slowed with a delayed return phase.

LABORATORY DATA. Her serum T_4 is 2.5 µg/dl, FT_4I 2.4, serum TSH is 80 µU/ml, and prolactin is 45 ng/ml.

QUESTIONS
1. Which of her clinical features suggest neurologic symptoms from a lack of thyroid hormone?
2. Which laboratory test shows that the patient has primary hypothyroidism rather than hypothyroidism secondary to pituitary disease? Would a head CT scan be indicated?
3. What is the most likely cause of her hypothyroidism, and what test would confirm this diagnosis?
4. What is the explanation for her amenorrhea?

Patient 2. A 26-year-old interior decorator complains of nervousness, weakness, and palpitations with exertion for the past 6 months. Recently, she has perspired excessively in her office and wants to sleep with fewer blankets than her husband. She has lost 5 kg while eating more than she did 1 year ago. She also complains of protrusion of her eyes, excessive lacrimation, and a sandy sensation in her eyes, but no diplopia. Menstrual periods have been regular but there is less bleeding. She has been taking birth control pills for 3 years.

PHYSICAL EXAMINATION. She appears anxious and hyperkinetic and is slender. Her pulse is 120/min, BP 130/60. Her skin is warm, moist, and smooth. She has lid lag, normal ocular motility, mild exophthalmos (though measuring only 18 mm bilaterally on the exophthalmometer; normal less than 20 mm), and slight periorbital swelling. The thyroid is diffusely enlarged to 60 g (3 times normal size), with a prominent isthmus and normal consistency. She has a bounding cardiac apical impulse, a pulmonic flow murmur, and a systolic bruit over the thyroid. She has a fine tremor and onycholysis of both fourth fingernails. The rest of the examination is unremarkable.

LABORATORY DATA. Serum T_4 is 22 mcg/dl, T_3 is 550 ng/dl, and serum TSH is <0.1 µU/ml.

QUESTIONS
1. What is the diagnosis? Are additional diagnostic tests indicated?
2. The thyroid hormone binding ratio is 1.20. Calculate the FT_4I and FT_3I.
3. What is the cause of the pulmonic flow murmur? Of the thyroid bruit?
4. What therapy would you prescribe, and what is her prognosis?
5. Is there any contraindication to pregnancy?

Patient 3. A 26-year-old hospital dietician had pharyngitis with a fever for 1 week. Two weeks later, she had a recurrence of a mild sore throat, noted swelling of her lower anterior neck, and moderate pain with swallowing.

PHYSICAL EXAMINATION. Her temperature was 38.5°C, pulse 100, BP 120/60. Her pharynx appeared normal. Her thyroid was enlarged to 40 g, the left lobe being slightly larger than the right; the entire gland was tender. There was no cervical lymphadenopathy.

LABORATORY DATA. Serum T_4 18.1 µg/dl, FT_4I 18, serum T_3 350 ng/dl, FT_3I 340, RAIU 2% at 24 hours.

QUESTIONS
1. What are the diagnosis and the cause of the condition?
2. Why is the RAIU so low?
3. What would her serum thyroglobulin be?
4. Is she hyperthyroid? What therapy would you recommend?
5. What clinical feature differentiates this condition from lymphocytic thyroiditis with hyperthyroidism?

Patient 4. A 22-year-old woman 4 months postpartum reports fatigue, depression, dry skin, and muscle cramps. She has continued to nurse her infant son. About 6 weeks postpartum, she was nervous, irritable, felt too warm, and noted palpitations. Her family attributed this to the stress of being a new mother.

PHYSICAL EXAMINATION. She has periorbital edema. Her pulse is 60, the thyroid gland is diffusely enlarged to 40 g (twice normal size), and she has delayed tendon reflexes.

LABORATORY DATA. Serum T_4 is 1.5 µg/dl, FT_4I is 1.4, and TSH is 60 µU/ml. Anti-microsomal antibody titer is 1:1600.

QUESTIONS
1. What is the current diagnosis and the cause of this condition?
2. What probably developed 6 weeks postpartum?
3. Why does the postpartum state predispose to this condition?
4. What therapy will you recommend?

Patient 5. A 40-year-old accountant comes to your office because he was found to have a small lump in his neck during a physical examination for life insurance. He recently learned from his mother that he had received x-ray therapy for recurrent tonsillitis at age 4.

PHYSICAL EXAMINATION. This examination is entirely normal except for a 2.5 cm firm oval nodule in the right lower lobe of the thyroid which moves well with swallowing. There is no cervical lymphadenopathy.

LABORATORY DATA. A thyroid scan shows that the nodule is cold. Serum T_4 is 9 µg/dl, serum TSH is 2µU/ml, and thyroid anti-microsomal antibody is negative.

QUESTIONS
1. What are the diagnostic possibilities?
2. Is the history of radiation to the neck important?
3. What additional diagnostic procedure would be helpful?
4. What therapy do you recommend?

Patient 6. A 32-year-old medical technologist had diarrhea for 3 months and had lost 10 pounds. Work-up of the diarrhea had not revealed any apparent cause. He had noted two lumps in his lower anterior neck recently that appeared to be increasing in size.

PHYSICAL EXAMINATION. He did not appear acutely or chronically ill. His pulse was 72, BP was 132/80. There were two firm nodules in the right lobe of the thyroid, one in the upper part and one near the midline, about 2 cm each. The left lobe was barely palpable. There were multiple pea-sized anterior cervical nodes on the right.

LABORATORY DATA. Complete blood count and routine blood chemistries were normal. Serum T_4 was 7 µg/dl, FT_4I 7.1, and TSH was 1.5 µU/ml. Thyroid anti-microsomal antibody was negative. Thyroid scan showed two cold regions in the right lobe corresponding to the palpable nodules.

QUESTIONS
1. What additional history would be important?
2. What tests would you suggest next?
3. Does the diagnosis revealed by these tests explain any other feature of his illness? Should be be screened for other conditions?
4. What are the implications in regard to his family?

SUGGESTED READING

General Reading

DeGroot, L.J., Larsen, P.R., Refetoff, S., and Stanbury, J.B. (eds): The Thyroid and its Diseases. 5th Ed. New York, John Wiley and Sons, 1984.

Hershman, J.M., and Bray, G.A. (eds.): The Thyroid. Physiology and Treatment of Disease. Oxford, Pergamon Press, 1979.
Van Middlesworth, L. (ed): The Thyroid Gland. A Practical Clinical Treatise. Chicago, Year Book Medical Publishers, 1986.

Physiology and Biochemistry
Engler, D., and Burger, A.G.: The deiodination of the iodothyronines and of their derivatives in man.Endocr Rev, 5:151, 1984.
Hershman, J.M., and Pekary, A.E.: Regulation of thyrotropin secretion. *In* The Pituitary Gland. Edited by H. Imura. New York, Raven Press, 1985.
Oppenheimer, J.H., and Samuels, H.H. (eds.): Molecular Basis of Action of Thyroid Hormone. New York, Academic Press, 1983.
Robbins, J., et al.: Thyroxine transport properties of plasma, molecular properties and biosynthesis. Recent Prog Horm Res, 34:477, 1978.

Hypothyroidism
Report of a Committee of the Clinical Society to Investigate the Subject of Myxedema. London, Longmans, Green, and Co., 1888.
Fisher, D.A., et al.: Screening for congenital hypothyroidism: results of screening one million North American infants. J Pediatr, 94:700, 1979.
Lever, E.G., Medeiros-Neto, G.A., and DeGroot, L.J.: Inheritied disorders of thyroid metabolism. Endocr Rev, 4:213, 1983.

Nonthyroid Illness
Brent, G.A., and Hershman, J.M.: Effects of nonthyroidal illness on thyroid function tests. *In* The Thyroid Gland. Edited by L. Van Middlesworth. Chicago, Year Book Medical Publishers, 1986.
Chopra, I.J., et al.: Thyroid function in nonthyroidal illness. Ann Intern Med, 98:946, 1983.
Wartofsky, L., and Burman, K.D.: Alterations in thyroid function with systemic illness: the "euthyroid sick syndrome". Endrocr Rev, 3:164, 1982.

Autoimmunity
Walfish, P.G., Wall, J.R., and Volpe, R. (eds.): Autoimmunity and the Thyroid. Orlando, Academic Press, 1985.
Weetman, A.P., and McGregor, A.M.: Autoimmune thyroid disease. Endocr Rev, 5:309, 1984.

Hyperthyroidism
Burman, K.D., and Baker, J.R., Jr.: Immune mechanisms in Graves' disease. Endocr Rev, 6:183, 1985.
Rappoport, B., et al.: Clinical experience with a human thyroid cell bioassay for thyroid-stimulating immunoglobulin. J Clin Endocrinol Metab, 58:332, 1984.
Trokel, S.L., and Jakobiec, F.A.: Correlation of CT scanning and pathologic features of ophthalmic Graves' disease. Ophthalmology, 88:553, 1981.
Volpe, R.: Thyrotoxicosis. Clin Endocrinol Metab, 7:1, 1978.
Walfish, P.G., and Chan, J.V.C.: Post-partum hyperthyroidism. Clin Endocrinol Metab, 14:417, 1985.
Woolf, P.D.: Transient painless thyroiditis with hyperthyroidism; a variant of lymphocytic thyroiditis? Endocr Rev, 1:411, 1980.

Thyroiditis
Fisher, D.A., et al.: The diagnosis of Hashimoto's thyroiditis. J Clin Endocrinol Metab, 40:795, 1975.
Greenberg, A.H., et al.: Juvenile chronic lymphocytic thyroiditis: clinical, laboratory, and histological correlations. J Clin Endocrinol Metab, 30:293, 1975.
Levine, S.N.: Current concepts of thyroiditis. Arch Intern Med, 143:1952, 1983.

Goiter and Carcinoma
Astwood, E.B., Cassidy, C.E., and Aurbach, G.D.: Treatment of goiter and thyroid nodules with thyroid. JAMA, 174:459, 1960.
DeGroot, L.J. (ed.): Radiation-Associated Thyroid Carcinoma. New York, Grune and Stratton, 1977.
Graze, K., et al.: Natural history of familial medullary thyroid carcinoma. N Engl J Med, 299:980, 1978.

Hershman, J.M., Blahd, W.H., and Gordon, H.E.: Thyroid Gland in Cancer Treatment. Edited by C.M. Haskell. Philadelphia, W.B. Saunders Co., 1985.

Mazzaferri, E.L., and Young, R.L.: Papillary thyroid carcinoma: a 10-year follow-up of the impact of therapy in 576 patients. Am J Med, 70:511, 1981.

Melvin, K.E.W., et al.: Studies in familial medullary thyroid carcinoma. Recent Prog Horm Res, 28:399, 1972.

Ramacciotti, C.E., et al.: Diagnostic accuracy and use of aspiration biopsy in the management of thyroid nodules. Arch Intern Med, 144:1169, 1984.

Rojeski, M.T., and Gharib, H.: Nodular thyroid disease. N Engl J Med, 313:428, 1985.

Stanbury, J.B., and Hetzel, B. (eds.): Endemic Goiter and Endemic Cretinism. New York, John Wiley and Sons, 1980.

ANSWERS TO QUESTIONS

Patient 1.

1. Her subtle loss of memory and mental slowness suggest reduced cerebration, which is difficult to quantitate. The delayed or "hung up" tendon reflexes are a sign of neuromuscular involvement.

2. The greatly elevated serum TSH indicates that the woman has primary hypothyroidism rather than pituitary or hypothalamic disease. A CT scan is unnecessary to make this differentiation. Some patients with primary hypothyroidism have an enlarged pituitary gland from hyperplasia of the thyrotrophs that may even cause enlargement of the sella turcica.

3. Hashimoto's thyroiditis is the most likely cause of the hypothyroidism. The firm lobulated thyroid gland also suggests this diagnosis. Significantly elevated titers of antimicrosomal antibodies would confirm the diagnosis, and are found in 3/4 of the patients.

4. Secondary amenorrhea may result from the hypothyroidism per se. Hypothyroidism itself may impair cyclic gonadotropin secretion by an upknown mechanism; the hyperprolactinemia, which is attributed to the hypothyroidism, may block gonadotropin secretion (see Chap. 2); another possibility is coexistent autoimmune ovarian failure, but this is quite rare. If the secondary amenorrhea is due to hypothyroidism, treatment with thyroxine should restore her menses.

Patient 2

1. She has classic Graves' disease with hyperthyroidism. Thyroid stimulating IgG should be abnormal, but this test is unnecessary to establish the diagnosis of Graves' disease. Although the hyperthyroidism could be due to lymphocytic thyroiditis with hyperthyroidism, which is associated with low thyroid radioiodine uptake, the exophthalmos indicates Graves' disease. Elevated RAIU and increased production of thyroid hormone is a reasonable assumption. To correct for the effects of an elevated TBG due to her birth control pills, a thyroid hormone binding ratio would be helpful.

3. $FT_4I = 22 \times 1.20 = 26.4$ $\qquad\qquad$ $FT_3I = 550 \times 1.20 = 660$

4. The pulmonic flow murmur, common in hyperthyroidism, is due to the increased cardiac output. The thyroid bruit indicates increased blood flow to the thyroid.

Because of the tachycardia and nervousness, a beta-adrenergic blocker is indicated. Her definitive therapy would be a long-term propylthiouracil or methimazole. When the hyperthyroidism is controlled by the antithyroid drug, the beta-blocker can be stopped.

After treatment for 1 year, she has nearly a 50% chance for a long-term remission. Because she is young, destructive forms of treatment are best avoided; therapy with ^{131}I or surgical thyroidectomy may be reconsidered if she relapses after stopping the antithyroid agent.

The prognosis concerning the exophthalmos is not predictable. Although most patients experience significant improvement, some become steadily worse.

5. Yes, but this contraindication is relative. Propylthiouracil and methimazole can be transmitted across the placenta and cause hypothyroidism and goiter in the fetus. Thyroid stimulating IgGs are also transmitted across the placenta and can cause neonatal hyperthyroidism. Pregnancy should be postponed for 1 year with the anticipation that the Graves' disease will be inactive, or at worst that the hyperthyroidism will be controlled on a low dose of antithyroid drug at that time.

Patient 3

1. The patient has all the clinical features of subacute granulomatous thyroiditis. The enlarged tender thyroid gland is the key to the diagnosis. Presumably, the cause is the same virus that caused the pharyngitis.

2. The inflammation of the thyroid gland interferes with normal biosynthesis including trapping and oxidative iodination. In addition, the release of hormone suppresses TSH secretion and lowers the thyroid uptake.

3. Her serum thyroglobulin would be considerably elevated because of the leak caused by the inflammation.

4. Features suggestive of hyperthyroidism could be explained in part by the local inflammatory disorder. However, her elevated serum T_4 and T_3 levels indicate chemical hyperthyroidism.

Because the disorder is self-limited, only rest, aspirin, and observation are indicated at this time. If the hyperthyroidism gets worse, a beta-blocker may be helpful. Corticosteroids reduce the inflammation of the thyroid and are given in worse cases in doses of 20 to 30 mg prednisone per day for 1 to 3 weeks.

5. Lymphocytic thyroiditis does not cause thyroid tenderness.

Patient 4

1. She has postpartum hypothyroidism. The positive anti-microsomal antibodies indicate that the cause is lymphocytic thyroiditis.

2. Her symptoms at 6 weeks postpartum suggest that she was hyperthyroid. The hyperthyroidism resolved spontaneously and then she underwent a transition to hypothyroidism which occurs in about half of the women who have postpartum thyrotoxicosis. The incidence of postpartum thyroiditis is about 5 to 7% based on surveys. Most cases are subclinical, as was her thyrotoxic phase.

3. During pregnancy there is a suppression of many immune responses, and postpartum there is a rebound enhancement of immunoreactivity leading to exacerbation or new onset of autoimmune thyroid disease.

4. She should be treated with a full replacement dose of thyroxine for 6 to 8 months. In most such patients, there is spontaneous recovery to a euthyroid state. Reduction of thyroid size and fall of antibody titers suggest remission of the thyroiditis. These women are predisposed to thyroiditis after a subsequent pregnancy.

Patient 5

1. All causes of thyroid nodules must be considered. The most common lesions in a cold single nodule are adenomas or differentiated carcinomas of the thyroid. Colloid nodule and lymphocytic thyroiditis are also possibilities, but the negative antibody test makes the latter unlikely.

2. The history of radiation to the neck is important because of the neoplasia that may develop 10 to 40 years later. In neck-irradiated patients, about 6% develop differentiated thyroid carcinoma. Of those with thyroid nodules removed surgically, nearly one-half are papillary or follicular carcinoma.

3. Fine-needle aspiration biopsy is recommended. This showed evidence of a follicular lesion; carcinoma could not be ruled out.

4. Thyroidectomy is recommended. At operation, a benign follicular adenoma was found and a left lobectomy was performed. The right lobe was entirely normal to inspection and was not removed. Because of the multicentricity of neoplasia in irradiated patients, some advocate total thyroidectomy. The counter argument is that occult microscopic carcinoma (<1 cm) does not alter the long-term prognosis. To prevent recurrent nodule formation by suppression of TSH secretion, the patient was placed on permanent thyroxine therapy post-operatively.

Patient 6

1. There was no history of irradiation in childhood or of familial thyroid cancer. His 4 younger siblings and parents were in good health.

2. Fine needle aspiration biopsy of the lesions and one of the lymph nodes showed polyhedral cells with amyloid stroma consistent with medullary thyroid carcinoma. His serum calcitonin was 32,000 pg/ml (normal <25).

3. About one-third of patients with medullary thyroid carcinoma have watery diarrhea, presumably due to a tumor product which is still unknown. Patients with familial medullary thyroid carcinoma may have bilateral pheochromocytoma and hyperparathyroidism. Although these conditions are unlikely in the absence of a positive family history, he should be screened for them.

4. His parents and younger siblings should be screened by measurement of serum calcitonin, before and after a provocative stimulus, such as calcium infusion or pentagastrin in order to discover the disease in an early treatable phase. Because of the lymphadenopathy and very high calcitonin level which indicate extensive disease, the prognosis for curative surgical resection in the patient is poor.

4

Adrenal Disease

Michael L. Tuck and Naftali Stern

ABBREVIATIONS

ACTH	corticotropin
beta-LPH	beta-lipotropin
alpha-MSH	alpha-melanocyte-stimulating hormone
CAH	congenital adrenal hyperplasia
CRF	corticotropin-releasing factor
CNS	central nervous system
CT	computed tomography
Compound S	11-deoxycortisol
DOC	11-deoxycorticosterone
17-KS	17-ketosteroids
17-OHCS	17-hydroxycorticosteroids
17-OHP	17-hydroxy-progesterone
18-OHB	18-hydroxy-corticosterone
POMC	proopiomelanocortin
PRA	plasma renin activity
VMA	vanillylmandelic acid

ADRENAL CORTEX

Physiology

Adrenal Steroidogenesis. The adrenal gland synthesizes three major classes of steroid hormones: glucocorticoids, mineralocorticoids, and sex steroids. Cortisol is the major glucocorticoid secreted by the adrenal gland and aldosterone is the major mineralocorticoid. Plasma levels of cortisol vary considerably due to diurnal variation and episodic secretion of cortisol. The daily production of cortisol, however, is rather constant. The metabolism of cortisol also determines its plasma concentration. Compared to other steroids, cortisol has a fairly long half-life in plasma. Once secreted, cortisol circulates bound to cortisol-binding globulin, transcortin, and is partitioned between free and bound fractions. Transcortin, a glycoprotein synthesized in the liver, binds many steroids but has the highest affinity for cortisol. Transcortin levels are increased by pregnancy and estrogen. Free cortisol is available to enter the cell and exert its physiologic effects. Cortisol is rapidly metabolized by the liver and excreted by the kidney. Several enzyme systems participate in the metabolism of cortisol yielding several urinary metabolites; only 1% of the cortisol pool is excreted unmetabolized or free in the urine.

The adrenal androgen/estrogen pathway is regulated by ACTH and other factors. This pathway makes only a small contribution to circulating testosterone and estrone/estradiol which are derived primarily from the gonads. The intermediate in this pathway, dehydroepiandrosterone sulfate, is slowly metabolized because of its high affinity for albumin; its plasma level serves as an indicator of adrenal androgen production. Adrenal androgen production can also be quantitated by measuring urine metabolites termed 17-ketosteroids.

MECHANISM OF STEROID HORMONE ACTION

Steroid hormones of all classes operate through almost identical cellular mechanisms of action. All steroids penetrate the cell wall by diffusion and bind to protein receptors that are specific for the type of steroid. The next step is a temperature dependent activation of the steroid receptor complex which enhances its affinity to combine with chromatin at a specific nuclear acceptor site. This process regulates the rate of transcription of messenger RNA from DNA for synthesis of specific enzymes and cell proteins.

The specificity of action for a given steroid depends on a functional receptor for the steroid in different tissues. Different receptors exist for the various steroid classes including glucocorticoid, mineralocorticoid, progesterone, estrogen and androgen. Receptor affinity also determines biologic activity and specificity; for example, glucocorticoids bind strongly to glucocorticoid receptors and weakly to mineralocorticoid receptors. Steroid receptors exist in two allosteric conformations, active and inactive; hormone binding induces a conformational change to the active form. Glucocorticoid receptors have been detected in most tissues. The nuclear acceptor sites bind the steroid-receptor and are present in excess so that saturation is never reached. The acceptor-receptor interaction increases the rate of transcription of specific genes and enhances the synthesis of proteins coded by them.

The mechanism of action of mineralocorticoids at the cellular level has some similarity to that of glucocorticoids. Target cells for aldosterone action are limited to distal tubular epithelial cells, sweat and salivary glands, and colonic epithelium. The major effect of aldosterone-induced newly synthesized proteins is an enhancement of electrolyte pump pathways to increase sodium movement into cells and potassium movement out of cells.

Glucocorticoids have a diversity of effects including metabolic, anti-inflammatory, and other actions. Glucocorticoids were named for their pronounced effect on inducing new enzyme synthesis in the liver to promote gluconeogenesis (Fig. 4–1). The catabolic effects of glucocorticoids lead to breakdown of amino acids in muscle (and fatty acids in adipose tissue) to supply increased amino acid substrate to the liver for support of gluconeo-

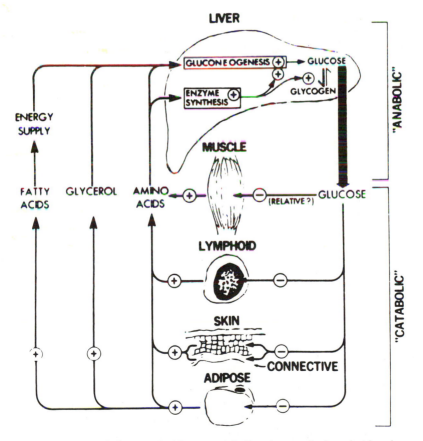

Fig. 4–1. Action of glucocorticoids on metabolism in muscle, lymphoid and connective and adipose tissue to increase substrate flow for hepatic gluconeogenesis. (From Baxter, J., et al.: Am J Med, *53*:573, 1972.)

genesis. Glucocorticoids are required for the normal action of epinephrine and glucagon in the liver to stimulate lipolysis, glycogenolysis, and gluco-neogenesis.

Pharmacologic amounts of glucocorticoids inhibit almost all components of the inflammatory reaction and may be important in regulating this process under stress conditions. During stress glucocorticoids increase cardiac performance and vascular pressor sensitivity to catecholamines. Glucocorticoids also influence calcium metabolism by decreasing gastrointestinal absorption and renal excretion of calcium and altering bone formation and turnover.

REGULATION OF STEROID SECRETION

Cortisol Secretion

Adrenocortical growth and steroid secretion are primarily controlled by the pituitary hormone, adrenocorticotropin (ACTH). Figure 4–2 shows the regulation of the hypothalamic-pituitary-adrenal axis. Corticotropin-releasing factor (CRF) is secreted by the paraventricular nuclei of the hypothalamus into the hypophyseal-portal system and, upon reaching the pituitary, causes release of ACTH. CRF is a 41-amino-acid peptide recently characterized and synthesized. ACTH is carried by the peripheral circulation to the adrenal where it is bound by specific receptors and causes steroid synthesis and secretion. Hypothalamic secretion of CRF is regulated by neural input from higher brain centers such as the limbic system. This neural input inhibits CRF synthesis and secretion resulting in a circadian rhythm of ACTH and cortisol secretion. ACTH and cortisol are released in secretory bursts that occur most frequently during the sixth to eighth hours of sleep and cease during the 2 hours prior to sleep.

The circadian rhythm is overcome by stress, such as surgical procedure, emotional situations, and hypoglycemia. Hormonal stimuli such as vaso-

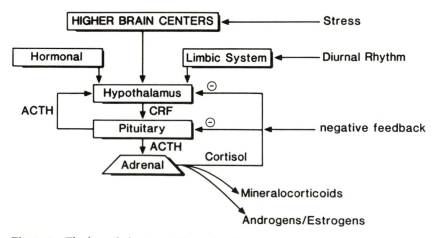

Fig. 4–2. The hypothalamic-pituitary-adrenal axis.

pressin, histamine, and angiotensin also release CRF and ACTH. Cortisol inhibits hypothalamic CRF and pituitary ACTH release; this negative feedback can be overcome by stress. ACTH also has a negative feedback effect on CRF release.

ACTH is synthesized from a larger precursor molecule known as proopiomelanocortin (POMC) which also forms the hormone beta-lipotropin (beta-LPH) in equimolar amounts to ACTH (Fig. 4–3). POMC has little ACTH activity. ACTH activates adrenal adenylate cyclase, increasing cyclic AMP, which stimulates phosphorylation of proteins leading to enhanced steroidogenesis. The major biosynthetic site of action of ACTH is conversion of cholesterol to pregnenolone, but it is also important for maintenance of several adrenal enzymes. The major extra-adrenal effect of ACTH is stimulation of melanocyte activity; excessive levels of ACTH cause hyperpigmentation.

ALDOSTERONE SECRETION

Aldosterone secretion is regulated by three or more control mechanisms: (1) the renin-angiotensin system, operating through volume-mediated changes; (2) potassium ion and (3) ACTH which operate independent of volume. Under most conditions the renin-angiotensin system predominates over the other control factors (Fig. 4–4). During volume depletion, renin, a proteolytic enzyme, is released from juxtaglomerular cells in the renal afferent arterioles. Two intrarenal receptor mechanisms control renin release. The juxtaglomerular cells respond to changes in renal perfusion pressure and the macula densa perceives changes in sodium delivery to the distal nephron. Released renin acts enzymatically on a circulating renin substrate molecule to produce the decapeptide, angiotensin I. Angiotensin I, which has no known major physiologic function, is rapidly converted by specific converting enzymes located mainly in the lung to angiotensin II. Angiotensin II stimulates the production of aldosterone in the zona glomerulosa of the adrenal cortex.

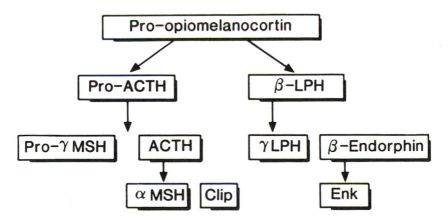

Fig. 4–3. Processing of ACTH and related peptides in the pituitary gland from proopiomelanocortin. (Enk = enkephalin)

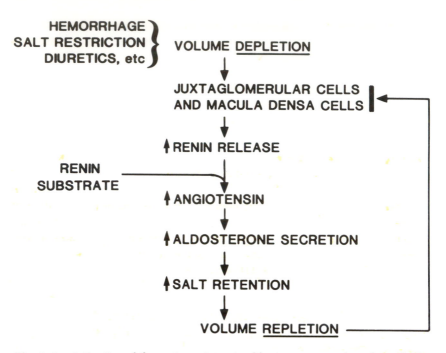

Fig. 4–4. Activation of the renin-angiotensin-aldosterone system by volume depletion and subsequent feedback effect of volume repletion to shut off the stimulus for renin release.

Released aldosterone acts on the distal tubule to increase sodium retention and restore effective blood volume, thereby shutting off the initial stimulus for renin release.

A second control factor for aldosterone is the potassium ion. Either infusion or oral ingestion of potassium increases aldosterone production, and depletion of potassium has the opposite effect. This effect is a direct action of potassium to stimulate aldosterone production in the zona glomerulosa and is quite sensitive to changes in serum potassium as small as 0.2 mEq/L. ACTH displays only modest effects on long-term aldosterone control. ACTH acutely stimulates aldosterone, but this response is not sustained. In the absence of ACTH, in hypopituitarism or steroid-suppressed subjects, aldosterone response remains relatively intact. Recently, factors such as dopamine and atrial natriuretic peptide have been shown to be inhibitors of aldosterone secretion. These factors may play a role in the modulation of aldosterone secretion.

Aldosterone is secreted from the zona glomerulosa cells of the adrenal cortex. With normal sodium and potassium intake, about 50 to 250 μg are secreted daily. Aldosterone is weakly bound to plasma proteins, and is rapidly inactivated by the liver and kidney. As a result, circulating aldosterone levels are low. The acid-labile metabolite of aldosterone measured in the urine represents approximately 10% of total daily aldosterone production. Plasma levels of aldosterone are measured by radioimmunoassay and are influenced by dietary sodium and potassium, posture, and time of day.

CUSHING'S SYNDROME

Definition

Cushing's syndrome refers to a diverse symptom complex due to excess steroid hormone production by the adrenal cortex (endogenous) or sustained administration of glucocorticoids. Endogenous Cushing's syndrome may be classifed by its site of origin which includes: (1) Pituitary-dependent (Cushing's disease) caused by a small pituitary tumor (microadenoma) producing excessive amounts of adrenocorticotropic hormone (ACTH); (2) Adrenal Cushing's syndrome caused by autonomous cortisol production by an adrenal tumor (adenoma, carcinoma, micronodular hyperplasia); and (3) Ectopic Cushing's syndrome due to ectopic ACTH production by a nonendocrine tumor. Cushing's syndrome is also classified as ACTH-dependent (Pituitary and Ectopic Cushing's) and ACTH-independent (Adrenal Cushing's). Table 4–1 gives the approximate incidence of the various forms of Cushing's syndrome.

Cushing's Disease. Hypercortisolism due to excess ACTH production from the pituitary is the most common cause of endogenous Cushing's syndrome comprising 70 to 80% of patients. Cushing's disease is more common in women, especially those of child-bearing age. Excess production of ACTH produces bilateral adrenal hyperplasia. The majority of patients (80%) have pituitary basophilic microadenomas, although tumors can be basophilic or mixed, usually located in the center of the anterior pituitary gland or rarely in the neurointermediate lobe of the pituitary. The majority of tumors are less than 10 mm in diameter, but about 10% of patients present with larger, invasive macroadenomas. In some cases, there is no histologic evidence of a pituitary tumor suggesting the possibility that excessive ACTH production is due to abnormal hypothalamic function with possible excessive release of corticotropin-releasing factor. Drugs that act on the central nervous system (CNS) lower ACTH and cortisol in some patients with this form of Cushing's syndrome. In addition, several abnormalities of CNS regulation of sleep and

Table 4–1.   Classification of Spontaneous Cushing's Syndrome

	Incidence (%)
ACTH dependent	
Cushing's disease	68
Ectopic ACTH-secreting tumor	15
ACTH independent	
Adenoma	5
Carcinoma	3
Nodular adrenal hyperplasia	9
Adrenocortical rest tumor	<1

hormonal release and high values of CRF in spinal fluid have been found in these patients. As the pathogenesis of the pituitary tumors in Cushing's disease is unknown, it is possible that most of the tumors arise from dysfunction of the hypothalamus and higher centers. An alternative hypothesis is that all patients with pituitary-dependent Cushing's syndrome have a pituitary ACTH-secreting tumor with some tumors being so small that they are undetectable. Plasma ACTH levels are normal or moderately elevated in this disorder in the presence of elevated plasma cortisol levels indicating decreased sensitivity to cortisol feedback suppression of ACTH.

Adrenal Cushing's Syndrome. Approximately 8% of cases of Cushing's syndrome are caused by adrenal adenomas or carcinoma. Adrenal tumors are more common in females than in males. The average size of adrenal adenomas is 5 to 8 cm in diameter; most tumors are unilateral and occur more frequently in the left adrenal. Cushing's syndrome in children is usually due to adrenal carcinoma, which is found in 65% of patients younger than age 15 years. Plasma ACTH is suppressed because of negative cortisol feedback at the hypothalamus and pituitary, and the normal adrenal tissue is atrophic. Adrenal carcinomas may secrete large amounts of other steroids, including androgens and estrogens. In males, increased estrogens cause feminization. Adrenal carcinoma may reach a large size, and metastasis is often present at diagnosis.

Nodular adrenal hyperplasia has been described in some cases of Cushing's syndrome. There is usually bilateral adrenal involvement and the glands contain both nodules and hyperplasia. Plasma ACTH is suppressed indicating autonomous cortisol production in these patients. However, the pathogenesis of this disorder may be pituitary-dependent Cushing's; the excess ACTH with time produces nodularity in both hyperplastic glands and ultimately autonomous cortisol secretion.

Ectopic Cushing's Syndrome. The ectopic ACTH syndrome is excessive production of biologically active ACTH by nonendocrine tumors arising most commonly from the lungs, but also from a variety of tumors (Table 4–2). Ectopic ACTH production accounts for 10 to 15% of cases of Cushing's syndrome; it is estimated that 2% of patients with small cell bronchogenic carcinoma have the clinical syndrome. Certain paraendocrine tumors, such as carcinoids and pheochromocytomas, can also produce ACTH. These tumors may originate embryologically from neural crest progenitor cells that have

Table 4–2.   Tumors Producing Ectopic Cushing's Syndrome

1. Oat cell carcinoma of the bronchus
2. Carcinoid tumors: Bronchial
                    Thymic
                    Pancreatic
3. Pancreatic islet cell tumors
4. Medullary carcinoma of the thyroid
5. Pheochromocytoma
6. Ovarian tumors
7. Miscellaneous

the capacity to synthesize and secrete peptide hormones or may arise from inactive DNA that becomes derepressed during neoplastic transformation. A high percentage of patients with lung cancer produce biologically inactive ACTH without biochemical Cushing's syndrome.

Plasma levels of ACTH uniformly exceed the normal range in the ectopic ACTH syndrome. These tumors are capable of synthesizing the common precursor of ACTH, POMC with release of several POMC-derived peptides such as beta-LPH, beta-endorphin and alpha-MSH. Some tumors may also produce corticotropin-releasing factor.

Signs and Symptoms

Cushing's syndrome represents an array of clinical features (Table 4–3) secondary to prolonged hypercortisolism and in some cases excess adrenal secretion of other steroids. Obesity is the most common finding with distribution predominantly in the face (moon facies), trunk, cervicodorsal (buffalo hump), and supraclavicular regions. However, obesity can be general without the typical centripetal distribution and may not be found in patients with the ectopic ACTH syndrome. The increase and redistribution of body fat in Cushing's syndrome is attributed to glucocorticoid effects on fatty acid turnover and enhanced lipogenesis secondary to hyperinsulinism.

There are several skin changes in Cushing's syndrome as the skin becomes increasingly thin and fragile. Ecchymosis and purpura due to loss of connective tissue are common and about half of the patients have wide purple striae located around the abdomen, hips, and axillary regions. These livid, wide striae differ from the paler, more superficial stretch marks of obesity. Increased skin transparency accounts for the plethoric appearance. Increased adrenal secretion of androgens can result in acne and mild hirsutism in women. Cortisol excess can produce lanugo-like hair growth over the body and face. Fungal skin infections such as tinea versicolor seem common. Hyperpig-

Table 4–3.   Incidence of Clinical Manifestations

	Incidence (%)
Obesity	90
Hypertension	85
Glucosuria and decreased glucose tolerance	80
Menstrual and sexual dysfunction	76
Hirsutism, acne, plethora	72
Striae, atrophic skin	67
Weakness, proximal myopathy	65
Osteoporosis	55
Easy bruisability	55
Psychiatric disturbances	50
Edema	46
Polyuria, polyphagia	16
Ocular changes and exophthalmos	8

mentation is sometimes found in patients with the ectopic ACTH syndrome caused by the melanocyte-stimulating properties of ACTH and the hormones associated with ACTH.

Weakness is a common presenting feature of patients with Cushing's syndrome, associated with a proximal myopathy and sometimes atrophy. The decrease in muscle mass is related to the protein catabolic effects of excess glucocorticoids and in some cases to hypokalemia.

Mild to moderate hypertension is almost uniformly present in Cushing's syndrome and has multiple etiologies. Markedly elevated levels of cortisol, because of its mineralocorticoid properties, produce sodium retention, volume expansion, and hypertension. Cortisol also has a direct effect on vascular reactivity and may enhance vascular sensitivity to pressor hormones such as norepinephrine. Excess cortisol also indirectly activates the renin-angiotensin system, mainly through enhancing hepatic production of renin substrate, a precursor for angiotensin II formation. However, measured levels of plasma renin activity in patients with Cushing's syndrome vary from low to high. The ectopic ACTH syndrome can be associated with excess production of the mineralocorticoid deoxycorticosterone, which produces hypokalemia and sodium retention. Surprisingly, hypertension is not as common in this form of Cushing's syndrome despite excess mineralocorticoid activity.

Osteoporosis sometimes associated with bone pain, kyphosis, and loss of height, is seen in adults with Cushing's syndrome. Glucocorticoids have multiple effects on bone and calcium metabolism. The protein catabolic effect of glucocorticoids on bone function includes direct inhibition of osteoblastic function, reduction in collagen synthesis, and enhanced bone reabsorption which may be secondary to increased parathyroid hormone activity. Glucocorticoids also cause a negative calcium balance by inhibiting calcium absorption from the gastrointestinal tract and by their action on the kidney to augment calcium excretion. This explains the high incidence of renal stones in Cushing's syndrome.

Glucocorticoids have multiple effects on carbohydrate metabolism, resulting in abnormal glucose tolerance in about 80% of patients, but clinical diabetes mellitus occurs in only a minority of patients. Glucocorticoids cause insulin resistance that may relate to effects on the insulin receptor or a postreceptor effect causing impaired insulin action. Glucocorticoids may also directly or indirectly influence hepatic gluconeogenesis and the other intracellular metabolic pathways for glucose metabolism.

Excess adrenal androgen production in some female patients with Cushing's syndrome can cause hirsutism and other signs of virilization. Generalized virilization with clitoromegaly occurs most frequently with adrenocortical carcinoma and sometimes adrenal-induced hyperandrogenism can occur without hypercortisolism. Hyperestrogenism can also be a manifestation of Cushing's syndrome occurring in children and men, and is nearly always due to adrenal carcinoma. Pathophysiologic mechanisms include increased estrogen production by the tumor or impaired androgen production or action.

Hyperpigmentation may occur in Cushing's syndrome due to prolonged elevation of ACTH and other POMC-derived peptides (beta-LPH, alpha-MSH) that can stimulate melanocyte function. Hyperpigmentation is most commonly associated with Cushing's syndrome due to ectopic ACTH production. Hyperpigmentation can be found in pituitary-dependent Cushing's syndrome and is especially prominent after bilateral adrenalectomy (Nelson's syndrome).

Mental changes are common in Cushing's syndrome and range from minor mood changes to severe psychosis. The psychiatric disturbance is greatest in patients with more severe hypercortisolism and includes changes in affect, cognitive function, and mood. Primary depressive disorders can be accompanied by hypercortisolism without clinical manifestations of Cushing's syndrome.

In children hypercortisolism leads to arrest of growth. Impaired immune response in Cushing's syndrome may explain the increased incidence of infections, particularly due to opportunistic organisms.

Diagnosis

Because of the large number of tests available to evaluate adrenal function, a stepwise and systematic approach divides the testing procedures into three phases: (1) conformation of hypercortisolism; (2) differentiation between the three forms of Cushing's syndrome; and (3) localization procedures.

Confirmation of Cushing's Syndrome

OVERNIGHT DEXAMETHASONE SUPPRESSION TEST. This test is based on the resistance to normal feedback suppression by exogenous steroids observed in Cushing's syndrome. In this outpatient screening test, 1 mg of dexamethasone is given orally at approximately 11:00 P.M. to midnight and a plasma cortisol is obtained at 8:00 A.M. the following morning. An 8:00 A.M. plasma cortisol level of less than 5 μg/dl almost always excludes Cushing's syndrome whereas patients with the disorder do not suppress plasma cortisol normally and have levels above 5 μg/dl. There are few false negative tests, but false positive results are not uncommon. Failure of subjects without Cushing's syndrome to suppress normally may be due to mental depression, alcoholism, or stress-related events. Variation in dexamethasone metabolism (due to anticonvulsant therapy) can give false-positive results. Exogenous estrogen administration also causes falsely high cortisol levels because estrogen increases cortisol-binding globulin.

URINARY FREE CORTISOL. This test is a direct measurement of the amount of cortisol not bound to plasma proteins. As plasma cortisol increases in Cushing's syndrome, less is bound because of saturation of binding sites that leads to an exponential increase in urinary free cortisol. The amplification effect of this test yields excellent discrimination in diagnosing hypercortisolism. Urinary free cortisol is elevated in over 95% of patients with Cushing's syndrome. As the test does not rely on excretion of metabolites of cortisol, it is unaffected by obesity and other conditions that alter cortisol metabolism. False-positive results may occur with depression, alcoholism, or acute stress.

An older urinary test of adrenal function is the Porter-Silber reaction for 17-hydroxycorticoid, which measures metabolites of cortisol. A limitation of the urinary 17-hydroxycorticoid measurement is the dependence of metabolite excretion on body weight leading to overlap between normals, patients with obesity and Cushing's syndrome. This problem can be partially corrected by expressing urinary 17-hydroxycorticoids per g of creatinine excretion.

DIURNAL VARIATION OF CORTISOL. Plasma cortisol values display diurnal variation, with levels being highest in the early morning and declining during the day to less than 50% of the 8:00 A.M. value at 4:00 P.M., and even less at 8:00 P.M. Loss of variation is highly suggestive of hypercortisolism. Caution in the sampling procedure is necessary because recent stress, exercise, and even venipuncture can transiently elevate plasma cortisol value. The test has sensitivity in mild to moderate cases of hypercortisolism. Circadian variation of cortisol, however, is not invariably lost in Cushing's syndrome, so caution must be exercised in the interpretation of this test.

LOW-DOSE DEXAMETHASONE SUPPRESSION. This test is highly reliable and perhaps the most definitive test for discriminating Cushing's syndrome from other conditions that might cause false positive results in other screening tests for this disorder. As originally described by Liddle in 1960, dexamethasone 2 mg per day (0.5 mg every 6 hours) is administered for 2 days; in normal subjects urinary 17-hydroxycorticoids are less than 3 mg per 24 hours (and urinary free cortisol is less than 20 μg per 24 hours).

Differential Diagnosis of Cushing's Syndrome

PLASMA ACTH. Plasma ACTH levels differ between the various types of Cushing's syndrome, being low in adrenal Cushing's, high in pituitary Cushing's and very high in ectopic Cushing's. An undetectable ACTH level with an increased cortisol level suggests adrenal Cushing's syndrome. In the ectopic ACTH syndrome, values are greater than 300 pg/ml in more than 60% of patients with high plasma cortisol values. In pituitary Cushing's syndrome, ACTH values are elevated in approximately 50% of patients; this elevation is mild to moderate (100 to 250 pg/ml). The normal levels of ACTH found in 50% of cases of pituitary Cushing's syndrome are inappropriately high in the presence of hypercortisolism.

Sampling for ACTH venous gradients during petrosal sinus catheterization in the areas of pituitary venous drainage may detect a central etiology of ACTH in the diagnosis of pituitary Cushing's syndrome. In special cases, chromatography of ACTH may reveal a larger molecular weight form of ACTH, favoring a diagnosis of ectopic Cushing's syndrome. These additional procedures are useful when 8:00 A.M. plasma ACTH levels are in the intermediate range of 100 to 200 pg/ml, suggesting either pituitary or ectopic Cushing's syndrome.

Beta-lipotropin is the major peptide cosynthesized with ACTH in equimolar ratios in normal individuals. In ectopic Cushing's syndrome, production rates are dissociated, causing greater beta-lipotropin than ACTH production, which results in higher plasma levels. Other POMC-derived peptides may be elevated in Cushing's syndrome so that measurement of molar ratios of these peptides may help to differentiate the type of Cushing's syndrome.

HIGH-DOSE DEXAMETHASONE TEST. This test is based on the observation that administration of large doses of a glucocorticoid will result in suppression of pituitary-adrenal function in cases of pituitary Cushing's syndrome, whereas there is no effect in cases of adrenal tumor and ectopic ACTH. Dexamethasone 8 mg per day (2 mg every 6 hours) is administered for 2 days; values for plasma or urinary cortisol will suppress by greater than 50% of baseline values in pituitary Cushing's syndrome. This test distinguishes pituitary Cushing's syndrome from other causes in approximately 90% of cases. Anomalous responses to high-dose dexamethasone include suppression of cortisol in cases of ectopic Cushing's syndrome due to bronchial adenoma, paradoxical increases in rare cases of pituitary Cushing's, failure of suppression in pituitary Cushing's associated with adrenal nodular hyperplasia.

Miscellaneous Tests

Insulin Tolerance Test. The majority of patients with Cushing's syndrome do not have a plasma cortisol response to insulin-induced hypoglycemia. This test is useful to distinguish Cushing's from other types of hypercortisolemia, such as depression or alcohol abuse where plasma cortisol responses to hypoglycemia are normal.

Metyrapone Test. Metyrapone blockade of 11-beta-hydroxylase activity and cortisol synthesis induces stimulation of ACTH release and enhanced steroidogenesis with increased production of 11-deoxycortisol (Compound S). Metyrapone is administered as 750 mg every 4 hours for 6 doses and serum cortisol and Compound S are measured at 8:00 A.M. the following morning. Patients with pituitary Cushing's syndrome have an augmented post-metyrapone response of Compound S, whereas adrenal and ectopic Cushing's patients have no response. Recent studies show that metyrapone testing may be more consistent than high-dose dexamethasone in distinguishing pituitary from adrenal Cushing's syndrome.

Corticotropin-releasing Factor (CRF) Stimulation Test. CRF, released from the hypothalamus, selectively stimulates the pituitary corticotrophic cells to increase ACTH secretion. Ovine CRF, administered as an intravenous bolus of 1 μg/kg body weight, increases ACTH and cortisol levels in patients with pituitary Cushing's syndrome; patients with ectopic and adrenal Cushing's syndrome have no ACTH or cortisol response. Initial experience suggested this test might differentiate pituitary from ectopic Cushing's syndrome as basal ACTH levels are elevated in both conditions, but exaggerated responses to CRF occur only in pituitary Cushing's. Cortisol and ACTH responses to CRF may be quite variable, however, in patients with pituitary Cushing's syndrome. The test may be useful in distinguishing depression-induced hypercortisolism from pituitary Cushing's. It appears unlikely that this rapid, simple procedure will attain sufficient diagnostic accuracy to replace the more detailed dexamethasone suppression testing procedures.

Localization Procedures

Pituitary Cushing's Syndrome. ACTH-producing pituitary microadenomas are generally small and do not alter sellar architecture. Thus, plain skull radiographs and sellar tomograms detect enlargement in only a small percentage of cases. Sellar computed tomographic scans and nuclear magnetic resonance scans may detect up to 70% of microadenomas in pituitary Cushing's; however, false-positive results do occur so that biochemical studies must support the diagnosis.

Adrenal Cushing's Syndrome. Adrenal computed tomographic scans enable noninvasive visualization of the adrenal glands in greater than 95% of cases. With such diagnostic accuracy, early use of adrenal CT scans with demonstration of a tumor may obviate further detailed testing to differentiate the etiology of Cushing's syndrome. Adrenal hyperplasia cannot be distinguished from normal glands by CT scanning. The CT scan of the adrenals has high sensitivity but less specificity.

Adrenal ultrasound imaging has almost equivalent diagnostic accuracy in adrenal Cushing's as the CT scan. For small adrenal tumors, special procedures such as angiography, adrenal retrograde venography, and radiocholesterol scanning may be useful.

Ectopic Cushing's Syndrome. Chest x ray will detect a lung lesion, usually oat cell carcinoma of the bronchus, in approximately 50% of patients. Lung tomography and CT may detect a higher percentage of ectopic ACTH secreting tumors in the thorax. Rarer sites of ectopic tumor production of ACTH such as pancreas, thyroid, neural crest neoplasm, and gastrointestinal tract require specialized procedures for diagnosis.

The extent to which patients should be evaluated to determine the etiology of Cushing's syndrome will depend somewhat on the difficulty in reaching that goal. In the case of Cushing's syndrome with high plasma ACTH, the majority of patients will have pituitary Cushing's rather than ectopic Cushing's syndrome. Cushing's syndrome with suppressed ACTH and a tumor on adrenal CT may need no further diagnostic testing. In other less clear-cut cases, the high-dose dexamethasone or metyrapone test is required to establish the etiology of hypercortisolism. Three conditions, depression, chronic alcoholism, and obesity can produce either a clinical or biochemical picture resembling Cushing's syndrome leading to confusion in interpretation of adrenal testing. Likewise, no single adrenal test is diagnostic; for example, high-dose dexamethasone will occasionally produce suppression of adrenal function in documented cases of adrenal or ectopic Cushing's syndrome.

Treatment

Without therapy to correct hypercortisolism, most cases of Cushing's syndrome progress, leading to severe complications and a fatal outcome. Treatment of Cushing's syndrome results in an overall successful outcome in over 85% of cases of benign adrenal and pituitary tumors. Adrenal carcinoma and ectopic Cushing's still have a poor prognosis. Treatment approaches are designed to correct hypercortisolism, eradicate tumor growth, and minimize deficiencies of other endocrine systems.

Pituitary Cushing's Syndrome. Transphenoidal resection of a pituitary adenoma is the treatment of choice in the majority of cases of pituitary Cushing's syndrome. Selective removal of a pituitary microadenoma will result in an overall initial remission rate of at least 85% of cases. Surgical outcome depends on tumor size; remission rates are high for microadenomas and much lower for large, more invasive tumors. The operative procedure is generally well-tolerated with low morbidity and mortality. Complications include diabetes insipidus, which is usually transient, rhinorrhea of cerebrospinal fluid, and hemorrhage. After a period of transient adrenal insufficiency requiring glucocorticoid replacement, the hypothalamic-pituitary-adrenal axis recovers and the function of other pituitary hormones remains intact. A special problem concerns patients with biochemical evidence suggesting pituitary Cushing's syndrome but with no roentgenographic evidence, and, in some cases, no surgical evidence of a pituitary tumor. In some cases in which total hypophysectomy has been curative, extremely small tumors were found on pathologic examination. Bilateral simultaneous inferior petrosal venous sinus catheterization and sampling for ACTH will lateralize a microadenoma and a hemihypophysectomy will result in a cure. In other situations, patients can be treated with neurotransmitter inhibitors of CRF and ACTH release such as cyproheptadine, a serotonergic antagonist.

Pituitary irradiation is another form of therapy for patients with pituitary Cushing's syndrome and is particularly useful in younger individuals. There is a long lag period before correction of hypercortisolism (12 to 18 months), and the remission rate in adults is only 20% compared with 70 to 80% in children. Radiation therapy with protons or alpha particles yields a higher remission rate and a shorter lag phase.

Adrenal Cushing's Syndrome. Surgery is the treatment of choice for benign unilateral adrenal adenomas. These cortisol-secreting tumors cause suppression of ACTH and atrophy of the contralateral adrenal gland requiring glucocorticoid replacement during surgery and for several months following tumor removal until the pituitary-adrenal axis recovers.

Surgery is the treatment of choice for adrenal carcinoma. For residual disease or inoperable carcinoma, mitotane can be used as a palliative drug.

Ectopic Cushing's Syndrome. Removal of the ACTH-secreting tumor is the treatment of choice but is usually not feasible due to the nature of the underlying process (e.g., oat-cell carcinoma of the lung). Adrenalectomy may be considered in cases of indolent, yet inoperable, tumors such as some medullary carcinomas of the thyroid.

Adrenal enzyme inhibitors are useful for reducing hypercortisolism. The decrease in plasma cortisol is not "sensed" by the autonomous ACTH-secreting tumor cells, and thus there is no compensatory increase in ACTH secretion (which might have overridden the effect of these drugs, as would be the case in pituitary Cushing's syndrome.) Metyrapone, an 11-hydroxylase inhibitor, at an average dose of 250 to 500 mg 3 times a day, provides an effective means of normalizing cortisol levels. Aminoglutethimide blocks the conversion of cholesterol to delta-5-pregnenolone and can also be used. Since hypoadrenalism can result, monitoring of therapy by measurements of plasma cortisol or urinary free cortisol (or both) is mandatory.

ADRENOCORTICAL INSUFFICIENCY

Adrenocortical insufficiency results primarily from deficient cortisol and in some cases deficient aldosterone and androgen production by the adrenal. Since the adrenal cortex is normally stimulated by ACTH, cortisol deficiency may result from adrenal disease (primary adrenal insufficiency) or from pituitary or hypothalamic disease (secondary adrenal insufficiency).

Primary Adrenal Insufficiency

Primary adrenocortical insufficiency was described by Addison in 1855 and included cases of idiopathic adrenal atrophy, tuberculosis and metastatic tumor. More than 90% of the cortex must be destroyed before clinical manifestations become evident. Currently, idiopathic adrenal atrophy, which is usually a form of chronic autoimmune adrenalitis, accounts for approximately 75% of cases and tuberculosis for approximately 20%.

That idiopathic adrenal atrophy is an autoimmune disorder is suggested by the following observations: (1) Presence of circulating antiadrenal antibodies (approximately 60% of cases) that may precede the clinical disease; (2) demonstration of adrenal cellular hypersensitivity and abnormal T-lymphocyte function; (3) association with certain histocompatibility antigens, especially HLA-B8, A1 or DW3; (4) association with other autoimmune endocrinopathies, resulting in "autoimmune polyglandular syndrome." *Type I polyglandular autoimmune syndrome* consists of hypoadrenalism (100%), hypoparathyroidism (76%), mucocutaneous candidiasis (73%), hypogonadism (17%), chronic active hepatitis (13%), and pernicious anemia (13%), and typically starts during childhood or adolescence. *Type II polyglandular autoimmune syndrome* consists of Addison's disease (100%), hypothyroidism (Hashimoto's thyroiditis or Graves' disease; 70%), and insulin-dependent diabetes mellitus (50%), the combination often referred to as Schmidt's syndrome. Association with HLA-A1, B8 and DW3 occurs in type II. *Vitiligo* (patchy loss of skin pigment) itself a probable manifestation of autoimmune abnormality, can be seen in both forms. Classification of the different causes of primary adrenal insufficiency is given in Table 4–4.

Secondary Adrenal Insufficiency

Secondary adrenal insufficiency is most commonly caused by corticosteroid administration, which suppresses CRH and ACTH secretion resulting in ad-

Table 4—4. Primary Adrenal Insufficiency

Chronic Adrenal Insufficiency
1. Autoimmune adrenal atrophy

2. Granulomatous disease:
   Tuberculosis
   Histoplasmosis
   Sarcoidosis

3. Neoplastic infiltration

4. "Metabolic" disorders:
   Amyloidosis
   Hemochromatosis
   Adrenoleukodystrophy
   Adrenomyeloneuropathy

5. Acquired immune deficiency syndrome

6. Congenital adrenal unresponsiveness to ACTH

7. Abdominal irradiation

8. Post-bilateral adrenalectomy

Acute Adrenal Insufficiency
1. Vascular:
   Adrenal Hemorrhage
     Infection
       Meningococcus
       Pseudomonas, etc.
     Anticoagulants
   Adrenal artery embolism
   Adrenal vein thrombosis

2. Post-bilateral adrenalectomy

renal atrophy and adrenal insufficiency after steroid withdrawal. Other causes include pituitary tumors and other conditions causing hypopituitarism (see Chap. 2).

Symptoms and Signs

Acute adrenal insufficiency is a potentially fatal medical emergency. Clinical features include muscular weakness, nausea, fever, shock, diarrhea, increased and then decreased temperature, hypoglycemia, hyponatremia, and hyperkalemia.

Cardinal signs of *chronic adrenal insufficiency* are weakness, weight loss, hyperpigmentation, hypotension, nausea, vomiting, diarrhea, and vitiligo. Other symptoms are salt craving, muscle cramps, flank tenderness, and loss of body hair especially in females. The ear cartilage may calcify in long-standing adrenal insufficiency.

Pathophysiology

The clinical features are due to deficient cortisol, aldosterone, and androgen effects in target tissues.

Glucocorticoid deficiency is manifested in both the primary and secondary forms and leads to weakness, hypoglycemia, weight loss and gastrointestinal discomfort. Hypoglycemia is related to removal of cortisol, a major "counter-hormone" to insulin, and impaired gluconeogenesis in the liver and kidney. Cortisol deficiency also leads to impaired ability of the kidneys to excrete an acute water load. It also causes impaired arterial vascular reactivity to pressor hormones, which, along with volume depletion mainly attributable to mineralocorticoid deficiency, contributes to the hypotension in adrenal insufficiency.

In primary adrenal insufficiency, lack of the inhibitory feedback effect of cortisol on ACTH and LPH secretion by the pituitary results in increased melanocyte-stimulatory activity that results in deposition of melanin in the skin. Increased pigmentation occurs in areas exposed to light or pressure such as the face, neck, knuckles, elbows, knees, mucous membranes, skin creases in the palms, and scars acquired after the onset of adrenal failure.

Aldosterone deficiency results in renal sodium loss from decreased sodium reabsorption in the distal tubule. This loss causes a decrease in total body sodium and plasma volume. In response, plasma renin activity increases markedly despite the concomitant reduction in the substrate for renin activity, angiotensinogen, secondary to glucocorticoid deficiency. Thus, in Addisonian patients, elevated plasma renin activity is an excellent marker for mineralocorticoid deficiency. The hypovolemic state may result in hypotension, particularly *orthostatic hypotension,* which is further aggravated by the reduced vascular reactivity to norepinephrine related to glucocorticoid deficiency. The lack of aldosterone also impairs renal secretion of potassium and hydrogen resulting in hyperkalemia and metabolic acidosis.

Androgen Deficiency. The adrenal androgens, dehydroepiandrosterone, dehydroepiandrosterone sulfate, and androstenedione, have weak biologic activity and are converted to testosterone, which has potent bioactivity. In the female, these androgens are mainly responsible for the growth of pubic and axillary hair. Deficiency of adrenal androgen results in the loss of body hair. In the male, where sexual habitus depends on testicular rather than adrenal secretion, loss of body hair implies associated hypogonadism, either primary (polyglandular syndrome) or secondary to generalized pituitary insufficiency.

Secondary adrenocortical failure is usually associated with deficiency of gonadotropins, GH and TSH. The isolated lack of ACTH from pituitary or hypothalamic lesions is rare. Suppression of ACTH secretion due to prolonged use of supraphysiologic doses of glucocorticoids is common. When the steroids are discontinued, the pituitary gland secretes little ACTH even though corticosteorid levels are low. Recovery of the hypothalamic-pituitary-adrenal axis may take months. The patient is consequently vulnerable to adrenal failure in times of stress during this period. The hypothalamus and pituitary must recover first; then the trophic effect of ACTH on the adrenal restores adrenal responsiveness to normal.

The clinical manifestations of secondary adrenocortical insufficiency differ from that of Addison's disease. First, the presentation may be that of generalized pituitary insufficiency with accompanying hypothyroidism (TSH deficiency) and hypogonadism (LH/FSH deficiency). Secondly, hyperpigmentation is not present because ACTH and beta-lipotropin levels are low. Finally, symptoms related to hypoaldosteronism are usually absent, since aldosterone is regulated predominantly by the renin-angiotensin axis and plasma potassium rather than by ACTH.

Acute adrenal crisis can be induced by acute pathologic processes in the adrenal cortex, such as bilateral hemorrhage (Table 4–4). Much more often, though, acute adrenal crisis evolves from any of the forms of chronic adrenal insufficiency. This is usually precipitated by stressful events such as severe infection, trauma, or surgical procedure during which the normal adrenal would maximize its glucocorticoid output to meet the acute metabolic need. With subnormal adrenal reserve, acute glucocorticoid (and mineralocorticoid) deficiency may ensue. Acute adrenal crisis usually presents as high fever, dehydration, nausea, vomiting, and hypotension that progresses rapidly to circulatory shock. Hyperkalemia and hyponatremia are seen if mineralocorticoid deficiency is also present. The dehydration leads to hemoconcentration, elevated blood urea nitrogen, and sometimes hypercalcemia that are readily reversible with fluid and electrolyte replacement.

Diagnosis

Plasma Cortisol. Plasma cortisol may serve as a one-sided test: low levels, particularly "inappropriately" low levels, are suggestive of hypoadrenalism, but normal levels do not exclude this condition. In general, a plasma cortisol of <10 μg/dl in the early morning (8:00 A.M.) when cortisol secretion should be at close to peak levels or during a stressful event that should normally lead to maximalization of cortisol secretion is suggestive of adrenal insufficiency. If plasma cortisol is <5 μg/dl under these circumstances, the diagnosis can be made with certainty.

Plasma ACTH. Baseline plasma ACTH is elevated in primary adrenal insufficiency (>250 pg/ml). Levels in secondary adrenal insufficiency are typically low (<50 pg/ml), but even levels within the normal range should be considered "inappropriately normal" if plasma cortisol is low. Thus, plasma ACTH may aid in differentiating primary from secondary hypoadrenalism.

ACTH Stimulation Test. The diagnosis of adrenocortical insufficiency is primarily based on the plasma cortisol determination during the ACTH stimulation test (Fig. 4–5). For this 1-hour test, 250 μg cosyntropin (the 1–24 amino acid sequence of ACTH) is given intravenously. Peak cortisol values occur at 30 to 90 minutes. A normal test consists of a baseline cortisol greater than 5 μg/100 ml, an increment between baseline and stimulated cortisol greater than 7 μg/100 ml, and a stimulated cortisol level greater than 18 μg/100 ml. An inadequate cortisol response to this test indicates adrenal insuf-

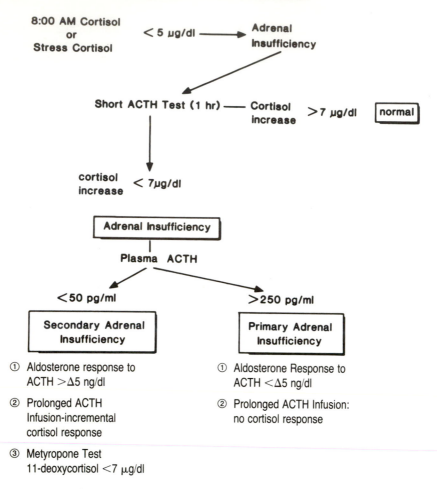

Fig. 4–5. Evaluation for adrenal insufficiency.

ficiency, and further tests are required to distinguish primary from secondary adrenal insufficiency.

Using samples already obtained during this test, it is then possible to evaluate the effect of ACTH on plasma aldosterone. In primary adrenal insufficiency, baseline aldosterone levels are low due to the diffuse destructive process in the adrenal gland that also affects the zona glomerulosa. For the same reason no significant increase in aldosterone is seen in these cases following ACTH administration. In secondary adrenal insufficiency, baseline aldosterone levels may be low or normal but aldosterone concentration increases by at least 4 ng/dl at 30 minutes after ACTH administration.

A *prolonged ACTH test* may be also used to differentiate between primary and secondary adrenal insufficiency. In secondary adrenal insufficiency, the adrenal response to ACTH may be initially blunted due to protracted ACTH deficiency. However, if the adrenal itself is intact, the response can usually be restored with prolonged stimulation. Following 3 consecutive days of administering ACTH (250 μg of cosyntropen) over 8 hours each day, the adrenal response as assessed by urinary 17-OHCS or plasma cortisol is normalized in secondary, but not in primary, adrenal insufficiency.

Metyrapone Test. The metyrapone test is also useful to assess pituitary ACTH reserve. Metyrapone inhibits the enzyme 11β-hydroxylase, during the final step in cortisol synthesis. The decrease in cortisol following 2 to 3 g metyrapone taken orally at 11:00 P.M. results in increased ACTH secretion; the adrenal responds by secreting 11-deoxycortisol (compound S). A normal response consists of a compound S value greater than 7 μg/100 ml at 8:00 A.M. Abnormal responses to metyrapone and hypoglycemia (see Chap. 2) with a normal response to ACTH confirm the diagnosis of secondary adrenocortical insufficiency.

Before undertaking this test, it is advisable to demonstrate normal cortisol response to ACTH. In patients with primary adrenal insufficiency, administration of metyrapone may be hazardous as adrenal crisis may be precipitated. If ACTH responsiveness is blunted (as expected with primary adrenal insufficiency), this test is superfluous. However, the combination of normal response to ACTH and abnormal metyrapone test strongly suggests the diagnosis of secondary adrenal insufficiency.

Treatment

Acute Adrenal Insufficiency. Acute adrenal insufficiency is treated by intravenous hydrocortisone: 100 mg injected as a bolus initially and then 100 mg every 6 hours for 24 to 48 hours. Fluid replacement is given as 5% glucose in saline solution, 4L over 4 hours; saline solution is administered to treat shock. From 20 to 40 mEq potassium may be added to the second and third liter to replace the total body deficit. As soon as the patient can tolerate oral fluids, glucocorticoids may be administered orally.

In addition to glucocorticoid therapy, a mineralocorticoid is usually required in the therapy of primary adrenal insufficiency. For example, 0.05 to 0.10 mg fludrocortisone (Florinef) may be added daily when oral glucocorticoid is begun. Mineralocorticoid replacement is not usually necessary in secondary adrenal insufficiency.

Chronic Adrenal Insufficiency. Prednisone (7.5 mg orally per day) or hydrocortisone (25 mg per day) and fluorocortisol (0.05 to 0.1 mg orally per day) are maintenance therapy. A normal diet is prescribed, with additional salt for excessive heat or humidity. The patient should carry prednisone or hydrocortisone for oral use, hydrocortisone hemisuccinate for intramuscular use in an emergency, and a medical identification card or bracelet stating diagnosis, medication, dosage, and physician's name and telephone number.

During stress, glucocorticoid dosage is increased to mimic normal function. For a "flu" syndrome with fever or a dental extraction, double the normal maintenance dosage for 2 to 3 days. For gastroenteritis with vomiting, patients should receive parenteral hydrocortisone.

For glucocorticoid coverage during surgical procedures, 100 mg hydrocortisone is given with preoperative medication, 100 mg intravenously during the surgical procedure, then 75 mg every 8 hours. Rapidly taper hydrocortisone to the normal dosage once the acute stress ends.

For mineralocorticoid replacement one may use plasma renin activity as a guide, the endpoint being reduction of the levels to the normal range.

CONGENITAL ADRENAL HYPERPLASIA

Definition

Congenital adrenal hyperplasia (CAH) comprises a group of genetically transmitted inborn errors of the enzyme systems involved in adrenal cortisol synthesis. Most defects are transmitted as autosomal recessive. Deficient cortisol synthesis leads to increased pituitary ACTH release, with hyperplasia of the adrenal glands and increased production of a number of steroids, including testosterone, in the virilizing syndrome.

Pathophysiology

Increased elaboration of testosterone in this syndrome exposes the fetus to excessive quantities of circulating testosterone and continued virilization after birth. In the female fetus, this condition leads to fusion of the labia and clitoral hypertrophy giving an appearance at birth of ambiguous external genitalia. The degree of fusion varies; in extreme cases a male-like phallus develops, and the urethra opens at the tip. The male fetus also undergoes virilization although abnormalities at birth are more difficult to detect. Untreated infants and children continue to show effects of virilization postnatally; manifestations are increased somatic growth; advancement of epiphyseal maturation; premature development of pubic, axillary, and facial hair; acne; lowering of voice pitch; and increased growth of the phallus. In spite of growth of the penis in boys, the testes generally do not grow in size to a concomitant degree, and spermatogenesis is diminished or absent. In the female, signs of puberty, such as breast development and menstruation, do not occur. Although virilization nearly always occurs, in rare forms of the syndrome testosterone cannot be produced and absence of fusion of the scrotal folds occurs, leading to feminization of the male fetus.

In addition to virilization (or rarely, feminization), other symptoms and signs develop because of excessive production of other steroids. Signs and symptoms of cortisol deficiency are rare because the enzymatic block is rarely complete, and under excessive ACTH stimulation, the adrenal cortex can produce adequate resting levels of cortisol. However, the adrenals are unable to produce the increased amounts of cortisol usually secreted under conditions of stress.

About half of the patients with 21-hydroxylase deficiency have aldosterone deficiency and develop life-threatening salt-losing crises, marked by lethargy, vomiting, dehydration, hyponatremia, and hyperkalemia. In patients with 11-hydroxylase deficiency, hypertension develops as a result of excessive production of 11-deoxycorticosterone.

In the 21-hydroxylase deficiency a linkage with certain HLA cell surface antigens has been found. The gene for 21-hydroxylase deficiency is located near the HLA-B locus. HLA genotyping allows prediction among family members of those who are heterozygote carriers of the gene. Other forms of CAH do not appear to be genetically linked to HLA.

21-Hydroxylase Deficiency. The most common type of deficiency is impairment of 21-hydroxylation leading to production of 21-deoxysteroids (Fig. 4–6). The steroid molecule can be hydroxylated at the 11 and 17 positions but not at the 21 position. As a result, the immediate steroid precursors to the 21-hydroxylase site, progesterone and 17-hydroxyprogesterone (17-OHP), accumulate in the blood and are used for diagnosis. Although elevated 17-OHP levels are in most cases diagnostic, a more reliable indicator is the excessive rise in 17-OHP after ACTH administration. ACTH (0.25 to 1.0

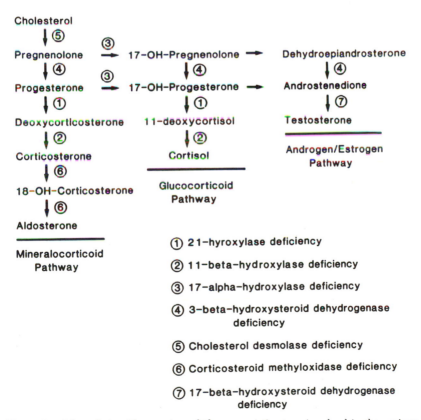

Fig. 4–6. Adrenal steroidogenesis and the enzymatic steps involved in the various forms of congenital adrenal hyperplasia.

mg) is administered as an intravenous bolus with sampling for 17-OHP at 0, 30, and 60 minutes.

In the simple virilizing form of 21-hydrolylase deficiency, there is virilization of the external genitalia in the genetic female fetus resulting in female pseudohermaphroditism (Chap. 5). The internal genitalia develop normally and female patients are born with a uterus and fallopian tubes. In male patients with 21-hydroxylase deficiency, the internal and external genitalia may be normal at birth and may go undetected until the postnatal period when manifestations of increased growth, accelerated epiphyseal closure and penile enlargement become apparent.

In about half the subjects, salt-losing crises may occur because of deficiency in aldosterone synthesis. Aldosterone is a 21-hydroxylated compound, and deficiency of 21-hydroxylase might naturally be expected to lead to aldosterone deficiency. Surprisingly, the non-salt-losers with 21-hydroxylase deficiency actually have normal or increased production of aldosterone. They do not develop signs of hyperaldosteronism because progesterone and 17-hydroxyprogesterone antagonize the renal response to aldosterone. A clear explanation of why some patients have aldosterone deficiency and others do not is not available. In the salt-wasting syndrome, the child may experience life-threatening adrenal crisis with hyperkalemia, hyponatremia and severe dehydration in the first few weeks of life requiring treatment for acute adrenal insufficiency. A late onset or acquired form of CAH with 21-hydroxylase deficiency has been described in women with onset in adolescence or early adulthood of virilization and menstrual disorders. Thus, there may be a spectrum of severity relating to differences in the extent of enzyme deficiency and variable signs of androgen excess.

11-Beta-hydroxylase Deficiency. In the second most frequent enzymatic defect, absence of 11-hydroxylation leads to formation of 11-deoxycortisol, which is physiologically inert, and 11-deoxycorticosterone, which is a potent retainer of sodium and may cause hypertension (Fig. 4–6). Patients with this form of the disorder are virilized because of the increased production of testosterone. Some are hypertensive but none are salt losers. The severity of hypertension is variable, and it is sometimes accompanied by hypokalemia. The diagnosis in these patients is made by finding increased amounts of 11-deoxycortisol, 11-deoxycorticosterone and 17-OHP in the plasma. Urinary tetrahydro-11-deoxycortisol is also elevated.

17-Alpha-hydroxylase Deficiency. In this rare form of CAH, there is a reduction in both the glucocorticoid and sex steroid pathways leading to shunting of steroid production to the mineralocorticoid pathway (Fig. 4–6). There is marked overproduction of corticosterone and 11-deoxycorticosterone (DOC) with the latter inducing salt retention, hypertension and hypokalemia. As the enzyme is also deficient in the gonad, there is a marked decrease in sex steroid production with sexual infantilism in females and pseudohermaphroditism in males.

3-Beta-hydroxysteroid Dehydrogenase Deficiency. In this syndrome pregnenolone cannot be converted to progesterone; therefore, cortisol, aldosterone, and testosterone cannot be formed (Fig. 4–6). Scrotal fusion does not occur in male fetuses, and because of impairment of aldosterone synthesis, salt-losing crises occur. High plasma levels of 17-OH-pregnenolone and dehydroepiandrosterone make the diagnosis. A milder, late-onset form has been described in hirsute females.

Cholesterol Desmolase Deficiency. Deficiency of the enzyme catalyzing the conversion of cholesterol to pregnenolone leads to severe adrenal insufficiency characterized by marked deposition of lipids in the adrenal and is referred to as lipoid adrenal hyperplasia (Fig. 4–6). Symptoms of aldosterone deficiency occur with hyponatremia and dehydration. Virilization does not occur.

Corticosteroid Methyloxidase Deficiency. In this rare syndrome, there is selective deficiency of enzymes in the zona glomerulosa region of the adrenal leading to reduced aldosterone production (Fig. 4–6). Glucocorticoid and sex steroid pathways are intact so ACTH levels and sexual development are normal. Profound salt wasting, dehydration, fever, failure to gain weight, hyponatremia, and hyperkalemia are the initial findings in children with this disorder.

The hydroxylation of corticosterone to form aldosterone is a two-step process and deficiencies of both steps (termed corticosteroid methyloxidase type I and II deficiencies) have been described. Reduced aldosterone and elevated corticosterone or 18-hydroxycorticosterone, expressed as a precursor-product ratio, establish this diagnosis.

17-Beta-hydroxysteroid Dehydogenase Deficiency. In this disorder the production of sex steroids is blocked but glucocorticoid and mineralocorticoid pathways are intact (Fig. 4–6). In males this deficiency causes pseudohermaphroditism with female external genitalia but with intact Wolffian duct derivatives. The defect in conversion of androstendione to testosterone may be more pronounced in the testes than in the adrenal glands. Diagnosis is made by demonstrating an abnormal ratio of plasma androstendione to testosterone.

Treatment

The major form of therapy for most forms of CAH is glucocorticoid administration which replaces the deficiency of cortisol and reduces ACTH overproduction. The reduction in ACTH production by glucocorticoid therapy reverses a major pathophysiologic abnormality in CAH by reducing the overstimulation of the adrenal glands. Excess androgen production is suppressed and progressive virilization is avoided. In the 11-hydroxylase and 17-hydroxylase deficiencies where hypertension is due to ACTH stimulation of 11-deoxycorticosterone, glucocorticoid replacement reverses the hypertension.

The dose of glucocorticoid recommended is higher than the usual daily secretory rate and can be as high as 20 mg/m^2/day of hydrocortisone although lower doses (10 to 15 mg/m^2/day) can be used in children. Daily dosage schedule is controversial with some experts advocating higher evening doses of glucocorticoids.

In those forms of CAH with mineralocorticoid deficiency, fludrocortisone (Florinef) is administered as 0.05 to 0.1 mg daily.

PRIMARY ALDOSTERONISM

Definition

Primary aldosteronism refers to excessive and autonomous adrenal production of aldosterone, the major adrenal mineralocorticoid. In various forms of secondary aldosteronism, the stimulus is extra-adrenal in origin. There are two major pathologic forms of primary aldosteronism with most cases of primary aldosteronism due to a single or, infrequently, multiple aldosterone-producing adrenal adenomas. Between 15 and 30% of all cases have bilateral adrenocortical hyperplasia as the source of excessive aldosterone production. In rare cases, primary aldosteronism is caused by (1) unilateral adrenal hyperplasia, (2) adrenal carcinoma or (3) glucocorticoid remediable hyperaldosteronism with bilateral adrenal hyperplasia in which excess aldosterone secretion can be normalized by dexamethasone.

Primary hyperaldosteronism is an uncommon cause of hypertension accounting for 0.1 to 0.5% of all cases of hypertension.

Pathophysiology

Almost all the pathophysiologic events in primary hyperaldosteronism can be explained by the effects of aldosterone on sodium and potassium transport. Aldosterone excess provides increased mineralocorticoid activity leading to increased reabsorption of sodium in exchange for potassium at the distal nephron. Increased sodium reabsorption results in increased total body sodium and *hypervolemia,* whereas enhanced urinary secretion of potassium leads to *hypokalemia and potassium depletion.*

Hypervolemia. Body fluid volume and total body sodium increase early in the course of mineralocorticoid excess. However, at a certain point, no further sodium retention occurs because proximal tubular sodium reabsorption decreases and sodium excretion increases. This mineralocorticoid *"escape phenomenon"* explains why patients with primary aldosteronism rarely exhibit progressive volume expansion or edema. The mechanisms underlying the "escape phenomenon" are poorly understood but may be related to the increased release of atrial natriuretic peptide from the atria and increased biosynthesis of renal dopamine during sodium-volume overload, both of which will promote sodium excretion. *Arterial hypertension* is the most obvious sequela of hypervolemia in primary hyperaldosteronism. Increased sodium content of blood vessel walls and increased vascular reactivity may also play a role in the pathogenesis of hypertension in primary hyperaldosteronism. All degrees of hypertension occur in this disorder, and contrary to previous beliefs severe hypertension may occur. Many patients with primary aldosteronism have hypertension only; they lack other discernible signs or symptoms. Thus, differentiation of this disease from the larger essential hypertensive population on a clinical basis may be difficult.

Hypervolemia in primary hyperaldosteronism also leads to marked suppression of the renin-angiotensin system. Thus, suppressed levels of plasma renin activity (PRA) are helpful in the diagnosis of this disease.

Hypokalemia and Potassium Depletion. A major function of potassium is to maintain excitability of nerve and muscle by contributing to the electrical potential difference across the cell membrane. Potassium depletion in primary aldosteronism results in muscle weakness and fatigue. Another consequence of potassium depletion is defective urinary concentration with nocturnal polyuria and polydipsia. The pathophysiology of kaliopenic nephropathy may be due to reversible alterations of distal tubule and collecting duct permeability to water. Chronic hypokalemia also alters the electrical potential of myocardial cells, leading to the electrocardiographic findings of U waves and widened Q-T interval. Hypokalemia causes diminished glucose tolerance or clinical diabetes mellitus in about 50% of patients with primary aldosteronism. Hypokalemia directly impairs insulin release from the pancreatic beta cell and may also influence the peripheral action of insulin. Aldosterone excess also increases hydrogen ion secretion, and metabolic alkalosis is found commonly in primary aldosteronism. The alkalosis is due to both a direct effect of aldosterone on the kidney and to the effect of hypokalemia on ammonia secretion.

Symptoms and Signs

Symptoms of primary aldosteronism include muscle weakness, fatigue, and nocturia. There are few typical physical stigmata of this disease. Moderate to severe arterial hypertension is a constant finding. Accompanying prolonged blood pressure elevation are hypertensive retinopathy and left ventricular hypertrophy. Edema is almost always absent.

Diagnosis

The diagnosis of primary hyperaldosteronism is suggested by:

1. *Arterial hypertension.*
2. *Hypokalemia with excessive urinary excretion of potassium.*

In the untreated hypertensive patient, a serum potassium of less than 3.5 mEq/L suggests primary aldosteronism. However, in the hypertensive patient population, one encounters diuretic-induced hypokalemia much more commonly than unprovoked hypokalemia. Urinary potassium excretion varies markedly with dietary content. However, 24-hour potassium excretion greater than 30 mEq *in the presence of serum K^+ less than 3.5 mEq/L* is inappropriately high. If the patient was not treated with diuretics, the diagnosis of a mineralocorticoid excess syndrome is likely.

In essential hypertensive individuals after stopping diuretic therapy, urinary potassium excretion should fall below 30 mEq/24 hours within 3 days if serum

K^+ is still <3.5 mEq/L, whereas patients with primary hyperaldosteronism continue to excrete an excess of potassium.

It is important to realize that serum potassium levels are a major determinant of aldosterone secretion. Thus, hypokalemia per se may turn off the secretion of aldosterone allowing reduced renal excretion of potassium and eventually various degrees of correction of the hypokalemia. Thus, hyperaldosteronism may exist in a normokalemic patient.

3. *Suppression of plasma renin activity.*

The next diagnostic step is to demonstrate suppression of plasma renin activity. In normal man, plasma renin activity increases with any form of volume depletion, such as sodium restriction, hemorrhage, upright posture, or diuretic administration. Likewise, volume expansion suppresses plasma renin activity, and the chronic hypervolemia of primary aldosteronism accounts for the suppressed levels seen in this disease. Several methods of volume depletion have been used to evaluate renin responsiveness. The most practical method of testing renin response is administration of a potent diuretic agent, such as furosemide (60 mg orally), with measurements of renin after upright posture. Although suppressed renin activity is found in most cases of primary aldosteronism, it is also present in 25% of the essential hypertensive population. Also, both basal and stimulated levels of PRA (with upright posture or diuretics) decline markedly with age, especially in patients with essential hypertension, which further hinders the usefulness of this test in older subjects.

Definitive diagnosis of primary hyperaldosteronism relies on the demonstration of elevated levels of aldosterone in plasma or urine. The majority of patients with primary aldosteronism demonstrate elevated baseline aldosterone levels, but levels in some patients overlap the normal range. Chronic hypokalemia may itself reduce aldosterone production by the adrenal tumor. To circumvent this problem, volume expansion is performed to test the suppressibility of aldosterone secretion. Volume expansion by several methods does not suppress aldosterone in primary aldosteronism due to the relative autonomy of the adrenal tumor. In contrast, in normal subjects or in other forms of hypertension, adequate volume expansion results in a 50 to 80% fall in aldosterone levels from baseline. Volume expansion may be performed by oral salt loading (200 to 300 mEq sodium intake for 5 days), infusion of normal saline solution (2 L for 4 hours), or administration of a potent mineralocorticoid (10 mg deoxycorticosterone acetate twice daily or 200 μg fludrocortisone thrice daily) for 3 days. Lack of aldosterone suppression in a hypertensive patient with hypokalemia and low renin is the final confirmation of the diagnosis of primary aldosteronism.

Captopril, an angiotensin converting enzyme inhibitor, may also provide a dynamic measurement of aldosterone in relation to renin. In normal subjects, the secretion of aldosterone is largely dependent on circulating angiotensin II. Thus, when the conversion of angiotensin I to angiotensin II is blocked by captopril, the decline in plasma angiotensin II levels leads to a large decline in plasma aldosterone and to a subsequent marked increase in plasma renin activity via removal of negative feedback. In patients with primary hyperaldosteronism, this sequence of events following oral captopril administration does not take place due to marked suppression of the renin-angiotensin axis. Further reduction in angiotensin II by captopril does not appreciably change plasma aldosterone or PRA levels. Two hours after captopril (25 mg orally), aldosterone levels greater than 15 ng/dl or aldosterone/plasma renin activity ratio greater than 50 are observed in primary aldosteronism and differentiate between patients with this disorder and subjects with essential hypertension or normal individuals.

Differential Diagnosis

The differential diagnosis of primary aldosteronism is given in Table 4–5. These disorders include those that resemble primary aldosteronism biochemically. Secondary aldosteronism is an elevation of aldosterone secretion due to increases in the renin-angiotensin system. Secondary aldosteronism is most conveniently divided into diseases with or without hypertension. The edematous disorders without hypertension cause most secondary aldosteronism and include the nephrotic syndrome, cirrhosis with ascites, and congestive heart failure. These underlying diseases lead to disturbances in circulating blood

Table 4–5. Differential Diagnosis of Primary Aldosteronism

	Plasma Renin	Plasma Aldosterone	Blood Pressure	Serum Potassium
Primary aldosteronism	low	high	high	low
Secondary hyperaldosteronism				
—edematous disorders	high	high	normal	low
—malignant hypertension	high	high	high	low
Renovascular hypertension	normal or high	normal or high	high	normal or low
Renin secreting tumors	high	high	high	normal or low
Congenital adrenal hyperplasia (11- and 17- hydroxylase deficiency)	low	low	high	low
Cushing's syndrome	low or normal	normal or low	high	low
Liddle's syndrome	low	low	high	low
Barter's syndrome	high	high	normal or low	low
Licorice ingestion	low	low	high	low
Low-renin essential hypertension	low	normal or low	high	normal
Ingestion of exogenous mineralocorticoids	low	low	high	low

volume, such as reduced central or "effective" blood volume (nephrotic syndrome, cirrhosis) or decreased renal perfusion, which stimulates the renin-angiotensin-aldosterone axis.

Secondary aldosteronism with hypertension is most commonly due to malignant or accelerated hypertension. This disorder has been associated with high levels of renin and aldosterone due to decreased renal perfusion and can be accompanied by hypokalemia and metabolic alkalosis. Renal vascular hypertension can be accompanied by secondary aldosteronism, but clinically significant hyperaldosteronism is uncommon in this disorder. Cushing's syndrome, especially the ectopic ACTH syndrome, can occur with hypertension and hypokalemia. In most cases, the classical physical stigmata of Cushing's syndrome direct attention toward the proper diagnosis. Certain forms of congenital adrenal hyperplasia, including the 11-beta-hydroxylase and 17-alpha-hydroxylase deficiency syndromes, result in hypertension and hypokalemia, which respond to glucocorticoid therapy. Liddle's syndrome, which is a familial disorder of increased sodium retention, results in hypertension and hypokalemia. This condition is attributed to increased activity of the nonaldosterone-dependent site for distal tubular sodium and potassium exchange. Other rare causes of hypertension and hypokalemia are tumors producing either renin or a mineralocorticoid. A familial form of primary aldosteronism with hypertension and hypokalemia responds to glucocorticoid therapy. Excessive ingestion of licorice can mimic primary aldosteronism by causing hypertension, hypokalemia, and renin suppression. Licorice contains glycyrrhizin, which in excess acts as a mineralocorticoid by binding to aldosterone receptor sites. Overdosage of fludrocortisone given for orthostatic hypotension or chronic exposure to nasal sprays that contain compounds with potent mineralocorticoid activities (alpha-fluroprednisolone) may result in hypertension and hypokalemia. Finally, approximately one-fourth of patients with essential hypertension may demonstrate low levels of plasma renin activity. However, the differential diagnosis rests on the fact that most of this group are normokalemic and have aldosterone levels in the normal to low range.

ADRENAL ADENOMA VERSUS HYPERPLASIA

Preoperative distinction between adrenal adenoma and bilateral hyperplasia is important because patients with hyperaldosteronism due to bilateral hyperplasia do not normalize blood pressure following bilateral total adrenalectomy. In contrast, in patients with aldosterone-producing adenomas, surgical removal of the adenoma leads to correction of hypertension. Differentiation between aldosterone producing adenoma and bilateral hyperplasia can be made based on the following tests.

Suggestive Tests

Degree of Hypokalemia. In general severe hypokalemia, especially K^+ <2.7 mEq/L is more likely to be associated with adrenal adenoma.

Posture Test. Aldosterone producing adenomas exhibit a sensitive response to ACTH and much less response to angiotensin, whereas the opposite is true for idiopathic hyperaldosteronism (bilateral adrenal hyperplasia). The normal response to upright posture (2 to 4 hours) consists of a rise in plasma renin activity that leads to a rise in plasma aldosterone via stimulation of angiotensin II formation. Like normals, patients with bilateral adrenal hyperplasia show increased aldosterone levels in response to upright posture accounted for by the partially normal renin response. However, subjects with adrenal adenoma show a paradoxical response, that is plasma aldosterone actually falls. This is probably related to the relative insensitivity of aldosterone producing adenomas to angiotensin II and the circadian decline in plasma aldosterone from the morning towards the noon hours that reflects the circadian rhythm of ACTH (or an ACTH-related compound). Nevertheless some patients with adrenal adenomas have a normal response to posture (aldosterone rises in response to upright posture).

Plasma 18-Hydroxycorticosterone. 18-hydroxycorticosterone (18-OHB) is the immediate precursor (or perhaps by-product) of aldosterone. It is secreted not only by the zona glomerulosa where aldosterone is being synthesized, but also by the zona fasciculata. High plasma levels of 18-OHB (in excess of 100 ng/dl) are found in patients with an aldosterone-producing adenoma, whereas in patients with bilateral adrenal hyperplasia, plasma 18-OHB concentrations are less than 90 ng/dl, but some overlap may occur.

Definitive Tests

Computed Tomography (CT) Scan. Once the biochemical diagnosis of primary hyperaldosteronism has been established, an abdominal CT scan should be ordered. Adenomas of 1 cm or larger are demonstrable. In bilateral adrenal hyperplasia, the adrenal glands may be normal or enlarged. The accuracy rate of CT scan in the diagnosis of hyperaldosteronism is approximately 90%.

Iodocholesterol Scans. Cholesterol is the precursor of all adrenal steroids. ^{131}I-labeled cholesterol is taken up by the adrenal cortex precursor of all adrenal steroids. With dexamethasone treatment [131]I-19-cholesterol uptake by normal adrenal tissue is minimized, but uptake by abnormal (hyperplastic or adenomatous) tissue continues.

Catheterization of adrenal veins may be performed if the other procedures do not resolve the question of adenoma vs. bilateral hyperplasia. Adenoma results in high aldosterone levels secreted into the adrenal effluent so that aldosterone levels are highest on the affected side, lower in the inferior vena cava, and lowest in the contralateral site where aldosterone production is completely suppressed secondary to suppression of the renin-angiotensin system. It is best to also obtain cortisol levels from each sampling site and use the *aldosterone/cortisol ratios* rather than aldosterone levels in order to circumvent the possible fortuitous effect of dilution of adrenal effluent with extra-adrenal venous blood at the sampling site.

Treatment

Surgical removal of an adenoma is recommended for patients with aldosterone-producing adenomas and medical therapy for bilateral adrenal hyperplasia. At operation, most adenomas are small, often less than 1 cm in diameter; however, the entire adrenal gland containing the tumor is usually excised. Surgical outcomes in the adenoma group result in 70% correction of hypertension and significant improvement in the remainder. Since ACTH and cortisol secretion are intact in primary aldosteronism, preoperative and postoperative steroid replacement is usually not needed. It is important preoperatively to replenish body potassium.

Medical therapy with spironolactone is the treatment of choice in patients with bilateral hyperplasia, but the results have been variable. In addition, long-term spironolactone treatment is frequently accompanied by impotence and gynecomastia in men and menstrual abnormalities in women. The antiserotonergic drug cyproheptadine has been useful in some cases. Improved understanding of the pathophysiology of bilateral hyperplasia is needed to permit more rational therapy. Amiloride, a potassium sparing diuretic, has been effective in controlling blood pressure and restoring normal plasma potassium levels in patients with primary hyperaldosteronism.

HYPOALDOSTERONISM

Pathophysiology

Hyporeninemic hypoaldosteronism occurs in patients with renal disease, commonly interstitial nephritis or nephropathy, particularly diabetic nephropathy. Hyperkalemia and metabolic acidosis result from aldosterone deficiency. Renal secretion of potassium and hydrogen ions is impaired; the resulting hyperkalemia further increases the acidosis by reducing renal ammonia production. Hypoaldosteronism appears to be due to decreased renin release by the kidney. The etiology of hyporeninemia in this disease may be related to destruction of the juxtaglomerular apparatus, impaired activation of renin, sympathetic nervous system defects, and reduced production of renal prostaglandins that enhance renin secretion.

Plasma concentrations of renin and aldosterone are low and do not increase normally in response to sodium restriction and upright posture. Aldosterone release does occur in response to ACTH or angiotensin II infusion, indicating that the adrenal glands are intact.

Diagnosis

In a patient with chronic hyperkalemia, hyperchloremic acidosis, and modest renal insufficiency, the diagnosis of hyporeninemic hypoaldosteronism is based on low plasma renin and aldosterone levels in response to sodium restriction and upright posture. Adrenal insufficiency should be excluded by demonstrating that the cortisol response to ACTH is normal.

Treatment

Hyperkalemia and acidosis respond to mineralocorticoid therapy with flu-drocortisone. Higher doses (usually 0.2 mg/day) are required to treat this disorder than are needed in adrenal insufficiency, perhaps because the diseased kidney is resistant to the steroid. Some patients, especially those with hypertension and increased fluid volume, may require therapy with a diuretic such as furosemide instead of (or in addition to) mineralocorticoid therapy to correct hyperkalemia and acidosis.

Other forms of hypoaldosteronism are less common and are summarized in Table 4–6.

THE ADRENAL MEDULLA

Physiology

The adrenal medulla is derived from primitive neural crest tissue. The major secretory products of the adrenal medulla and the sympathetic nerve endings are the catecholamines, epinephrine and norepinephrine. A third member of this group, dopamine, appears to be most important within the central nervous system. These dihydroxylated phenolic compounds have diverse functions, including regulation of the neural and cardiovascular systems.

Table 4–6. Syndromes of Hypoaldosteronism Excluding Hyporeninemic Hypoaldosteronism

Entity	Mechanisms	Comments
Addison's disease	Diffuse destruction of the adrenal cortex including the zona glomerulosa	
Heparin treatment	Direct effect of heparin on aldosterone secretion	Usually after prolonged therapy
After resection of aldosterone-producing adenoma	Suppression of aldosterone secretion in normal cortical tissue by adenoma with delayed recovery after surgery	Can be prevented by spironolactone treatment before surgery
Hyperreninemic hypoaldosteronism	Selective injury to the adrenal zona glomerulosa during hypotensive episodes in critically ill patients	Cortisol secretion is intact. Presents with hyperkalemia in ICU patients
Congenital adrenal hyperplasia with methyloxidase type II defect	Enzymatic block in the conversion of 18-OHB to aldosterone	
Pseudohypoaldosteronism	Decreased responsiveness to aldosterone: mineralocorticoid receptor defect	Aldosterone levels are higher

The following biotransformations are involved in the synthesis of catecholamines:

1. Tyrosine   tyrosine hydroxylase   →   Dihydroxyphenylalanine (dopa)
2. Dopa   dopa decarboxylase   →   Dopamine
3. Dopamine   dopamine beta oxidase   →   Norepinephrine
4. Norepinephrine   N-methyltransferase   →   Epinephrine

The postganglionic sympathetic nerves and adrenal medulla contain all the
enzymes to synthesize catecholamines from the amino acid, tyrosine. The
first step requires the microsomal enzyme, tyrosine hydroxylase, which is
rate-limiting for the entire biosynthetic sequence. The second reaction involves
the cytoplasmic enzyme, dopa-decarboxylase, to produce dopamine, which
is taken up by active transport into cytoplasmic storage granules. Within these
granules, dopamine is oxidized to norepinephrine by dopamine beta oxidase.
The last transformation, yielding epinephrine, involves the enzyme phenyl-
ethylamine N-methyl transferase, present only in the adrenal medulla and the
organ of Zuckerkandl. Thus, in the adrenal medulla, epinephrine constitutes
about 75% of the end-product, whereas norepinephrine is the major extra-
adrenal product. Evidence suggests that the last enzymatic reaction is regulated
by glucocorticoids. Because of the close anatomic relationship between the
adrenal cortex and medulla, drainage through the adrenal portal system results
in high steroid concentrations in the medulla.

Catecholamine release involves migration of the cytoplasmic storage granules to the cell surface where they are discharged by exocytosis. Upon stimulation and membrane depolarization, the granules discharge not only catecholamines, but also ATP and the enzyme, dopamine-beta-oxidase. The fate
of released catecholamines is complex. Some catecholamines are bound to
specific alpha and beta adrenergic receptors in various target tissues to initiate
their diverse physiologic effects. A major portion of released catecholamines
is taken up by the neuron for storage in new cytoplasmic granules. This
reuptake transport pathway serves as an efficient, economical process to reuti-
lize these amines. The third fate of these compounds is metabolic inactivation
and excretion in the urine. Two primary enzyme systems are responsible for
inactivation of catecholamines (Fig. 4–7). The primary enzyme is catechol-
O-methyl transferase, present in most tissues, especially liver and kidney.
The resulting inactive methylated amines, metanephrine and normetanephrine,
are either excreted in the urine or further metabolized by oxidative deamination
by the enzyme, monoamine oxidase. The final metabolic product is vanillylmandelic acid. Under normal conditions, vanillylmandelic acid comprises
about 75% of total urinary catecholamines, and metanephrines about 10%.
Finally, about 1% consists of free catecholamines, which are excreted unaltered in the urine.

PHEOCHROMOCYTOMA

The most common tumor of sympathetic origin in adults is pheochromocytoma, which derives from chromaffin cells in the adrenal medulla or extra-

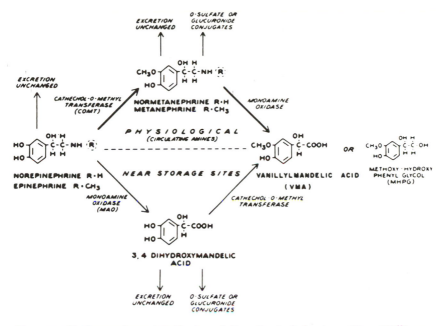

Fig. 4–7. Pathways for metabolic degradation of catecholamines. (From Williams, R: Textbook of Endocrinology. (5th Ed. Courtesy of W.B. Saunders Co., 1974.)

adrenal ganglia. Other rare neoplasms of sympathetic origin include neuroblastoma, ganglioneuroma, and chemodectoma. Although the incidence of pheochromocytoma is only 0.1% of all patients with hypertension, this disorder represents a curable form of hypertension, which is potentially lethal if untreated.

The tumor occurs with almost equal frequency in both sexes and has been found at all ages from infancy to the eighth decade. Pheochromocytomas occurring in childhood are frequently bilateral, more often malignant, and commonly familial. Because of their neural crest origin, these tumors can occur at any location along the primitive chromaffin system. Most commonly, they arise in the adrenal medulla or sympathetic ganglia along the abdominal aorta. Less than 5% of these tumors are extra-abdominal, usually in the thoracic sympathetic chain or rarely in the bladder wall. About 15% of pheochromocytomas are multiple and 10% are malignant.

Pathophysiology

Most findings in pheochromocytoma can be attributed to the pharmacologic action of the major catecholamines, epinephrine and norepinephrine. The effects of these sympathomimetic amines are partially determined by their receptor-binding affinity to target tissues. The adrenergic nervous system has two types of receptors, alpha and beta, which can be further divided into alpha 1 and 2 and beta 1 and 2 subtypes. Alpha-adrenergic receptors are predominantly involved in maintenance of peripheral circulation, with additional effects on gastrointestinal sphincter constriction, pupil dilatation, and sweating. Beta-adrenergic receptors increase cardiac rate and contractility and also cause peripheral vasodilation, bronchodilation, and decreased gastrointestinal motility. Norepinephrine has predominantly alpha effects, whereas epinephrine acts on both alpha and beta-adrenergic receptors. Adrenergic action is effected when receptor binding activates the cell membrane enzyme, adenylate cyclase, to change intracellular cyclic AMP levels.

Hypertension in pheochromocytoma is predominantly an alpha-adrenergic effect related to excess norepinephrine and is the most consistent manifestation of this disorder. Blood pressure elevation may be sustained or paroxysmal, depending on the nature of the catecholamine release. Sustained hypertension is seen in approximately half of the cases, but dramatic fluctuations in blood pressure are characteristic of this disease. Orthostatic hypotension associated with postural tachycardia is an important finding occurring in over 60% of patients with pheochromocytoma. The postural fall in blood pressure may be volume-related, but more likely reflects attenuation of normal circulatory reflexes. In addition, a few patients can have severe hypotension and shock, presumably related to high production of epinephrine.

Table 4–7 outlines the various modes of presentation of pheochromocytoma, emphasizing the differential diagnosis from several common illnesses. Classic findings with pheochromocytoma, in order of decreasing frequency, are hypertension, headache, sweating, palpitations, pallor, nausea, tremor,

Table 4–7.   Modes of Presentation in Pheochromocytoma

Disorder	Symptoms
Paroxysmal attack	Hypertension, headache, sweating, pallor, palpitation, nausea, chest and abdominal pain, tremor
Sustained hypertension	Symptoms mild or nonspecific, suggesting essential hypertension
Hypermetabolism	Tremor, sweating, weight loss, increased basal metabolic rate, suggesting hyperthyroidism
Increased blood glucose	Suggesting diabetes mellitus
Decreased gastrointestinal motility	Suggesting abdominal obstruction or Hirschsprung's disease
Hypertension in pregnancy	Mimics toxemia of pregnancy with hypermetabolism and psychic changes
Anxiety syndromes	Orthostatic dizziness, palpitations, paresthesias, and tremor, suggesting psychoneurosis or hyperventilation syndrome
Abdominal mass	Patient may be relatively free of symptoms if large tumor rapidly metabolizes catecholamines
Hypotension	May mimic any of the more common forms of shock
Congestive heart failure	Catecholamine-induced cardiomyopathy may mimic more common causes of congestive heart failure

weakness, flushing with heat intolerance, epigastric and chest pains, and paresthesias. Paroxysmal attacks are often precipitated by postural changes, smoking, palpation of the abdomen, overeating, induction of anesthesia, urination, exercise and certain drugs. Attacks may occur a number of times per day or several months apart, followed by symptom-free intervals.

The hypermetabolic features of pheochromocytoma incude tremor, weight loss, heat intolerance, and increased basal metabolic rate. Catecholamines block insulin release and increase gluconeogenesis and fatty acid mobilization, accounting for the high incidence of abnormal glucose tolerance, fasting hyperglycemia, and glycosuria in this disease. Catecholamines drastically reduce gastrointestinal motility and increase sphincter tone, leading to nausea, abdominal pain, and, at times, symptoms of intestinal obstruction. Because certain symptoms, including sweating, headache, hypermetabolism, and emotional lability, are common in pregnancy, the onset of hypertension in pregnancy often leads to the diagnosis of toxemia. Pheochromocytoma in pregnancy, if unrecognized, leads to morbidity and mortality in both mother and fetus. Autonomic nervous system abnormalities, such as postural hypotension, sweating, palpitations, and chest pains may suggest psychoneurosis. Many patients with essential hypertension have one or more features suggesting pheochromocytoma; yet only a small percentage of this group have the disease. A rare patient with pheochromocytoma has a large abdominal mass without symptoms of catecholamine excess; these large tumors degrade catecholamines within the tumor, yielding low or normal catecholamine levels but high levels of inactive metabolites. Cathecholamine excess can also produce a specific myocarditis and myocardial necrosis. In this setting, the patient may manifest signs of severe, refractory congestive heart failure masking the more common findings in this disease. Myocardial damage may reflect a direct inflammatory effect of catecholamines on cardiac tissue. Pheochromocytoma in children may result in impaired growth along with sustained hypertension, clinical symptoms of diabetes mellitus, and hypermetabolism. Rarely pheochromocytoma can involve the bladder wall and cause palpitations, headache, and sweating during or immediately after voiding.

ASSOCIATED FAMILIAL DISORDERS

Although the majority of pheochromocytomas occur sporadically, they also show a familial occurrence with autosomal dominant inheritance. Pheochromocytoma can be associated with medullary carcinoma of the thyroid. The relationship of these two diseases is based on their common embryonic origin from neural crest cells. This disorder, termed multiple endocrine neoplasia (MEN IIa) has a high incidence of bilateral pheochromocytoma. There may be associated parathyroid gland hyperplasia or adenomas. The coexistence of mucosal neuromas, thickened corneal nerves, gastrointestinal tract ganglioneuromas and marfanoid habitus with the above is designated MEN IIb.

Pheochromocytoma is frequently associated with other neuroectodermal syndromes, particularly neurofibromatosis, in 5 to 10% of patients. Other neurocutaneous findings in pheochromocytoma include cafe-au-lait spots, hyperpigmentation, and axillary freckling. Associated neuroectodermal disorders include Lindau's disease, Sturge-Weber syndrome, and tuberous sclerosis.

Symptoms and Signs

The symptomatic triad of pheochromocytoma consists of sweating, tachycardia and headache. In the presence of hypertension, this complex has high diagnostic specificity. The absence of these three symptoms in hypertensive subjects usually excludes pheochromocytoma. Flushing episodes, mistakenly thought to be characteristic, are extremely rare in pheochromocytoma. When symptoms of pheochromocytoma occur in paroxysms, the attacks are discrete with symptom-free intervals, which help to distinguish pheochromocytoma symptoms from chronic anxiety.

Hypertension in pheochromocytoma is usually severe and grade 3 or 4 hypertensive retinopathy is common. Also, the hypertension may be resistant to standard hypertensive therapy; in fact, certain antihypertensive agents such as beta-blockers may produce a paradoxical increase in blood pressure. The patients are often thin with a forceful heartbeat. Examination of the skin may reveal sweating, pallor, cafe-au-lait spots, but cool, moist extremities. The veins of the dorsum of the hand may not be apparent due to intense venoconstriction. Catecholamine-induced myocarditis may manifest itself as arrhythmias, gallop rhythms, and signs of congestive heart failure. A palpable abdominal tumor is found in 10 to 15% of cases, and palpation may elicit an attack. Quite frequently the patient has hypertension and a generally negative physical examination, so specific laboratory testing is needed. In this setting, indications for laboratory evaluation include all cases of severe hypertension, all children with hypertension, and patients with onset of hypertensive episodes during labor or anesthesia.

Diagnosis

Measurement of basal levels of norepinephrine and epinephrine and their metabolites in plasma and urine offer high specificity and sensitivity in the detection of pheochromocytoma (Table 4–8). Because of ease of performance

Table 4–8.   Normal Values

Plasma Concentrations	
Catecholamines: Epinephrine (supine)	$\leq$75 ng/l
Norepinephrine (supine)	50–440 ng/l
Urinary Excretion Rates	
Catecholamines	$\leq$100 µg/24 hr
Metanephrines	$\leq$1.2 mg/24 hr
Vanillylmandelic acid	$\leq$6.5 mg/24 hr

and availability, the urine test of catecholamines and their metabolites has been most widely employed.

URINARY CATECHOLAMINES AND METABOLITES

Metanephrines and Normetanephrines. These 3-methoxy metabolites can be measured by a relatively simple photometric method, usually expressed as total metanephrines. Many consider this the most reliable assay because it is virtually free from major interfering substances and specific and sensitive. Monoamine oxidase inhibitors, chlorpromazine, benzodiazepines, and alpha-methyldopa will falsely elevate urinary metanephrines. Normal values are less than 1.2 mg/day.

Total Free Catecholamines. This assay measures the sum of norepinephrine and epinephrine excreted unaltered in the urine and is best quantified by high-pressure liquid chromatography (HPLC). This separatory procedure fractionates norepinephrine and epinephrine for purposes of localizing adrenal and extra-adrenal tumor sites. Several pharmacologic compounds produce a false positive elevation of catecholamines, the most common being the antihypertensive agent, alpha-methyldopa. Since this sensitive procedure is expensive and technically more difficult than the other assays, it should not be used for routine screening. The normal adult secretion of free catecholamines is less than 100 µg/day.

Vanillylmandelic Acid (VMA). This acid is the final product of catecholamine metabolism. It is measured by organic extraction, conversion to vanillin, and spectrophotometric assay. This procedure is quite specific. However, some VMA screening tests are nonspecific because they measure phenolic acids in such foods as bananas, coffee, nuts and chocolate. In addition, the monoamine oxidase inhibitors and alpha-methyldopa result in a misleading decrease in VMA excretion. Normal values are less than 6.5 mg/day.

Plasma Catecholmines

Measurement of supine resting plasma norepinephrine and epinephrine offer high diagnostic utility in the diagnosis of pheochromocytoma. Some studies have suggested that plasma catecholamines when collected properly are more reliable than measurements of urinary VMA and metanephrine. However, sampling conditions must be rigorously standardized as plasma catecholamine levels vary acutely with stress, volume status, time of day, posture, meals, exercise, smoking and chronically change with body weight and age and other conditions. For sampling, patients should be fasting, supine for 30 minutes with a needle inserted intravenously 20 minutes before sampling.

In general, if the urinary assays are done by correct methods, the vast majority of cases of pheochromocytoma show an elevation of free catecholamines (99%) or total metanephrines (97%). Therefore, in routine screening of hypertensive patients, the best recommendation is a single measurement of total metanephrines and confirmation of abnormal levels by assay of total free catecholamines. Traditionally, most measurements have been done on

24-hour urine specimens, a procedure that is plagued by the problem of inaccurate collection. To circumvent this problem, either a timed 2-hour to 3-hour single-voided specimen or a random urine sample expressed per milligram of creatinine is useful if collected during or immediately after an attack. The plasma catecholamine assays have advantages in situations around or following an acute attack or sampling during provocative testing.

Pharmacologic Tests

Before the availability of accurate plasma and urinary tests for pheochromocytoma, the monitoring of blood pressure during administration of pharmacologic agents that stimulated or blocked catecholamine release was utilized to diagnose this disease. Today, with accurate tests of catecholamine levels, these potentially hazardous and relatively inaccurate procedures are rarely employed. However, an occasional patient may have normal or equivocal catecholamine levels; then a provocative test using glucagon may be carried out in conjunction with obtaining plasma specimens for catecholamines. Glucagon is given as an intravenous bolus (1 mg intravenously) with rapid measurement of blood pressure and sampling for plasma catecholamines 1 to 3 minutes after drug administration. A positive test includes a rise in blood pressure of 20/15 mm Hg above the baseline blood pressure and at least a 3-fold increment in catecholamine levels over baseline.

The clonidine suppression test has been proposed as a means of differentiating pheochromocytoma from essential hypertension. Clonidine causes a diffuse inhibition of sympathetic nervous system outflow with suppression of plasma norepinephrine levels in normals and patients with essential hypertension. Patients with catecholamine-producing tumors, which bypass the normal control mechanisms of catecholamine release, do not suppress plasma norepinephrine after clonidine. Clonidine as a 0.3 mg single oral dose is administered to the patient in the supine resting position, and samples for plasma norepinephrine and epinephrine are obtained before and 3 hours after clonidine administration. In most patients with essential hypertension, plasma catecholamine levels will decrease below 500 ng/l after clonidine, whereas levels in patients with pheochromocytoma will remain above this level.

Tumor Localization

Prior to surgery, tumor localization is an absolute requirement because of the diversity of location of pheochromocytoma tumors. Computed tomography is the procedure of choice for detection and localization of pheochromocytoma as it is highly accurate (96% localizing precision) and noninvasive, thereby avoiding the potential hazards of arteriography. Tumors of 1.0 cm or larger can be detected. CT scanning can also detect some extra-adrenal tumors, including intrathoracic and intracranial lesions. In small adrenal tumors, extra-adrenal tumors, or multiple tumors, selective catheterization with vena caval sampling for catecholamines has proved to be highly accurate as a localizing procedure.

The recently-described imaging technique using metaiodine-^{131}I-iodobenzylguanidine, a substance that is specifically taken up in neoplastic chromaffin tissue, has proven useful in localizing small occult tumors.

Treatment

Proper preoperative management has dramatically reduced the morbidity and mortality of surgical procedures. Phenoxybenzamine (10 mg orally twice daily) is administered preoperatively and increased to 40 to 100 mg daily until symptoms are controlled. Phentolamine, a shorter acting alpha-blocker, is used to control more severe paroxysms. A high-sodium diet may be given preoperatively to counteract volume depletion. Beta blockade should not be used preoperatively unless cardiac arrhythmias occur.

Therapy during surgical procedure should include monitoring of pulse, arterial and venous pressure, and electrocardiogram throughout the procedure. During the operation when the tumor is localized, it is important to ligate the venous drainage before excision to prevent excessive catecholamine release. Immediately after removal of the tumor, the blood pressure may fall precipitously; administration of a plasma expander before tumor removal usually prevents this complication. Surgical results are extremely rewarding; in fact, normotension resumes in the early postoperative period. A check of urinary catecholamines should be made the week after the operation to document complete tumor removal.

For inoperable pheochromocytoma, chronic medical therapy is necessary; the drug of choice is the inhibitor of tyrosine hydroxylase, alpha-methyltryosine. Unfortunately, for most cases of malignant pheochromocytoma, medical therapy is the only choice since these tumors respond poorly to antitumor therapy such as radiation or cytotoxic agents.

CLINICAL PROBLEMS

Patient 1. This 37-year-old white woman was admitted to the clinic with severe weakness. Her history dates back 10 years, when she noted that her fingers had areas of loss of pigmentation. Over the past year, she developed total body alopecia, including loss of head, axillary, and pubic hair. She also noted increased pigmentation and freckling of the face, back, hands, elbows, and knees. Four months before admission she became severely fatigued, nauseated, and weak. She was diagnosed as having the "flu" and placed on bedrest for 3 weeks without improvement. During this time she had a 15-pound weight loss, extreme weakness, abdominal pain, and anorexia. She was only able to retain liquids; solid foods caused epigastric pain, vomiting, and left lower quadrant cramping. Upon standing she had lightheadedness, palpitations, dyspnea, and fullness in her ears. There was no history of fever, chills, sweats, cough, or exposure to tuberculosis. She had a past history of goiter and had complaints of cold intolerance, dry skin, somnolence, and constipation. There was no family history of endocrine disorder, tuberculosis, or alopecia.

PHYSICAL EXAMINATION. This revealed a thin, pale, chronically ill woman. Blood pressure (BP) supine was 100/60; on standing no BP could be auscultated, only a systolic pressure by palpation. Pulse rate went from 84 to 120 upon standing. Total alopecia of the scalp accompanied increased pigmentaiton along her wig line. Increased freckling and vitiligo were apparent around the eyes. No mucosal pigmentations were noted. The thyroid was slightly enlarged, firm, and irregular without discrete nodules. She had dark pigmentaiton around the nipples. There was no axillary or pubic hair. Heart examination revealed tachycardia without abnormal sounds or murmurs. The abdomen was normal in the left lower quadrant with no rebound tenderness. There were no masses; liver and spleen were not palpable. Vitiligo covered the hands. Deep tendon reflexes were symmetrical with normal relaxation phase.

LABORATORY DATA. Hematocrit (HCT), 39%; white blood count (WBC), 6900 with 87 segs, 9 lymphocytes, 3 monocytes, and 1 undifferentiated cell. Serum Na, 135 mEq/L; K, 6.7 mEq/L; Cl, 99 mEq/L; CO_2, 24.8 mEq/L; glucose, 118 mg/100 ml; creatinine, 1.0 mg/100 ml; blood urea nitrogen (BUN), 18 mg/100 ml. Serum, calcium, magnesium, and liver function tests were normal. Electrocardiogram showed peaked T waves suggestive of hyperkalemia. Chest x ray was normal.

Serum cortisol, 1.0 μg/100 ml; after ACTH stimulation, cortisol remained 1.0 μg/100 ml. Serum aldosterone, 1.7 ng/100 ml (normal, 6 to 30 ng/100 ml in upright position).

Plasma ACTH, 310 pg/ml (normal, 8:00 A.M. 30 to 120 pg/ml). Serum vitamin B_{12}, 993 pg/ml (normal, 300 to 1025 pg.ml); T_4, RIA, 7.2 μg/100 ml; T_3, 103 ng/100 ml; TSH, 2 μU/ml.

QUESTIONS
1. What is the pathophysiology of the patient's symptoms?
2. What is your diagnosis, and what is the cause of the disease?
3. What other diseases are associated with this disorder?
4. What therapy would you initiate at the time of diagnosis?

Patient 2. This 5-year-old boy was first seen with complaints of excessive growth, pubic hair, and acne (Fig. 4–8). At 3 weeks of age he was admitted to the hospital with complaints of poor feeding, failure to gain weight, and vomiting. Physical examination revealed evidence of dehydration; serum sodium, 110 mEq/L; serum potassium, 9.5 mEq/L; urine sodium, 72 mEq/L; urine potassium 15 mEq/L; 17-ketosteroids 4.2 mg/24 hours (normal, less than 0.5 mg/24 hours); pregnanetriol, 3.2 mg/24 hours (normal, less than 0.5 mg/24 hours). He was treated with intravenous fluids, deoxycorticosterone acetate, 1 mg/24 hours, and cortisone, 10 mg/day. One week later he was discharged with serum Na, 142 mEq/L; K, 4.8 mEq/L; urine 17-ketosteroids, 0.5 mg/24 hours; and pregnanetriol, 0.3 mg/24 hours.

At the age of 11 months he was readmitted to the hospital with recurrence of vomiting, dehydration, and evidence of pneumonia. Serum Na, 115 mEq/L; K, 9.4 mEq/L; urine 17-ketosteroids, 5.8 mg/24 hours, and pregnanetriol, 2.4 mg/24 hours. Bone age was 1 year. Cortisone dosage was increased to 15 mg/day. Florinef (9α-fluorohydrocortisone), 0.1 mg daily, was substituted for deoxycorticosterone. Cortisone was given only intermittently because parents thought it was responsible for hyperpigmentation.

At the age of 3 years he had an upper respiratory infection and was seen at the hospital. Dehydration was no longer evident; 17-ketosteroids, 10.1 mg/24 hours (normal, less than 2.0 mg/24 hours); pregnanetriol, 12.5 mg/24 hours; serum Na, 130 mEq/L; K, 5.8 mEq/L. Cortisone dosage was increased to 20 mg/day. Parents were unable to understand the need for cortisone and Florinef. They were skeptical of the need for cortisone and one day took him to a physician who told them nothing was wrong with the boy's adrenals.

At age 5, he was referred to UCLA's clinic at the insistence of the school nurse who had noted his large size, hoarse voice, increased muscularity, acne, pubic hair, enlarged penis, and hair growth on the upper lip. Physical examination confirmed these findings, his height was 131 cm (about 6 SD above the mean), and his weight was 31 kg (also 6 SD above the mean). Serum sodium was 140 mEq/L; serum K was 4.6 mEq/L. Although the penis was greatly enlarged, the testes were normal in size for his age. Bone age was 12 years.

Over the next few years, his height continued well above the ninety-fifth percentile. He continued to take his medications sporadically. At age 9½, serum testosterone was 440 ng/100 ml, FSH and LH were unmeasureable. 17-ketosteroids were 84.8, and pregnanetriol was 18 mg/24 hours. Serum 17-hydroxyprogesterone was 640 ng/dl (normal, less than 90 ng/dl), and post-ACTH value was 42,000 ng/dl.

QUESTIONS
1. Which tests support the diagnosis of congenital adrenal hyperplasia?
2. What are the reasons for his salt loss? What enzymatic defects are associated with salt retention?
3. How does the urinary pregnanetriol and serum 17-hydroxyprogesterone establish the enzymatic defect?
4. Why is this boy tall? What will his adult height be—normal, short, or tall?

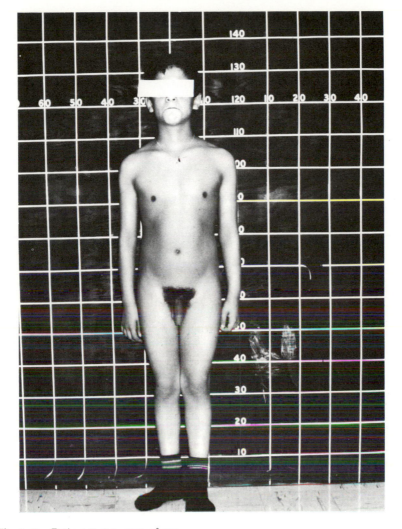

Fig. 4–8. Patient 2 at 5 years of age.

Patient 3. A 40-year-old woman described development of protruding abdomen, rounded face, increased facial hair, calf cramps, weakness, and recent leg ulcers that would not heal. She gave a history of hypertension recently diagnosed, menstrual irregularity, and swelling of her hands and feet for 2 years. Friends had commented that she looked older and had round rosy cheeks. She denied visual symptoms, acne, stria, or increased thirst or urination.

PHYSICAL EXAMINATION. BP, 155/100; P, 80 reg.; R, 15; T, 98.0. She was a well-developed white woman, with plethoric round face and protuberant abdomen. Skin was dry and thin, with bruises over her lower extremities. Soft downy hair was heavy over mustache area and chin. Visual fields were normal. Supraclavicular and dorsal fat pads were enlarged. Examination of the chest and heart was normal. The abdomen had increased fat centrally. Extremities had no pitting edema. Neurologic examination was normal.

LABORATORY DATA. Complete blood count, urinalysis, and electrolytes were normal. Oral glucose tolerance test was mildly diabetic, with fasting glucose of 100, 1 hour of 200, 2 hours of 150, and 3 hours of 120 mg/100 ml. Plasma cortisol at 8:00 A.M. after 1.0 mg of dexamethasone at 11:00 P.M. the night before was 16 μg/dl. Urinary free cortisol was 260 μg per 24 hours.

	Plasma cortisol (μg/dl)		Urinary 17-hydroxycorticosteroids mg/24 hrs.
	A.M.	P.M.	
Basal	22	18	18.3
	25		17.9
2 mg dexamethasone/day	24		12.7
	21		15.5
8 mg dexamethasone/day	15		6.3
	10		4.5

Plasma ACTH, 140 pg/ml.
Skull and sella films were normal.
Chest x-ray: mild demineralization of ribs with two old fractures.
CT scan pituitary sella: 8mm microadenoma in the pituitary; no suprasellar extension.
CT scan adrenal: normal
CRF Test: ACTH: basal 130
       (pg/ml) peak 460
       Cortisol: basal 18
       (μg/dl) peak 32

QUESTIONS
1. What physical findings indicate glucocorticoid excess?
2. What laboratory data help diagnose Cushing's syndrome and its cause in this case?

Patient 4. This 36-year-old white male was admitted for progressive, generalized weakness of 3 years' duration. He had been hypertensive for 4 years and was treated with thiazide diuretics. For the past 2 years, he had experienced nocturia getting up 3 to 4 times nightly, but did not have increased thirst. Recently, the weakness had progressed from intermittent to constant and was associated with muscle cramps. There was no family history of hypertension or muscular disease. He denied excessive licorice ingestion or use of steroids.

PHYSICAL EXAMINATION. The examination revealed a well-developed man. BP, 190/110 supine, 176/96 upright; pulse, 80/minute supine, 92/minute upright; respiration (R), 20/minute; temperature (T), 99.4°. Funduscopic examination disclosed mild arteriolar attenuation. Cardiac examination revealed an S4 gallop at the apex. Abdomen was without masses, or bruits. Pulses were palpable and equal; extremities had no edema. Generalized weakness to muscle testing was noted.

LABORATORY DATA. Hematocrit (HCT), 44% and WBC, 8700 with normal differential. Urinalysis, specific gravity, 1.007; pH, 6.0. Serum creatinine, 1.2 mg/100 ml; BUN, 18 mg/100 ml; creatinine clearance, 80 ml/min.

Electrolytes	Serum (mEq/L)				Urine (mEq/24 hrs)	
	Na	K	Cl	CO$_2$	Na	K
	144	2.6	104	33	62	69

		Plasma renin activity	
		Patient (ng/ml/hr)	Normal Range (ng/ml/hr)
10 mEq Na intake:	Supine	0.5	1.8–8.2
	Upright	0.9	2.2–12.3
4 hours postdiuretic: (60 mg furosemide)	Upright	0.8	1.8–6.4

Urine aldosterone excretion-33 μg/24 hours (normal, 10 to 24 μg/24 hours)

Plasma aldosterone (ng/100 ml)		Patient	Normal Range
120 mEq Na intake:	Supine	22	2–5
	Upright (4 Hrs.)	16	3–16
200 mEq Na intake:	Upright Supine	20	1–5
Saline infusion	pre	20	50–80% suppression
(2 L normal	post	17	from baseline
saline/4 hrs)			

Plasma 18-hydroxycorticosterone 120 ng per dl (normal 10–25 ng/dl).
EKG—suggests left ventricular hypertrophy, prolonged QT interval, flattening of T waves.
Chest x-ray—mild left ventricular hypertrophy
Rapid sequence IVP-normal

QUESTIONS
1. What symptoms suggest aldosteronoma?
2. What is the pathophysiology of these symptoms?
3. How would serum and urine potassium determinations in the basal state aid in the diagnosis of the patient?
4. What present and further diagnostic procedures would aid in clarification of the pathology and in the decision for surgical procedure versus medical therapy in this case?

Patient 5. This 38-year-old white male for the past 6 months had noted sudden onset of an intense frontal headache with sweating and tightness in the chest, coming on after sudden changes in position. He ascribed the symptoms to ''nerves,'' as he had recently separated from his wife. He also noted postural dizziness and a nauseated feeling, which he related to recent constipation. On one occasion, he sought medical help and was told that his BP was high. He was given a sedative, but did not return for follow-up as instructed. Two weeks prior to admission, he began to experience mild exertional dyspnea and noted ankle swelling. At this time, he had one episode of rapid heart rate diagnosed in a local emergency room as atrial tachycardia, which responded to digitalis and propranolol therapy. Because of a BP of 220/130 noted on that visit, he was referred for further evaluation. His mother and one brother had hypertension. The patient's past medical history revealed excellent health, and he was taking no medication.

PHYSICAL EXAMINATION. The examination revealed a thin man who appeared nervous and tremulous. BP 185/125 supine, 145/112 upright; R, 16/minute; T, 98°; pulse, 96 supine, 108 upright. Examination of the fundi showed grade III arteriolar narrowing. The thyroid gland was normal in size. Carotid pulses were equal and strong. His skin was moist. The lungs had bilateral rales. Cardiac examination revealed normal rhythm; point of maximal impulse was forceful and sustained; a third heart sound was heard at the apex. Pulses were all strong and equal, with no bruits. Abdominal examination revealed no tenderness, masses or organomegaly. Extremities had 1 + pitting edema.

LABORATORY DATA. Hgb, 15.2; HCT, 44%; WBC, 8500 with normal differential. Na, 142; K, 4.1; HCO3, 28; Cl, 96 mEq/L; creatinine, 1.2 mg/100 ml; BUN, 18 mg/100 ml; FBS, 125 mg/100 ml; Ca, 9.6 mg/100 ml; P, 3.3 mg/100 ml; cholesterol, 256 mg/100 ml.
Oral glucose tolerance test mildly diabetic.
Serum thyroxine, 6.4 μg/100 ml.
Chest x-ray, moderate left venticular hypertrophy and increased vascular markings in upper lung fields.
EKG normal sinus rhythm.
Urine metanephrine, 3.1 mg/24 hours
Total free catecholamines, 280 μg/24 hours; urine norepinephrine 196 μg/24 hours.
Plasma norepinephrine (supine) 1820 pg/ml
3 hours after Clonidine (0.3 mg) 1642 pg/ml
Abdominal CT scan; mass in left adrenal gland.

QUESTIONS
1. What is the pathophysiology of the patient's symptoms?
2. What is the significance of a 30% ratio of epinephrine to total catecholamines?
3. What further diagnostic studies would rule out endocrine disorders associated with pheochromocytoma in this patient?
4. What effect would propranolol have on the patient's blood pressure?

SUGGESTED READING

Cushing's Syndrome

Aron, D.C., et al.: Cushing's syndrome: problems in diagnosis. Medicine *60*:25, 1981.

Baxter, J.D., and Tyrell, J.B.: The adrenal cortex. *In* Endocrinology and Metabolism. Edited by P. Felig, J.D. Baxter, A.E. Broadus, and L.A. Frohman. 2nd Ed. New York, McGraw-Hill, 1987.

Beierwaltes, W.H., Sisson, J.C., and Shapiro, B.: Diagnosis of adrenal tumors with radionuclide imaging. Spec Top Endocrinol Metab, 6:1, 1984.

Boggan, J.E., Tyrrell, J.B., and Wilson, C.B.: Transsphenoidal microsurgical management of Cushing's disease: Report of 100 cases. J Neurosurg, *59*:195, 1983.

Carey, R.M., Varma, S.K., Drake, C.R., Jr., et al.: Ectopic secretion of corticotropin-releasing factor as a cause of Cushing's syndrome: A clinical, morphological and biochemical study. N Engl J Med, *311*:13, 1984.

Chrousos, G.P., Schuermeyer, T.H., Doppman, J., et al.: Clinical applications of corticotropin-releasing factor. Ann Intern Med, *102*:344, 1985.

Crapo, L.: Cushing's syndrome. A review of diagnostic tests. Metabolism *28*:955, 1979.

Dunlap, N.E., Grizzle, W.E., and Siegel, A.L.: Cushing's syndrome: Screening methods in hospitalized patients. Arch Pathol Lab Med *109*:222, 1985.

Findling, J.W., et al.: Selective venous sampling for ACTH in Cushing's syndrome. Differentiation between Cushing's disease and the ectopic ACTH syndrome. Ann Intern Med, *94*:647, 1981.

Gold, E.M.: The Cushing syndromes: changing view of diagnosis and treatment. Ann Intern Med, *90*:829, 1979.

Henley, D.J., Van Heerden, J.A., Grant, C.S., et al.: Adrenal cortical carcinoma: A continuing challenge. Surgery, *94*:926, 1983.

Howlett, T.A., Rees, L.H., and Besser, G.M.: Cushing's syndrome. *In* Clin Endocrinol Metab. Edited by G.M. Besser and L.H. Rees. The pituitary-adrenal axis *14*:911, 1985.

Oldfield, E.H., Chrousos, G.P., Schulte, H.M., et al.: Preoperative lateralization of ACTH-secreting pituitary microadenomas by bilateral and simultaneous inferior petrosal venous sinus sampling. N Engl J Med, *312*:100, 1985.

Orth, D.N.: Metyrapone is useful only as adjunctive therapy in Cushing's disease. Ann Intern Med, *89*:128, 1978.

Snell, M.E., Lawrence, R., Sutton, D., et al.: Advances in the techniques of localization of adrenal tumors and their influence on the surgical approach to the tumor. Br J Urol, *55*:617, 1983.

Stern, N., and Tuck, M.: The adrenal cortex and mineralocorticoid hypertension. *In* Manual of Endocrinology and Metabolism. Edited by N. Lavin. Boston, Little Brown and Co., 1986.

White, F.E., White, M.C., Drury, P.L., et al.: Value of computed tomography of the abdomen and chest in investigation of Cushing's syndrome. Br Med J, *284*:771, 1982.

Adrenal Insufficiency

Burke, C.W.: Adrenocortical insufficiency. *In* Clin Endocrinol Metab. Edited by G.M. Besser and L.H. Rees. The pituitary-adrenocortical axis. *14*:947, 1985.

Green, L.W., Cole, W., Greene, J.B., et al.: Adrenal insufficiency as a complication of the acquired immunodeficiency syndrome. Ann Intern Med, *101*:497, 1984.

Irvine, W.J., and Toft, A.D.: Diagnosing adrenocortical insufficiency. Practitioner, *218*:539, 1977.

Leshin, M.: Acute adrenal insufficiency: Recognition, management and prevention. Urol Clin North Am, *9*:229, 1982.

Loriaux, D.L.: The polyendocrine deficiency syndromes. N Engl J Med, *312*:1568, 1985.

Nelson, D.H.: The Adrenal Cortex: Physiological Function and Disease. Philadelphia, W.B. Saunders Co., 1980.

Nerup, J.: Addison's disease—clinical studies. A report of 108 cases. Acta Endocrinol, *76*:127, 1974.

O'Connell, T.X., and Aston, S.J.: Acute adrenal hemorrhage complicating anticoagulant therapy. Surg Gynecol Obstet, *139*:355, 1974.

Primary Aldosteronism

Bravo, E.L., et al.: The changing spectrum of primary hyperaldosteronism. Am J Med *74*:641, 1983.

Carey, R.M., Sen, S., Dolan, L.M., et al.: Idiopathic hyperaldosteronism: A possible role for aldosterone-stimulating factor. N Engl J Med, *311*:94, 1984.

Ganguly, A.: New insights and questions about glucocorticoid suppressible hyperaldosteronism. Am J Med, *72*:851, 1982.

Guerin, C.K., Wahner, H.W., Gorman, C.A., et al.: Computer graphic scanning versus radioisotope imaging in adrenocortical diagnosis. Am J Med, *75*:653, 1983.

Hunt, T.K., Schambelan, M., and Biglieri, E.G.: Selection of patients and operatve approach in primary aldosteronism. Ann Surg, *182*:353, 1975.

Kem, D.C., Tang, K., Hanson, C.S., et al.: The prediction of anatomical morphology of primary aldosteronism using serum 18-hydroxycorticosterone levels. J Clin Endocrinol Metab, *60*:67, 1985.

Lyons, D.F., Kem, D.C., Brown, R.D., et al.: Single dose captopril: A diagnostic test for primary aldosteronism. J Clin Endocrinol Metab, *57*:892, 1983.

Melby, J.C.: Primary aldosteronism. Kidney Int, *26*:769, 1984.

Streeten, D.H.P., Tomycz, N., and Anderson, G.H.: Reliability of screening methods for the diagnosis of primary hyperaldosteronism. Am J Med, *67*:403, 1979.

Weinberger, M.H., et al.: Primary hyperaldosteronism: Diagnosis, localization and treatment. Ann Intern Med, *90*:386, 1979.

Pheochromocytoma

Bravo, E.L., et al.: Circulating and urinary catecholamines in pheochromocytoma. Diagnostic and pathophysiologic implications. N Engl J Med, *301*:682, 1979.

Bravo, E.L., and Gifford, R.W., Jr.: Pheochromocytoma: Diagnosis, localization and management. N Engl J Med, *305*:12, 1983.

Cryer, P.E.: Diseases of the adrenal medullae and sympathetic nervous system. *In* Endocrinology and Metabolism. Edited by P. Felig, J.D. Baxter, A.E. Broadus, and L.A. Frohman. 2nd Ed. New York, McGraw-Hill, 1987.

Engelman, K.: Phaeochromocytoma. Clin Endocrinol Metab, *6*:769, 1977.

Francis, I.R., Glazer, G.M., Shapiro, B., et al.: Complementary roles in CT and ^{131}I-MIBG scintigraphy in diagnosing pheochromocytoma. Am J Radiol, *141*:719, 1983.

Juan, D.: Pheochromocytoma: Clinical manifestations and diagnostic tests. Urology, *17*:1, 1981.

Kirkendahl, W.M., Liechty, R.D., and Culp, D.A.: Diagnosis and treatment of patients with pheochromocytoma. Arch Intern Med, *115*:529, 1965.

Manger, W., and Gifford, R.W., Jr.: Pheochromocytoma. New York, Springer-Verlag, 1977.

Teply, J.J., and Lawrence, G.H.: Pheochromocytoma. Am J Surg, *140*:107, 1980.

ANSWERS TO QUESTIONS:

Patient 1

1. Symptoms of anorexia, nausea, vomiting, abdominal cramping, and weight loss result from cortisol deficiency in the cells of the gastrointestinal tract. Somnolence and fatigue result from cortisol deficiency in brain cells, and extreme weakness results from lack of cortisol effect in muscle cells. Light-headedness, palpitations, dyspnea, and fullness in the ears on standing upright are the result of total body sodium and volume depletion from aldosterone deficiency and also lack of the normal response of arterioles to the vasoconstrictor effect of catecholamines in cortisol deficiency. Dry skin probably is due to both volume depletion and lack of cortisol in the skin and appendage cells. Alopecia of the head and vitiligo are probably a result of autoimmune-mediated disease of the melanocytes and hair follicles, and loss of axillary and pubic hair is the result of adrenal androgen deficiency. Increased skin pigmentation and freckling are caused by chronic elevation of ACTH and LPH.

2. The diagnosis of primary adrenal insufficiency is made by the low serum cortisol, which does not respond to ACTH stimulation and the elevated plasma ACTH level. Low serum aldosterone is also consistent with primary rather than secondary adrenal insufficiency. The cause of the adrenal disease is most likely autoimmune adrenalitis resulting in adrenal atrophy. Vitiligo is associated with idiopathic adrenal atrophy in 17% of patients. A negative tuberculin skin test and positive serum antiadrenal antibodies would confirm the diagnosis. Hashimoto's thyroiditis is suggested by the thyroid examination. The diagnosis would be confirmed by finding a significant titer of antithyroid antibodies in the serum.

3. Idiopathic hypoparathyroidism, pernicious anemia, diabetes mellitus, thyroiditis (Hashi-

moto's and Graves' disease), and ovarian atrophy are all associated with idiopathic (but not tuberculous) adrenal atrophy.

4. The patient's chronic adrenal insufficiency will be corrected by replacement doses of glucocorticoid (prednisone, 7.5 mg daily; or hydrocortisone, 30 mg daily) and mineralocorticoid (fludrocortisone, 0.1 mg daily).

Patient 2

1. Elevated urinary 17-ketosteroids and pregnanetriol, elevated urinary sodium excretion, decreased potassium excretion in the presence of decreased serum sodium, and elevated serum potassium confirm the diagnosis of congenital adrenal hyperplasia. The high serum 17-hydroxyprogesterone after ACTH suggest 21-hydroxylase deficiency.

2. Salt loss occurs from a failure to secrete adequate quantities of aldosterone, particularly when salt intake is diminished as a result of intercurrent illness and sodium conservation does not occur. Failure to secrete adequate quantities of aldosterone occurs with 21-hydroxylase deficiency, 3β-dehydrogenase deficiency and 20, 22-desmolase deficiency. Retention of sodium occurs in 11-hydroxylase deficiency, because of increased secretion of 11-deoxycorticosterone, a potent mineralocorticoid.

3. 17-hydroxyprogesterone is the plasma precursor of pregnanetriol in the urine, and both are increased in 21-hydroxylase deficiency.

4. The patient is tall because of excessive growth stimulation by androgenic substances such as testosterone produced by the adrenals. Because his bone age is 15 years, he only has 3 years of skeletal maturation left before his epiphyses fuse completely to arrest growth. His height is average for a 12-year-old at a chronologic age for 9 years. He will be short as an adult.

Patient 3

1. Thinning of skin, muscle weakness, mild hypertension, centripetal fat deposition, bruises, light facial hair, altered facial appearance, and poor healing result from chronic excessive glucocorticoid secretion.

2. Cushing's syndrome was diagnosed by lack of circadian rhythm of plasma cortisol, lack of cortisol suppression by the low-dose dexamethasone test, and elevated urinary 17-hydroxycorticosteroids. Mildly elevated plasma ACTH and greater than 50% suppression of urinary 17-hydroxysteroids by the high dose of dexamethasone are indicative of pituitary dependent Cushing's. This was confirmed on CT scan of the sella.

Patient 4

1. Hypertension combined with muscle weakness, cramps, and nocturia suggest mineralocorticoid excess.

2. Chronic sodium retention from aldosterone excess results in hypertension. Potassium depletion from persistent mineralocorticoid action at the distal tubule of the nephron causes inability to concentrate the urine, muscle weakness, and cramps.

3. Basal urinary K^+ greater than 40 mEq/24 hours in the presence of hypokalemia (K^+ less than 3.5) indicates mineralocorticoid excess. Increased Na^+ delivery to the distal tubule in the presence of nonsuppressible aldosterone secretion enhances urinary K^+ excretion and induces further hypokalemia, whereas in the normal state Na^+ load does not alter K^+ excretion markedly.

4. The most useful tests are adrenal CT scan, [131]I-19-iodocholesterol adrenal scanning and adrenal venography with bilateral adrenal vein sampling for aldosterone levels. If aldosterone levels were elevated and similar bilaterally and the venogram confirmed bilateral hyperplasia, or if both adrenals were visualized on CT scan and iodocholesterol adrenal scan, medical therapy would be recommended; whereas if an aldosteronoma were localized by unilaterally elevated aldosterone levels and an adrenal tumor on venogram or CT scan, the patient would potentially be cured by surgical removal of the tumor. An elevated plasma 18-hydroxycorticosterone favors the diagnosis of an aldosterone-producing adenoma, as does the fall in plasma aldosterone after 4 hours upright posture.

Patient 5

1. Episodic catecholamine secretion is suggested by sudden headache, sweating, tachycardia, and tightness in the chest precipitated by change in position. Chronic catecholamine excess produces postural drop in blood pressure, nausea, and constipation.

2. Secretion of 30% of catecholamines as epinephrine is characteristic of a pheochromocytoma located in the adrenal gland because the synthesis of epinephrine requires high concentrations of cortisol.

3. Basal and calcium-stimulated calcitonin measurements would screen for associated medullary carcinoma of the thyroid. Parathormone and calcium levels would exclude hyperparathyroidism.

4. Propranolol blocks beta adrenergic receptors and thus blocks the vasodilating effect of catecholamines. Thus beta blockade in the presence of elevated plasma catecholamines results in unopposed alpha-mediated vasoconstriction and increased blood pressure.

5

Sexual Differentiation and Development

Barbara Lippe

ABBREVIATIONS

Compound S	11-deoxycortisol
DOC	deoxycorticosterone
FSH	follicle-stimulating hormone
GnRH	gonadotropin-releasing hormone
hCG	human chorionic gonadotropin
HPA	hypothalamic-pituitary axis
HPGA	hypothalamic-pituitary-gonadal axis
IGF-1	insulin-like growth factor-1 (somatomedin C)
LH	luteinizing hormone
MIS	Müllerian inhibiting substance
17-OHP	17-hydroxy-progesterone

SEXUAL DIFFERENTIATION OF THE FETUS

The sequence of embryonic and physiologic changes controlling sexual differentiation of the fetus begins with germ cell formation and fertilization, and then proceeds by a series of staged modifications of embryonic tissue primordia. The steps can be viewed as levels of development and the factors that influence each level as mechanisms encompassing the disciplines of anatomy, biochemistry, enzymology, endocrinology, and genetics. These levels and the key factors that influence development are shown diagrammatically in Figure 5–1.

Fertilization and Gonadal Development

The first level of sexual differentiation is zygote formation. Fertilization confers to the zygote so-called genetic sex, with the 46,XX karyotype normally being female, and the 46,XY karyotype being male. With successive mitotic cell divisions, the somatic cells and germ cells of the fetus usually express the same karyotype as the zygote. Abnormality in the sex chromosomes, such as mosaicism, monosomy, or polysomy, may occur at the time of maternal or paternal germ cell formation (for example, meiotic non-dysjunction resulting in an XY bearing sperm), at the time of fertilization (multiple fertilizations resulting, for example, in a 47,XXY, 47,XXX, or 48,XXXY zygote), or during an early mitotic division (with subsequently derived cell lines expressing different karyotypes).

The second level is that of gonadal development. The first differentiating events occur during the fourth week of fetal gestation (fertilization age) when the gonadal ridges begin to differentiate. The gonadal ridges are paired proliferations of coelomic epithelium and mesenchyme, which have the potential to develop into either testes or ovaries. The epithelium first proliferates, invades the mesenchyme, and begins to form undifferentiated sex cords. Then the germ cells, which originate in the yolk sac, migrate by amoeboid movement along the dorsal mesentery (under as yet unknown control mechanisms) and, by the sixth week, invade the genital ridges. The interaction between the differentiating somatic cells of the gonad and the germ cells determines the fate of the gonad(s). Three events must occur:

1. Germ cells must reach each genital ridge for a fertile gonad to develop. At this point the concept of laterality becomes important because subsequent embryonic events are dependent, in part, on processes occurring in each gonad, independently, and may or may not be the same on each side.
2. The chromosomal component that the germ cell confers should be the same on each side if the same type of gonad is to be induced on each side.
3. The somatic components of the gonad must be "induced" to form a testis, or else an ovary will form.

In the normal male, there appears to be a specific gene or genes, carried

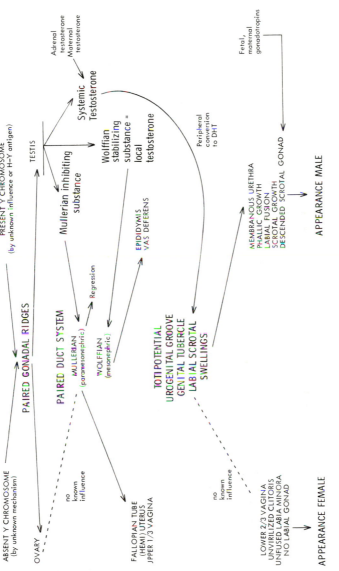

DEVELOPMENT OF THE GENITAL TRACT

ABSENT Y CHROMOSOME
(by unknown mechanism)

PRESENT Y CHROMOSOME
(by unknown influence or H–Y antigen)

PAIRED GONADAL RIDGES

OVARY

TESTIS

no known influence

PAIRED DUCT SYSTEM

MULLERIAN
(paramesonephric)

Regression

Mullerian inhibiting substance

WOLFFIAN
(mesonephric)

Wolffian stabilizing substance = local testosterone

Systemic Testosterone

Adrenal testosterone
Maternal testosterone

FALLOPIAN TUBE
(HEMI) UTERUS
UPPER 1/3 VAGINA

EPIDIDYMIS
VAS DEFERENS

TOTIPOTENTIAL
UROGENITAL GROOVE
GENITAL TUBERCLE
LABIAL SCROTAL
SWELLINGS

Peripheral conversion to DHT

no known influence

LOWER 2/3 VAGINA
UNVIRILIZED CLITORIS
UNFUSED LABIA MINORA
NO LABIAL GONAD

MEMBRANOUS URETHRA
PHALLIC GROWTH
LABIAL FUSION
SCROTAL GROWTH
DESCENDED SCROTAL GONAD

Fetal, maternal gonadotropins

APPEARANCE FEMALE

APPEARANCE MALE

Fig. 5–1. Development of the genital tract. This diagram outlines the factors that influence the development of each level of sexual differentiation.

on the Y chromosome and regulated by a gene or genes on the Y, the X or an autosome, which are responsible for testicular induction. The prime candidate for this gene product has been the H-Y antigen, a male specific cell-surface antigen originally defined by skin grafting experiments and measured by serologic tests using antisera raised against male cells. The hypothesis was that in the clinically demonstrated or putative Y-bearing fetus (that is, whether or not the Y chromosome could be identified in the peripheral karyotype), this H-Y material was synthesized and secreted by numerous tissues and bound by specific cell-surface receptors. In the developing genital ridge, the presence of cell surface H-Y antigen was believed to be responsible for somatic cell-to-cell interaction resulting in testicular tubule formation. Furthermore, it was proposed that its presence, as a consequence of secretion by some Y-bearing cells, could induce a testis even if the karyotype of the gonad ridge cells themselves was not Y bearing (gonadal sex-reversal). The H-Y antigen hypothesis also suggested that if it was not produced in "normal" quantities (presumably from a developing embryo in whom all cells do not bear the appropriate genetic message to synthesize the material), only part of a genital ridge, or one but not both ridges, would be induced to become a testis. Finally, the hypothesis proposed that in the normal female fetus, or the fetus not capable of synthesizing H-Y antigen, the gonadal ridge would develop into an ovary; that is, the ovary was the unmodified gonad of the fetus.

While this hypothesis could explain the clinical gonadal status of the normal XY male, the normal XX female, the many variations in gonadal development associated with mosaic or abnormal karyotypes, or XX karyotypes in which H-Y antigen could be detected, the H-Y antigen hypothesis of gonadal induction is now being questioned. Most recent experimental data, obtained from a strain of mice that inherit a variant mutation that allows for sterile testes development but not H-Y antigen expression (the so-called XX Sxr' mouse), suggest that the testis-induction factor may not be identical to H-Y antigen. The newly emerging data are being interpreted to indicate a role for H-Y antigen in spermatogenesis but not in testis induction. Thus, the molecular and genetic origin of the actual testis inducer remains to be determined. Similarly, roles for regulatory steps in inducer action, such as receptors or post-receptor mechanisms, are yet to be documented. Nevertheless, the concept of a Y-programmed testis inducer, the absence of which results in ovarian development, remains valid.

As germ cells penetrate the differentiating gonad, another regulatory step may occur. If the sex chromosome composition of the germ cell is different from that of the gonad (i.e., an XX germ cell in a developing testis), the germ cell will usually not survive and the gonad will be sterile. However, in some cases, evidence suggests that the XY germ cell may act as a second inducer and may direct an XX genital ridge into testicular differentiation.

The rates at which the testis and ovary develop are markedly disparate. Testicular development is rapid and complete by the 9th week, whereupon the testicle begins to function. There is some evidence that testosterone secretion may be stimulated by chorionic gonadotropin (hCG) since fetal gonadal receptors for LH-hCG develop early and the concentration of fetal serum hCG peaks between the 10th and 14th week. Fetal pituitary gonadotropins do not begin to rise significantly until the second trimester, so if they have a role in testicular function it is later in gestation. Ovarian organogenesis occurs at a much slower rate. It involves continued development of cortical cords from the germinal epithelium and continued invasion by primordial germ cells. When the maximum number of germ cells is attained, the medulla begins to take on a cord-like appearance and the germ cells group around the cords, enter the first meiosis, and follicles and stroma develop. This recognizable ovarian structure may not be present until 17 to 20 weeks of fetal gestation. The role in this process of either hCG or fetal pituitary gonadotropins remains to be determined. Unlike the testis, which tends to retain its structure whether germ cells are viable or not, the structure of the ovary tends to be determined by the state of the primordial follicles. If rapid follicular atresia occurs, as happens in many patients with X-chromosome monosomy (Turner's syndrome, 45,X and its variants), then fibrosis occurs. This postulated mechanism may explain the streak ovary in many of these patients. Conversely, it explains why a few Turner's patients may actually be fertile, since a follicle in its first meiosis contains a haploid chromosome number and only one X. Thus, a normal karyotype is not necessary for induction of the ovary, but a normal number of follicles is necessary for its continued preservation.

Internal Genital Duct Formation

During the earliest stage of fetal development, series of paired mesodermal ducts appear. The first, the pronephric ducts, are present by 3 weeks and degenerate soon thereafter. The metanephric ducts develop into the kidneys. The internal genital ducts develop from two other sets of mesodermal duct-like structures. Both develop alongside each gonadal ridge and their development (or regression) depends on two sets of control mechanisms. The mesonephric (Wolffian) ducts are present in close proximity to the gonadal ridges by 4 weeks, while the paramesonephric (Müllerian) ducts develop at 5 weeks in a more lateral position.

Once testicular organogenesis begins, Müllerian inhibiting substance (MIS) [also called anti-Müllerian hormone or Müllerian regression factor] is detectable. This substance is of Sertoli cell origin. The human and bovine genes for MIS have recently been isolated and cloned. The human MIS has been identified as a precursor protein of 560 amino acids, and the mature protein of 535 amino acids (mol. wt-57,000 daltons) then undergoes glycosylation and dimerization. MIS appears to be secreted locally or in such low concentrations that the product of one testis appears to affect the Müllerian structures on that side only. When present, it causes the regression of the Müllerian ducts adjacent to the developing testis at a critical time (prior to 8 weeks of gestation). Should a testis not be present (as in the normal female or the Turner's female) or should there fail to be production or action of MIS even when a testis is present (as in some conditions of mixed gonadal dysgenesis, hermaphroditism, and in the genetic condition of the XY male with uterii hernia inguinali), then these ducts develop into a fallopian tube, hemiuterus [to fuse later with the contralateral side (if present)], and the upper $\frac{1}{3}$ of the vagina. The ovary does not directly influence the process of maintaining the Müllerian structures. Because of its more lateral position, there is no direct contact between the paramesonephric duct and the gonad for which it is the potential excretory unit. Thus, excreted ova must pass freely into the peritoneum to reach the fimbriated end of the fallopian tube.

The Wolffian ducts also require active testicular secretion for their stabilization and subsequent differentiation. This stabilization is effected by locally secreted testosterone of Leydig cell origin (not systemic testosterone). Once the duct is stabilized, testosterone (acting prior to the development of 5-alpha reductase activity, thereby being the active hormone) then causes Wolffian differentiation into epididymis, vas deferens, seminal vesicle, and common ejaculatory duct. This process of male internal genital ductal development is obvious by 9 weeks and may be complete by 14 weeks. Because of its more medial location, the mesonephric duct is directly in contact with the gonad, and, when stabilized, becomes the integral excretory unit for sperm. In the absence of locally secreted testosterone, the Wolffian (mesonephric) ducts passively degenerate (leaving only residue such as Gartner's duct). Thus, the normal female internal genitalia (presence of Müllerian ducts and regression of Wolffian ducts) occur if a testis is absent. Normal male internal development requires two secretory products of the testis.

External Genital Development

The development of the external genitalia involves two complex embryonic mechanisms: the development of the excretory units of both the alimentary and urogenital systems and their subsequent sexual differentiation. The first steps occur identically in the fetus of both sexes and are not hormonally mediated. At about 3 weeks gestation, the cloacal membrane, which closes the hindgut, is already present. Cloacal folds develop around the cloacal membrane and unite cephalad to form a single genital tubercle and develop into lateral genital folds. The cloacal membrane then divides into urogenital and anal membranes (6 weeks), and finally into an anterior urogenital groove and a posterior anorectal canal (8 weeks). The genital folds divide into medial urethral folds (surrounding the urogenital groove) and lateral labioscrotal swellings. All these embryologic events occur in the fetus of either ''sex'' and result in common indifferent primordia for subsequent ''sexual differentiation.'' (This stage is schematically depicted in Fig. 5–2A.) Congenital anomalies such as imperforate anus, extrophy of the cloaca, agenesis of the phallus, or penoscrotal transposition all occur during the undifferentiated time. When seen, they indicate to the clinician that an early embryogenic defect has occurred rather than one mediated by an abnormality in gonadal development or hormone action.

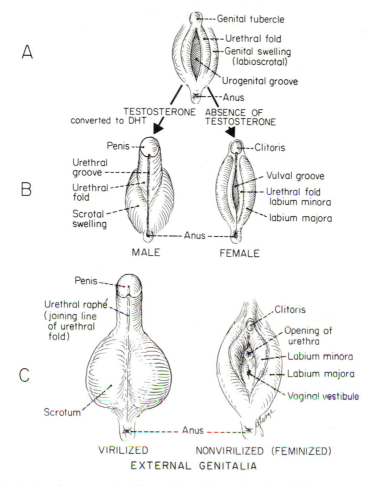

A

--- Genital tubercle

-- Urethral fold

-- Genital swelling
(labioscrotal)

Urogenital groove

-- Anus

TESTOSTERONE
converted to DHT

ABSENCE OF
TESTOSTERONE

B

Penis --

Urethral
groove ----

Urethral --
fold

Scrotal --
swelling

--- Clitoris

-- Vulval groove

-- Urethral fold
labium minora

-- labium majora

----- Anus -----

MALE   FEMALE

C

Penis---

Urethral raphé
(joining line
of urethral
fold)

Scrotum

--- Clitoris

-- Opening of
urethra

-- Labium minora

-- Labium majora

-- Vaginal vestibule

------ Anus ------

VIRILIZED   NONVIRILIZED (FEMINIZED)

EXTERNAL GENITALIA

Fig. 5–2. Development and differentiation of the external genitalia.

After 8 weeks of gestation, sexual divergence of the external genitalia begins with the ability of systemically circulating testosterone to masculinize the genital tubercle (elongation and lengthening of the anogenital distance). Masculinization continues as the labioscrotal swellings move caudally and fuse in the midline to form the scrotum and the urethral folds fuse to form the cavernous portion of the penile urethra (12 to 14 weeks) (Fig. 5–2B, left panel). Subsequently, labioscrotal fusion can no longer occur or progress (regardless of concentrations of testosterone), but the phallus (or clitoris) continues to elongate under androgen stimulation. Therefore, degrees of incomplete fusion of the male or fusion of these structures in the female are as they appear at 14 weeks. However, in the male, the final formation of the glandular urethra (to the tip of the phallus) does not appear to be a direct part of this masculinization process. Instead, it occurs later, during the 4th month, as an invagination of penile ectoderm to reach the urethral lumen. This may explain the occurrence of minor degrees of hypospadias (displacement of the urethral meatus) in the absence of known disorders of testosterone secretion or dihydrotestosterone action. Finally, the testes do not descend into the scrotum until late in the third trimester (Fig. 5–2C left panel). In the normal male, the testosterone is of Leydig cell origin. Leydig cell steroidogenic activity may initially begin without stimulus of gonadotropin, but it is primarily first under hCG and then pituitary LH stimulation. Regardless of origin (testis, adrenal, or exogenous), testosterone is converted to dihydrotestosterone by the presence of high concentrations of peripheral 5-alpha-reductase activity. Dihydrotestosterone preferentially binds to androgen receptors and effects androgen action at the level of the nucleus. It is therefore primarily dihydrotestosterone that is the fetal masculinizing hormone.

Development of the vagina begins to occur in the fetus of both sexes at 9 weeks. It begins as a proliferation of the dorsal wall of the urogenital sinus at a point contacted by the caudal tip of the fused Müllerian duct (which will contribute to the upper $\frac{1}{3}$ of the vagina in the female) or between the opening of the Wolffian ducts (in the male). The epithelial proliferation gives rise to a mass of cells (vaginal cord) that, in the female, grows caudally along the urethra, undergoes cavitation, and opens separately on the perineum relatively late in gestation (16 to 18 weeks). In the male, or in the female exposed to androgen, caudal growth is inhibited and the canalized portion develops as either the prostatic utricle or a portion of the lower $\frac{2}{3}$ of the vagina that fails to reach the perineum. Thus, normal female external differentiation is a relatively unmodified embryologic state (Fig. 5–2B right panel). The genital swellings remain as the unfused labia majora, the urethral folds as the labia minora, and the urogenital (vulval) groove as the vestibule for the cavitating vagina (Fig. 5–2C right panel).

PATHOGENESIS AND DIFFERENTIAL DIAGNOSIS OF AMBIGUOUS GENITALIA

Ambiguity of the external genitalia at birth is a consequence of either a developmental anomaly during or after the formation of the genitalia or the result of a derangement in the hormonal environment of the fetus or its ability to respond normally to hormonal stimuli. Thus, the differential diagnosis of the infant with ambiguous genitalia tends to fit into one of the following four pathophysiologic categories:

1. Virilization of the ovary-bearing XX female (female pseudohermaphroditism)
2. Incomplete masculinization of the testis-bearing XY male (male pseudohermaphroditism)
3. Gonadal intersex (where some degree of mixed gonadal structures has occurred)
4. Anatomic disruption of normal female or male structures

The methods of clinical and laboratory diagnosis of these conditions are summarized below:

Virilization of the Ovary-Bearing XX Female

A major clue that an infant with ambiguous genitalia may be a virilized female is absence of palpable inguinal or labio-scrotal gonads. While virilization is usually not complete (Fig. 5–3) it can progress to the extreme of a complete penile urethra. However, the ovaries will almost always be in their normal pelvic location and the fallopian tubes, uterus, and at least the upper ⅓ of the vagina will be normally placed. A contrast urogram will often fill the vaginal structure, may show the impression of the cervix, and can sometimes delineate the uterine cavity and the tubes. Ultrasonography may show the presence of a uterine structure between the bladder and the rectum. The most common causes are the virilizing forms of congenital adrenal hyperplasia (Chap. 4). The 21-hydroxylase deficiency form is the most frequent form (90%) with the 11-hydroxylase deficiency form much less common (10%). Elevated plasma 17-alpha-hydroxyprogesterone concentrations, obtained after the first 36 hours of age (when high neonatal values have started to fall), are

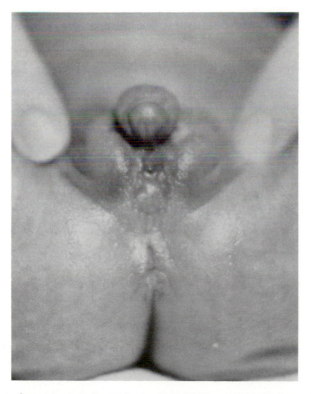

Fig. 5–3. Ambiguous genitalia. Note the empty labioscrotal folds, the enlarged clitorophallic structure, and the posterior labial fusion with a small introitus.

usually diagnostic of 21-hydroxylase deficiency, and high 11-deoxycortisol levels (Compound S) are diagnostic of the 11-hydroxylase deficient form. Urinary 17-ketosteroids will elevate over time in both, and urinary pregnanetriol will increase in the 21-hydroxylase form. In about half of the patients with 21-hydroxylase deficiency, severe salt loss occurs as a result of aldosterone deficiency. In the other half, salt-wasting may be subtle and demonstrated only under physiologic stress or with biochemical testing. Why there are two distinct clinical forms of this condition remains to be determined. In 11-hydroxylase deficiency, hypertension occurs in about one half of the patients and salt loss in a smaller number.

Other causes of virilization of the female fetus are rare. These include maternal ingestion of androgens or virilizing progestational agents (such as Norlutin), or maternal virilizing conditions such as luteoma of pregnancy. Idiopathic virilization is a diagnosis of exclusion since some Leydig tissue may be present as the only evidence of a remnant dysgenetic testis in a 46,XX infant with virilization and normal Müllerian structures. Thus, stimulation tests or laparotomy may be needed.

Incomplete Masculinization of the Testis-bearing XY Male

The major clue to this category of patients can be the presence of bilateral inguinal or scrotal gonads since they preclude simple virilization of a female and suggest either a form of male pseudohermaphroditism or gonadal intersex (Fig. 5–4). While an XX or a mosaic-bearing karyotype will favor the latter (since 80% of true hermaphrodites are XX), an XY karyotype is consistent with an incompletely masculinized male. However, not all neonates with male pseudohermaphroditism have bilaterally descended testes, so the finding is useful only when present. There are 4 subgroups within this category that will be summarized below: (1) enzymatic deficiencies in the pathway of testosterone synthesis or its conversion to dihydrotestosterone; (2) receptor or post-receptor abnormalities in testosterone action; (3) testicular dysgenesis or dysfunction leading to insufficient testosterone production [with or without defects in production of MIS]; and (4) hypothalamic-pituitary dysfunction with insufficient LH stimulation of Leydig cells.

1. *Enzymatic deficiencies in the pathway of testosterone synthesis or its conversion to dihydrotestosterone:* there are 5 steps in testicular testosterone biosynthesis (involving eight enzymatic conversions), three steps of which also may involve the adrenal gland and the synthesis of cortisol and can be considered part of the spectrum of congenital adrenal hyperplasia. Degrees of adrenal insufficiency with or without clinical salt loss can occur, and, as a consequence of the cortisol deficiency, activation of the hypothalamic-pituitary adrenal axis will result in excess of precursors at steps proximal to the block. The first of these is the conversion of cholesterol to pregnenolone (the 3 steps are carried out by a single P450 enzyme and the deficiency is called 20,22 desmolase deficiency or side-chain cleavage enzyme deficiency), followed by the conversion of pregnenolone to progesterone (involving two

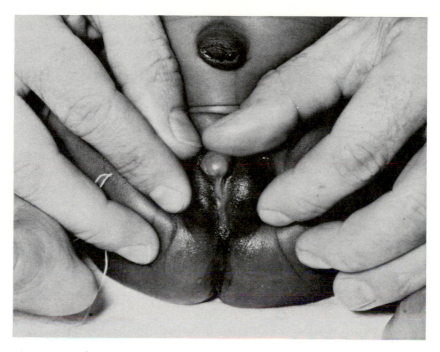

Fig. 5–4. Ambiguous genitalia. Note bilateral scrotal gonads. The remainder of the anatomy appears the same as the infant in Figure 5–3.

enzymes, 3-beta-hydroxysteroid dehydrogenase and a delta-4-5 isomerase), and then the hydroxylation of both the delta-4 steroid (progesterone) and the delta-5 steroid (pregnenolone) at the 17 position by 17-alpha hydroxylase. The next step in testosterone synthesis separates the adrenal corticosteroids (which retain their C-21 side chain) from the androgens (C-19 steroids) by cleaving the side chain of both the delta-4 and delta-5 with a 17-20 desmolase or lyase. Thus, deficiency of this enzyme does not involve the adrenal. The final step is reduction at the 17-keto position of both the delta-4 and delta-5 steroids by 17-ketosteroid reductase or 17-beta-hydroxysteroid dehydrogenase. This enzyme is also responsible for the interconversion of estradiol to estrone (C-18 steroids). Finally, virilization of the male is accomplished following the peripheral converison of testosterone to dihydrotestosterone by the enzyme 5-alpha reductase. Thus, this deficiency can be included in the group of enzymatic deficiencies that lead to undervirilization. Differential diagnosis of all the conditions in this category depends on the basal and stimulated concentrations of plasma and/or urinary steroids.

2. *Receptor or post-receptor abnormalities in testosterone action:* Testosterone and dihydrotestosterone act by binding to an intracellular androgen receptor protein, forming a complex that then interacts with acceptor sites in nuclei and brings about synthesis of new messenger RNA and proteins. Genetic deficiencies in receptor concentration or binding kinetics lead to various

degrees of male pseudohermaphroditism. The classical, and most extreme form, is the complete testicular feminization syndrome. This is a consequence of a gene defect on a region of the short arm of one X chromosome, carried by phenotypically normal females, and transmitted to those male offspring receiving the putative abnormal X. At birth these XY infants are phenotypic females, without genital ambiguity. The testes are usually intra-abdominal, although they may herniate into the inguinal or labial region anytime during childhood. Müllerian structures are absent, since Müllerian inhibiting substance is normally produced, but the lower two-thirds of the vagina is present, albeit ending blindly. In adult women, pubic and axillary hair are absent or sparse. Wolffian structures are absent or rudimentary as testosterone action is required for stabilization. Diagnosis can usually be made on clinical grounds. Measurement of androgen receptor may or may not be helpful since there are families of complete testicular feminization in which receptor binding is normal and the defect is either as yet undefined or at a post-receptor step. Treatment is to maintain and support the female gender assignment and to perform gonadectomy.

There is a second group of XY individuals who represent the heterogeneous entity of partial androgen resistance. This entity also appears to be an X-linked recessive trait, and pedigrees have been described by, and named after, Lubs, Gilbert-Dreyfus, Rosewater, and Reifenstein and are often called Reifenstein syndrome. These patients and families differ from complete testicular feminization because they are usually phenotypically ambiguous or significantly masculinized at birth and within a family there can be a marked variability of phenotype. Diagnosis is difficult when there is no family history of a similarly affected individual, since, in the prepubertal child, hormonal studies may be normal. In early infancy and again in adolescence, an increased plasma testosterone coupled with an increased LH concentration may assist in diagnosis. Androgen receptor binding studies may or may not be abnormal, and the degree of binding abnormality does not necessarily correlate with the degree of virilization. Similarly, phallic response to a short trial of testosterone in infancy may not predict responses at puberty. Breast development may occur in some patients at puberty, and fertility has not been observed. Treatment (which, in the infant, involves assigning a gender) has varied from case to case. In most families in which there are multiple affected members, gender choice has been male, and treatment involves surgical reconstruction, where indicated. High-dose androgen therapy to try to increase the degree of virilization has not generally been effective. In suspected or proven cases, some have had gonadectomies and been reared as females.

3. *Testicular dysgenesis or dysfunction leading to insufficient testosterone production (with or without defects in production of MIS):* There are a group of XY individuals with ambiguous genitalia and some persistence of Müllerian structures who have bilateral dysgenetic testes. These appear similar to streak gonads; because of a high risk for gonadoblastoma formation, they should be removed. The Müllerian structures may be left in situ if the infant is reared

as a female. These patients differ from those with the syndrome of hernia uterii inguinali (persistent Müllerian structures), in which ambiguity, if present at all, is limited to unilateral or bilateral cryptorchidism. In these XY male patients, there appears to be a failure of Sertoli cell production of MIS, while Leydig cell production of testosterone is normal. Thus, virilization and stabilization of Wolffian structures are normal. These patients are always reared as males, the cryptorchidism is corrected surgically, and the Müllerian structures are removed if they present in a hernia or are otherwise symptomatic. There is a third group of XY males in whom Müllerian structures persist but the external genitalia are female. The syndrome is called true XY gonadal dysgenesis (or Swyer syndrome) and appears to be transmitted as an X-linked mutant gene. While the female genitalia suggest total lack of androgen production by the fetus, the gonadal streaks are at risk for gonadoblastoma formation. This contrasts to the XX form of pure familial gonadal dysgenesis (which, when it occurs with sensorineural hearing loss, is called Perrault syndrome) and which does not appear to have a risk of gonadoblastoma. Finally, phenotypically normal, well-virilized XY males may be born without evidence of any testes at all. They present with cryptorchidism, castrate levels of gonadotropins in infancy and again during puberty, and, when evaluated radiologically and surgically, fail to have testes. The epididymis and vas are present (demonstrating Wolffian stabilization by testosterone) and Müllerian structures are absent (demonstrating that MIS was produced). Thus, functional Leydig and Sertoli cells were present initially, and the testes then underwent regression. The mechanism for this sporadic occurrence is unknown.

4. *Hypothalamic-pituitary dysfunction with insufficient LH stimulation of Leydig cells:* Fetal Leydig cell steroidogenesis may begin autonomously, but is soon under hCG control, and the pattern of testosterone secretion during early gestation follows that of hCG. Thus, early male sexual differentiation occurs independently of LH. However, pituitary LH of fetal origin appears to be necessary for the continued growth and function of the fetal testis. Therefore, microphallus, underdeveloped scrotum, and cryptorchidism have all been described in conditions of hypopituitarism or syndromes associated with hypothalamic gonadotropin deficiency (such as Kallmann syndrome or the Prader-Willi syndrome). Associated features in those infants who are subsequently diagnosed as having hypopituitarism might include neonatal hypoglycemia or hypothyroidism. In both these and the isolated gonadotropin group, there would be failure of the postnatal surge of LH and testosterone. Sex of rearing is usually male since phallic growth can usually be achieved with exogenous testosterone.

Gonadal Intersex

This group includes patients with true hermaphroditism (defined as patients bearing gonads which contain ovarian follicles and testicular tubules, Fig. 5–5), and those with mixed or asymmetric gonadal dysgenesis (defined as patients having a testis and a streak gonad with preservation of most of the

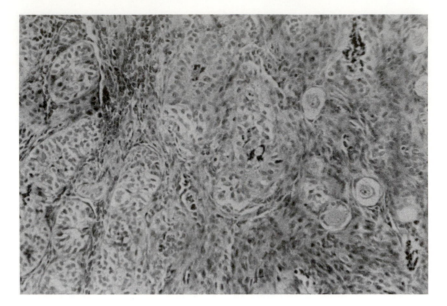

Fig. 5–5. Microscopic appearance of an ovotestis. This gonad was present in an infant with ambiguous genitalia. It demonstrates the existence of both testicular tubules (left) and ovarian follicles (right).

Müllerian structures). The karyotype of the true hermaphrodites is most often 46,XX followed by 46,XX/46,XY mosaicism, while that of mixed gonadal dysgenesis is most often 46,XY/45,X. However, multiple other karyotypes have been observed in each condition, and the status of either the gonads or the internal structures cannot be necessarily predicted from the karyotype. Thus, unless both gonads can be surgically examined in the inguinal area, the management of these patients almost always includes an exploratory laparotomy. Sex of rearing is most often determined by the predicted degree of functionally correctable anatomy. In both conditions, if sex of rearing is male, the intact testes must be exteriorized but need not be removed. However, if a gonadal streak or dysgenetic testis is found, it should be removed. The uterus, fallopian tubes, and any ovarian tissue are also removed. If the infant is reared as a female, all testicular and streak tissue are removed but ovarian tissue (an intact ovary, or the clearly demarcated ovary section of an ovotestis with no evidence of testicular tissue at the hilus, may be left in situ even if there is a Y chromosome in the karyotype).

Anatomic Disruption of Normal Female or Male Structures

Disorders of embryogenesis affecting the genital tubercle, urogenital sinus, rectum, or bladder may all present with ambiguous external genitalia. These include disorders such as extrophy of the cloaca or bladder, complete agenesis of the phallus with a fistula for urinary excretion, and penoscrotal transposition. While the endocrinologist is often called upon to evaluate these infants, the mechanism does not involve the sex chromosomes or hormones of sexual differentiation. Nevertheless, involvement with these patients is necessary since decisions concerning gender assignment may involve measures such as sex reversal and removal of the testes in a male without the potential for phallic reconstruction.

GONADAL FUNCTION FROM BIRTH TO PUBERTY

The mechanisms that control gonadal function actually begin in the fetus. Fetal hypothalamic-pituitary activity can be demonstrated in the second trimester and there is evidence suggesting that a component of fetal gonadal activity is directly stimulated by fetal pituitary gonadotropins. Toward the end of gestation, fetal gonadotropin secretion decreases. This decrease is believed to be a consequence of negative feedback inhibition on the hypothalamic-pituitary-axis (HPA) from increasing circulating levels of sex steroids of fetal and placental origin. At birth, there is a rapid decline in these circulating steroids following placental separation and a consequent reactivity of the HPA with a subsequent increase in gonadally derived hormones. In the male infant during the first 3 months of life, gonadotropins increase and plasma testosterone concentrations may rise to levels as high as those detected in mid-puberty. In the female infant, the rise in estradiol is less striking, but gonadotropins are increased and ovarian follicular development may occur. In infants without gonads, or in males with androgen insensitivity, the HPA responds as it does in the castrate adult, with high levels of gonadotropins. The gonadotropins are secreted in a pulsatile fashion, suggesting that the hypothalamic "pulse generator," which is responsible for pulses of gonadotropin-releasing hormone (GnRH), is active in the infant.

The mechanisms that account for the decline in activity of the "pulse generator" to its prepubertal level of activity are not clear at this time. It is known that gonadal steroid feedback inhibition may play some role, since gonadally intact infants revert to a prepubertal pattern of gonadotropin secretion faster than do castrate children. Nevertheless, the fact that, even in the absence of gonads, the gonadotropins decline in childhood implies other mechanisms of inhibition. Similarly, the mechanisms that are responsible for reactivation of the system as puberty is initiated are also unknown. However, as the pubertal pattern begins, there is a circadian pattern of increased GnRH pulses, the amplitude of the pulses first rising at night, during the first few hours of sleep. This is reflected by pubertal concentrations of LH during sleep, while daytime concentrations are still prepubertal. As the process progresses, daytime pulses develop and finally the adult pattern of similar day and night secretion is reached. A component of this reactivation of the HPA is described as a shift from negative inhibition to positive feedback by gonadal steroids. However, the mediators for the change are yet to be defined. Factors as diverse as genetic family patterns, nutritional status, and neurotransmitter concentrations probably all play a role. The role of changing frequency of the GnRH pulses has been examined for the ovulatory cycle, but has not been well studied in the initiation of puberty in man. The most common frequency of pulses in primates is every 60 to 90 minutes.

The clinical implications of the gradual changes that occur in the hypothalamic-pituitary-gonadal axis (HPGA) in the prepubertal and early pubertal child are now considered. When one evaluates a single blood sample to assess a child or adolescent with a possible problem in sexual development:

1. Hormonal concentrations vary with age and span a spectrum of normal which can range from low (prepubertal) to high (fully pubertal) values. Therefore, single determinations of estradiol, testosterone, FSH, or LH are often not helpful in assessing, describing, or diagnosing a clinical state. For example, basal serum FSH and LH determinations from normal children between the ages of 1 and 11 or more years of age may be low, but still in the so-called normal range for the agonadal child or for the child with hypogonadotropic hypogonadism. Thus, they might not distinguish these states. In the child with precocious puberty, a single determination could be high and suggest the diagnosis, but if it were low it would not preclude the diagnosis.

2. Single levels of estradiol or testosterone often lag behind the clinical features of puberty and are frequently more helpful in confirming the clinical impression of "delayed" puberty than they are in making an etiologic or appropriate diagnosis (such as early puberty). That is, the normal nocturnal rise of testosterone in the pubertal male would be missed by a daytime sample as might the rise in the child with precocious puberty. Only high, and reproducible levels tend to be diagnostic.

When one is considering the physical examination:

1. The physical changes that occur during puberty in the male and female have been divided into visible stages that reflect the sequential nature of the process. While the age of onset of the earliest pubertal changes is highly variable, the rate of progression of change thereafter is less variable. Therefore, a standard nomenclature for describing each stage allows the observer to evaluate the rate and degree of progression of change. In the female, the most commonly used physical standards are those of Tanner and Marshall for breast and pubic hair development. In that system, Tanner stage I is prepubertal and Tanner stage V is adult. The mean age of onset of breast budding (Tanner II) is 10.5 years with 2 standard deviations being 8.5 to 12.5. Since full maturity may take as long as 4.5 years, the number of years during which normal changes in breast development can occur is quite long. Pubic hair development, which in the female is a consequence of the interaction of gonadal and adrenal steroids, spans a slightly narrower range (11.7 ± 2.5 to 14.4 ± 2.2), although wider variations are possible. Changes in the ovaries and uterus cannot be easily assessed clinically, but may, in fact, demonstrate the earliest effects of activation of the HPGA.

The changes that occur in the male can also be staged according to the standards of Tanner as they apply to pubic and axillary hair and phallic and scrotal development. These are available in most pediatric texts. Another helpful schema is illustrated in Figure 5–6. Stage 1 is prepubertal, stage 5 is

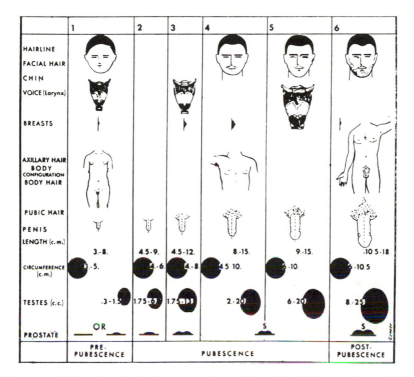

Fig. 5–6. Male pubertal development. (From Schonfeld, W.A.: Am J Dis Child, *65*:535, 1943.)

fully pubertal, and stage 6 represents further changes which may not occur until the middle of the third decade. A key to male pubertal staging is testicular size [and best described as a volumetric measurement (in cc) since the testis is an ellipsoid organ]. The first physical change in the male is the beginning enlargement of the testis as the gland responds to increased gonadotropin secretion. Enlargement from 2 cc or less (the prepubertal state) begins at 11.5 ± 2.0 years. It may take 1 year to reach 6 cc before which no other physical signs of puberty may be present. The physical changes thereafter are primarily a consequence of testicular Leydig cell androgen secretion. Further testicular enlargement is mainly testicular tubule development. In the male with Klinefelter's syndrome (47,XXY), masculinization may be normal at puberty, since Leydig cell secretion remains partially intact. However, the tubules are hyalinized and the volume of the testis usually remains at 6 cc or less. Gynecomastia, or unilateral or bilateral development of breast tissue in the male, is a normal response during puberty, occurring in as many as 70% of males at some time during the process. The development of the breast tissue may be due to the high ratio of estradiol to testosterone secreted by the testis during early and mid-puberty. It is usually transitory, lasting 1 to 2 years and undergoes resolution as the ratio reverses itself with increasing testosterone production. Excessive size or persistence of tissue beyond adolescence may necessitate surgical removal for cosmetic reasons, but the tissue is usually normal. However, post-pubertal development of gynecomastia signals an abnormality in hormonal secretion or milieu and needs evaluation. There are a number of pathologic conditions which may have associated pubertal gynecomastia. Klinefelter's syndrome is the most common, since it may occur in 1/1000 males and gynecomastia appears to occur in about 50% of affected individuals. The characteristic clinical clue to the diagnosis will be testicular volumes that are small in the face of progressive signs of androgenization. Rare conditions resulting in pubertal gynecomastia include syndromes of partial androgen insensitivity, excess peripheral aromatase activity, and exposure to exogenous estrogens. In addition, the same drugs and medical conditions that result in gynecomastia in adults can result in gynecomastia in the adolescent male.

2. Menarche (for which there is no easily documented parallel event in the male), while not an actual physical finding, is a definable recordable point in the pubertal process. While it is a consequence of increasing ovarian estrogen production, uterine growth, and endometrial proliferation, it usually does not reflect complete maturation of the HPGA since most first menses are not the result of an ovulatory cycle. It occurs at a mean interval of 2.3 years after breast development is first noted and in American girls is currently reported to be at 12.8 years. Its occurrence is helpful in assessing the progress of a given individual, but its absence is not helpful in assessing the physiologic reasons for a disorder in pubertal development.

3. Statural growth and changes in growth rate are two other physical and dynamic components of puberty that reflect the changes that are occurring primarily in the HPGA. In girls, peak growth velocity occurs between breast and pubic hair stages II and III (preceding menarche). However, the intensity of the so-called "growth spurt" seems related to the time of occurrence; i.e., in the year preceding menarche, early developers gain more height than do late developers. This accounts for the lack of a significant difference in the adult heights of "early and late growers" in spite of the anecdotal impression that early developers "end-up" short. In the male, the pubertal growth spurt period is longer than that in the female. The peak velocity is reached at a mean age of 15.5 years, and while it is less intense than that of the female, its extended time period contributes to ultimately taller stature. Since, in both, the onset of the growth spurt and puberty are related and correlated with skeletal maturation (bone age), assessment of puberty and its consequent hormonal changes is a requisite for the evaluation of growth during this time interval. The role of hormones other than those of the HPGA, such as growth hormone and somatomedin-C (IGF-I), are currently being investigated.

Thus, when one is considering which dynamic tests of the HPA or HPGA to use in evaluating the child or adolescent with a disorder of growth or pubertal development, the above factors make clear why tests that are applicable in adults may not apply:

1. Clomiphene, an anti-estrogen which probably acts by blocking the neg-

ative feedback effect of estrogen and may be useful in estrogenized but non-ovulating women and mildly hypogonadal men, does not usually stimulate an LH surge in the prepubertal child and cannot, therefore, be used reliably to distinguish hypogonadotropic hypogonadism from delayed puberty.

2. GnRH administration, as a single bolus or a short term infusion, elicits only modest LH and FSH responses in the prepubertal child and, therefore, does not necessarily distinguish between delayed puberty and conditions such as hypogonadotropic hypogonadism. Similarly, failure of FSH or LH to respond to GnRH does not necessarily implicate a primary pituitary problem, since pituitary gonadotropin release often requires pulsatile GnRH priming. However, in the child with central precocious puberty, the GnRH test is useful, since the FSH and LH responses are usually exaggerated.

3. In the male, the hCG stimulation test can be useful because the testis is capable of responding to hCG with testosterone production at any age and with little or no priming.

4. Progesterone, given to a woman to convert an estrogenized proliferative uterine lining to a secretory lining, and then stopped (Progesterone-withdrawal test) to induce uterine sloughing (bleeding), will be helpful only in girls who have progressed to a stage of sufficient breast development to suggest that estrogen production has taken place.

CLINICAL CONDITIONS OF ABERRANT GROWTH AND PUBERTAL DEVELOPMENT

The interrelationships between the maturation of the HPA, gonadal responses, and pubertal growth and development make it necessary to consider disorders of growth and pubertal development together in the adolescent.

Delayed Growth and Puberty

Based on the mean age +2 SD for the onset of pubertal changes, 2% of girls fail to exhibit breast development by age 13 years, and 2% of boys fail to have testicular enlargement by 13.5 years. The majority of these children progress into puberty within 1 to 2 more years and have no demonstrable somatic or hormonal abnormalities. Uncharacterized genetic factors may be responsible for the time of initiation of puberty as pubertal delay tends to run in families. In such individuals, the bone age is usually 1 to 2 years delayed and tends to be in line with the height of the individual. This pattern of delayed growth and puberty is called *constitutional growth delay.*

Following is a list of the kinds of conditions that can be responsible for the small fraction of children with pubertal delay (with or without growth delay) that are not *constitutional.*

Systemic Disorders
1. Generalized—infectious, inflammatory, neoplastic
2. Specific organ system—cardiovascular, respiratory, gastrointestinal, renal, neuromuscular. Of clinical note is that the pathologic process, such as inflammatory bowel disease, can be subtle and manifest only as pubertal delay
3. Endocrine—undiagnosed or poorly controlled conditions

4. Nutritional—anorexia nervosa, "athletic amenorrhea," willful dieting, malnutrition

Hypothalamic Dysfunction
1. Generalized—postinfectious, inflammatory, postradiation, traumatic
2. Specific—lesion or process causing dysfunction
   a. Congenital malformation—midline defect or cleft syndrome associated with failure to produce releasing hormones
   b. Craniopharyngioma with suprasellar extension
   c. Infiltrative lesion—histiocytosis X
   d. Hypothalamic tumor
3. Syndromes—associated with dysfunction
   a. Kallmann's—anosmia and hypogonadotropic hypogonadism
   b. Prader-Willi—mental retardation, hypogonadism, hypotonia, obesity
   c. Laurence-Moon-Bardet-Biedl—mental retardation, hypogonadism, retinitis pigmentosa, polydactyly
   d. Cryptorchidism—alone or with a syndrome in which hypothalamic dysfunction may be implicated
4. Idiopathic or familial—failure to produce or secrete GnRH

Pituitary Dysfunction
1. Generalized—infectious, granulomatous, vascular (insufficiency, infarct, compression), autoimmune destruction
2. Specific lesion or process
   a. Congenital malformation—aplasia or hypoplasia
   b. Craniopharyngioma—with pituitary destruction
   c. Adenoma
   d. Histiocytosis X
3. Syndromes associated with primary pituitary gonadotropin deficiency

Gonadal Dysfunction
1. Generalized—gonadal failure as a consequence of a systemic condition such as cystic fibrosis (male) or galactosemia (female), or secondary to an autoimmune destructive process
2. Specific
   a. Congenital or Genetic
      Ovarian or pure (46,XX) gonadal dysgenesis in the female
      Uterine—congenital absence (presents with primary amenorrhea)
      Testicular—anorchia or "vanishing testis"
      Swyer's syndrome—46,XY gonadal dysgenesis with somatic sex reversal (female phenotype)
      Testicular feminization syndrome—46,XY androgen insensitivity and its variants (female phenotype and primary amenorrhea)
      Other enzymatic causes of sex-hormone insufficiency
   b. Chromosomal
      Ovarian—45,X gonadal dysgenesis (Turner's syndrome and its other chromosomal variants)
      Testicular—47,XXY Klinefelter's syndrome and its variants
   c. Infectious, inflammatory, traumatic
      Ovarian—secondary to pelvic inflammatory disease, torsion or therapeutic radiation, or chemotherapy
      Uterine—secondary to pelvic inflammatory disease, traumatic abortion or idiopathic
      Testicular—cryptorchidism, secondary to orchitis, torsion, vascular insufficiency (after orchiopexy or herniorrhaphy), following radiation or chemotherapy
   d. Miscellaneous
      Ovarian—insensitivity to gonadotropin syndrome
      Testicular—associated with neuromuscular disease such as myotonic dystrophy

CONDITIONS OF PRECOCIOUS SEXUAL DEVELOPMENT

Precocious puberty is defined as the progressive development of secondary sexual characteristics in a female prior to the age of 8 years and in a male prior to the age of 9 years. Isosexual precocity denotes characteristics appropriate for the gender of the child (feminization of the female and virilization of the male). When the characteristics are at variance with gender (virilization of the female or feminization of the male), the patients usually have a "pseudo" form of precocity. The following are the general categories into which most of the causes of isosexual and "pseudo" precocity fall:

1. True isosexual precocity—due to early activation of the HPGA
   a. Idiopathic—80% in females; less than 50% in males—When assessed, the pulsatile nature of gonadotropin secretion is present. The treatment for this condition is the use of analogs of GnRH that functionally block the effect of the endogenous GnRH.
   b. Secondary to a CNS lesion (see 2a below), trauma, infection, or malformation. This can occur with gliomas in patients with neurofibromatosis
   c. Part of the "overlap syndrome" of long-standing untreated primary hypothyroidism
   d. Acquired—following maturation of the HPA due to systemic sex steroids—as occurs in McCune-Albright's polyostotic fibrous dysplasia (where ovarian cysts first produce sexual precocity and then the HPA matures early)—or after the treatment of virilizing adrenal hyperplasia
2. Isosexual precocity—independent of activation of the HPA
   a. Gonadotropin releasing hormone produced from a hamartoma of the tuber cinerium (accessory hypothalamus)
   b. Ectopic hCG secretion
   c. Pituitary lesion with autonomous LH/FSH production (rare)
   d. Gonadal autonomy—ovarian cyst or tumor; testicular tumor (the hormones can be androgens, estrogens or both); testicular malregulation of testosterone secretion; "familial testotoxicosis"
   e. Extragonadal hormone production—usually adrenal—can be congenital adrenal hyperplasia, adrenal adenoma, adrenal carcinoma—the hormones can be androgens, estrogens, or both
   f. Exogenous hormone exposure
   g. Factitious—local vaginal bleeding that is nonhormonal in origin (infectious, traumatic, tumor, or actually from urinary tract)
3. "Pseudo" precocious puberty—this usually results from the abnormal production or exposure to androgen or estrogen. The most common causes are abnormal production or exposure to androgen or estrogen independent of the HPA as in 2 d to f (above).

When precocious secondary sexual characteristics are present, do not progress, and no pathologic process is found, the following conditions may be defined:

1. Female with precocious thelarche—usually occurs in a child 6 to 36 months of age. Breast development usually stabilizes at Tanner II–III.

The causes are believed to be transient estrogen secretion from an ovarian cyst, transient activation of the HPA, increased sensitivity to endogenous estrogen, or exogenous estrogen.

2. Male with prepubertal gynecomastia. A search for a feminizing lesion must be made, but in its absence this rare condition is benign and nonprogressive.

3. Precocious adrenarche—Defined as pubic and/or axillary hair in a girl prior to age 8 and a boy prior to age 9. The condition is much more common in females. When "idiopathic," it is characterized by concentrations of circulating weak adrenal androgens similar to those at the time of Tanner stage II–III. A search should be made for virilizing conditions such as mild or atypical forms of congenital adrenal hyperplasia.

CLINICAL PROBLEMS

Patient 1

You are called to the newborn nursery to consult on the gender identification of a full-term infant born with ambiguous genitalia.

PHYSICAL EXAMINATION. The infant appears healthy, and has no other abnormal findings apart from the genitalia. A photograph of the infant appears in Figure 5–7. A midline organ looks like an enlarged clitoris or a phallus with hypospadias. Midline fusion from the rectum anteriorly is incomplete, ending in a single orifice that looks like an introitus. Urine appears to emanate from within it. The labioscrotal folds are somewhat ruggated and are asymmetric. One appears empty while the other contains a palpable gonad-like structure.

The family history, obtained from a distraught father, appears to be negative, as does the history of the pregnancy.

You order the following laboratory tests:

1. Contrast genitogram and pelvic ultrasound, Figure 5–7B and C.
2. Serum (to be obtained at or after 36 hours of age) for testosterone, dihydrotestosterone, 17-alpha-hydroxyprogesterone, DHEA, androstenedione, 11-deoxycortisol. The results are all in the normal neonatal range, including the testosterone that is appropriate for a male infant.
3. A peripheral leukocyte karyotype. The results were available on day 5 of life and were 45,X/46,XY.

QUESTIONS
1. What did you tell the family initially?
2. Did you allow them to name the child immediately?
3. What is the likely internal anatomy?
4. What recommendations did you make to the family about sex assignment?

Patient 2

A 13-year-old female is brought to your office with a complaint of pain in her lower belly. On physical examination you note a mass in the right groin which appears to be a hernia. The remainder of her genital examination is unremarkable for a prepubertal girl. There is no pubic hair or clitoromegaly. She does have Tanner III breast development but has not had a menses. The mass is reducible but you feel surgical repair is indicated. Preoperatively, you obtain a plasma testosterone, which is 110 ng/dl [3.8 nmol/L]; this is the level of a Tanner II male and high for a prepubertal female. The dihydrotestosterone was appropriate for the level of testosterone.

QUESTIONS
1. What other tests might be helpful?
2. What are the likely diagnoses?
3. What do you tell the family?

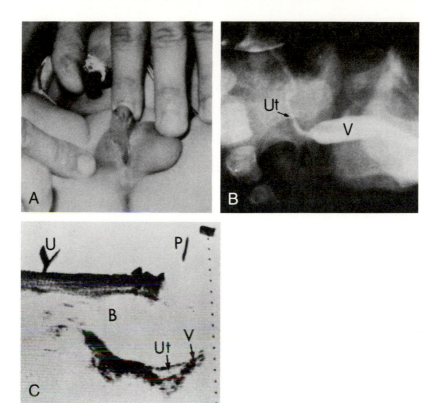

Fig. 5–7. *A.* An infant with ambiguous genitalia and an asymmetric appearance;
B. A contrast genitogram demonstrating the presence of a vagina (V) and a uterine cavity (Ut);
C. A longitudinal pelvic ultrasound demonstrating a uterine structure (Ut) and vagina (V) below the fluid filled bladder (B). (U = umbilicus; P = pelvis.)

   4.   What kind of surgery will you suggest to the surgeon?

Patient 3
   A 2-year-old boy is referred to you (a pediatric endocrinologist) because his pediatrician thought he had a form of precocious puberty. On his most recent physical examination, she noted his penis was enlarging and there were a few pubic hairs. She obtained a serum testosterone which was 110 ng/dl [3.6 nmol/L]. On your physical examination, you note he is quite tall, muscular, and healthy appearing. His penis is the size of a mid-pubertal male, and there are some curly pubic hairs. The scrotum is loose and rugated; each testis is 1 cc in volume. The remainder of the physical examination is unremarkable, except he cried and was uncooperative so you are not sure if his blood pressure determination of 140/90 is accurate. A bone age x-ray reveals advanced skeletal maturation. The first laboratory tests you obtain are a serum 17-alpha-hydroxyproges-terone (17-OHP) and a serum 11-deoxycortisol.

QUESTIONS
   1.   What suggested that you begin the evaluation with adrenal steroid precursors and not gonadotropins?
   2.   If the 17-OHP is high and the 11-DOC low, what is the likely diagnosis?
   3.   If the 11-DOC is abnormally high, what is the likely diagnosis?
   4.   If these steroids are normal what other tests would you do?

SUGGESTED READING

Sexual Differentiation of the Fetus

Cate, R.L., et al.: Isolation of the bovine and human genes for Müllerian inhibiting substance and expression of the human gene in animal cells. Cell, *45*:685, 1986.

Griffin, J.E., and Wilson, J.D.: The syndromes of androgen resistance. N Engl J Med, *302*:198, 1980.

Jirasek, J.E.: Development of the Genital System and Male Pseudohermaphroditism. Baltimore, Johns Hopkins Press, 1971.

McLaren, A., et al.: Male sexual differentiation in mice lacking H-Y antigen. Nature, *312*:552, 1984.

Wachtel, S.S.: The dysgenetic gonad: aberrant testicular differentiation. Biol Reprod, *22*:1, 1980.

Pathogenesis and Differential Diagnosis of Ambiguous Genitalia

Kaplan, S.A.: Disorders of the adrenal cortex II: Congenital Adrenal Hyperplasia. Pediatr Clin North Am, *26*:77, 1979.

Lippe, B.M.: Ambiguous genitalia and pseudohermaphroditism. Pediatr Clin North Am, *26*:91, 1979.

Sanger, P.: Abnormal sex differentiation. J. Pediatr, *104*:1, 1984.

Gonadal Function from Birth to Puberty

Grumbach, M.M.: The neuroendocrinology of puberty. *In* Neuroendocrinology. Edited by D.T. Krieger and J.C. Hughes. Sunderland, MA, Sinauer Associates, 1980.

Penny, R.: Disorders of the testes. *In* Clinical Pediatric and Adolescent Endocrinology. Edited by S.A. Kaplan. Philadelphia, W.B. Saunders Co., 1982.

Rosenfeld, R.L.: The ovary and female sexual maturation. *In* Clinical Pediatric and Adolescent Endocrinology. Edited by S.A. Kaplan. Philadelphia, W.B. Saunders Co., 1982.

Clinical Conditions of Aberrant Growth and Pubertal Development

Frasier, S.D.: Pediatric Endocrinology. New York, Grune and Stratton, 1980.

Pescovitz, O.H., et al.: The NIH experience with precocious puberty: Diagnostic subgroups and response to short-term luteinizing hormone releasing hormone analogue therapy. J Pediatr, *108*:47, 1986.

ANSWERS TO QUESTIONS

Patient 1

1. It is best to tell the family exactly what you are thinking in language they can understand. I usually say that the messages that determine the sex of a child come from both parents, and that the genitalia develop as a result of the messages; it is, therefore, possible to get two sets of messages and to then develop part of the appearance like a male and part like a female. The important thing is that you, the doctor, will work as quickly as possible to tell the family how and why their baby has developed its present appearance (through the tests you do) and then you will work with them to decide which set of messages are "stronger" so they actually participate in the later decision about sex of rearing. You can tell them to tell their relatives that the baby was born underdeveloped and therefore the doctors have to do tests to know which way the development will finish.

2. NO!! They have been waiting 9 months for a certain child (such as Kathy or John). In several days you will make a decision and give them that child. If you give the baby a "neuter" name (such as Terry), when you make the "right" decision, they will still have the "wrong" baby.

3. Since the most likely diagnosis is mixed gonadal dysgenesis, the internal anatomy is likely to be a streak ovary (as in Turner's syndrome) on the right side, next to which is a fallopian tube attached to a semi-uterus which goes down to a cervix. The left side is a testis that has an epididymis and blind-ending vas.

4. There is no correct answer. Many endocrinologists would rear this child as a female, removing the testis and the streak gonad and reducing the size of the phallic structure (in infancy). Later, the vagina can be enlarged. Some would rear the child as a male, removing the streak ovary and the uterus, tube and vagina, then do a series of urethral reconstructions

to move the opening onto the phallic structure. In either case the child, as an adult, will be sterile. The keys are the anatomy of the individual child (potential for reconstruction for normal sexual function), the number of surgeries that would be involved, and the understanding of the parents.

Patient 2
1. Chromosomes (likely to be 46,XY), an LH (likely to be high), and a pelvic ultrasound (likely to show testes-like structures in both inguinal canals, a blind ending vagina, no cervix, and no uterus).
2. The complete form of androgen resistance (Testicular Feminization syndrome). In this form, androgen receptor binding would be absent (this test is done on fibroblasts cultured from genital skin so it is not routinely performed and not necessary to make the diagnosis). One of the incomplete forms is possible (although there is usually more virilization).
3. I tell the family what the condition is, and why this really makes this child a girl (even with the XY and the gonads that are like testes); I emphasize that if the tissues don't "see" testosterone and can never be made to "see" it, then this is a girl.
4. I recommend removing the testes at the time of hernia repair and giving the girl estrogen.

Patient 3
1. Since the testes were not enlarged, it is likely the testosterone is coming from the adrenal. In the picture of gonadotropin mediated sexual precocity, the testes are the source of the androgen and should enlarge.
2. The most common form of virilizing congenital adrenal hyperplasia, the 21-hydroxylase deficient form. Since the child did well until now, it is the non-salt losing variant.
3. The rare 11-hydroxylase deficient form of congenital adrenal hyperplasia. About half of these individuals have hypertension.
4. One would have to find the source of the testosterone by imaging the adrenals to look for a tumor and/or by stimulating the adrenals and collecting venous effluent from both sides. A testicular tumor is most unlikely. Sources of exogenous testosterone are rare.

6

Female Reproductive Disorders

Glenn D. Braunstein

ABBREVIATIONS

CAH	congenital adrenal hyperplasia
DHEA-S	dehydroepiandrosterone sulfate
E_2	estradiol
FSH	follicle-stimulating hormone
GH	growth hormone
GnRH	gonadotropin-releasing hormone
LH	luteinizing hormone
P	progesterone
TEBG	testosterone-estradiol-binding globulin

DEVELOPMENT OF THE FEMALE REPRODUCTIVE SYSTEM

Between 6 and 8 weeks of fetal development, the ovaries become morphologically distinct and rapid proliferation of oogonia takes place. The number of germ cells in the ovaries increase rapidly, reaching a peak of 6 to 7 million at approximately 20 weeks of gestation. At the time of birth, however, the ovaries only contain 1 to 2 million eggs, the others having been depleted by the process of follicular atresia (Fig. 6–1). The process of atresia continues throughout the next 50 years.

During childhood, the hypothalamic-pituitary-ovarian axis remains relatively quiescent. The serum levels of the pituitary gonadotropins, follicle stimulating hormone (FSH), and luteinizing hormone (LH) are low, and minute quantities of estrogens are capable of further suppressing FSH and LH secretion. The pituitary during this period is relatively unresponsive to an exogenous injection of the hypothalamic decapeptide, gonadotropin-releasing hormone (GnRH). Between ages 6 and 8 years, the serum concentrations of FSH increase and at approximately 10 years of age, the serum levels of LH and estradiol (E_2) rise. The rising E_2 concentration stimulates the secondary sexual organs to develop leading to uterine, vaginal, and breast enlargement. Although the events that initiate puberty are unknown, it is clear that during this period, the sensitivity of the hypothalamus and pituitary to feedback inhibition by gonadal steroids decreases, resulting in increased secretion of GnRH and thus LH and FSH, which in turn results in greater secretion of gonadal steroids. The end result is the establishment of pulsatile GnRH, LH, and FSH secretion and normal menstrual cycles.

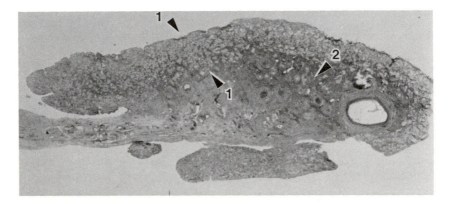

Fig. 6–1. Premature Ovary. Section of ovary from a female fetus demonstrating the cortex and medulla of the ovary. 1. The ovarian cortex is filled with numerous primordial follicles containing primitive germ cells. 2. The ovarian medulla is adjacent to the cortex and includes connective tissue and blood vessels. The hilum of the ovary is contiguous to the medulla in the picture (×10 magnification).

THE NORMAL MENSTRUAL CYCLE

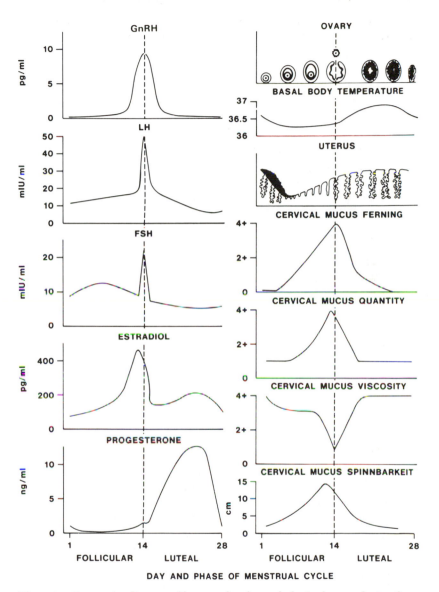

Fig. 6–2. Composite diagram of hormonal and morphologic changes during the normal menstrual cycle.

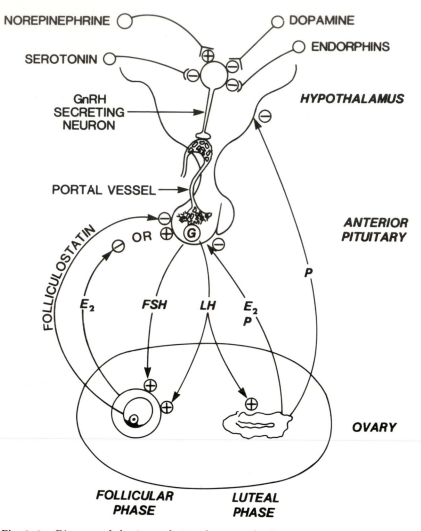

Fig. 6–3. Diagram of the interrelations between the hypothalamus, pituitary, and ovary during the normal menstrual cycle. See text for discussion. (G: gonadotrope, GnRH: gonadotropin-releasing hormone, E_2: estradiol, P: progesterone, +: positive feedback or stimulation, and −: negative feedback or inhibition).

NORMAL MENSTRUAL CYCLE

Between menarche and menopause, the reproductive organs of most women undergo a series of closely coordinated changes at approximately monthly intervals; together these actions comprise the normal menstrual cycle. A menstrual cycle begins with the first day of genital bleeding (day 1) and ends just prior to the next menstrual period. The following discussion describes the individual changes that take place in the hypothalamus, pituitary, ovaries, and sexual accessory organs during the normal cycle. Figures 6–2 and 6–3 depict these events; for illustrative purposes, the depicted menstrual cycles are 28 days long, although normal cycle length varies from 25 to 34 days.

Hypothalamus

The area of the central nervous system above the pituitary and surrounding the third ventricle contains numerous nuclei that control a variety of bodily processes. GnRH is synthesized within the medial basal hypothalamus, primarily in the arcuate nucleus. GnRH is released into the hypothalamo-hypophyseal portal system in a pulsatile fashion every 1 to 3 hours. The secretion of GnRH appears to be regulated primarily by biogenic amines interacting with the arcuate nucleus. Norepinephrine stimulates GnRH release, while dopamine and serotonin inhibit GnRH secretion. In addition, endogenous opioids appear to modulate GnRH secretion by directly inhibiting GnRH release from the arcuate nucleus. A rise in portal blood GnRH levels has been found at midcycle (approximately day 14).

Pituitary

The glycoprotein gonadotropic hormones, LH and FSH, are synthesized in the same basophilic cells, the gonadotropes. Under the influence of GnRH, both LH and FSH are synthesized and secreted by these cells in an episodic pattern with a midcycle surge. The amplitude and frequency of secretion are modulated by the gonadal steroid concentrations and by the frequency of GnRH pulses.

During the first half of the follicular (proliferative) phase, when the estradiol (E_2) levels are low, FSH gradually rises owing to decreased negative feedback. The FSH levels decrease during the second half of the follicular phase under the influence of increased negative feedback by E_2 and possibly folliculostatin (inhibin), a nonsteroidal, specific FSH inhibitor that has been identified in follicular fluid. At midcycle there is a surge of FSH that results both from the midcycle rise of GnRH and from enhanced sensitivity of the gonadotropes to the effects of GnRH. This enhanced sensitivity is probably due to a positive feedback effect of gonadal steroids. The negative feedback suppression by the high levels of E_2 plus progesterone (P) during the luteal (secretory) phase results in suppression of FSH release until a few days before menstruation begins, when the FSH levels begin to rise owing to a fall in the E_2 and P concentrations.

The LH levels during the follicular phase gradually rise, initially through decreased negative feedback by the low E_2 levels and then by apparent positive E_2 feedback. As with FSH, a midcycle surge of LH occurs secondary to GnRH stimulation and enhanced sensitivity of the gonadotropes to GnRH. A progressive decline of LH during the first two-thirds of the luteal phase is due to the negative feedback effects of the gonadal steroids, both on GnRH release and on gonadotrope sensitivity to GnRH. Just prior to the beginning of the next menstrual cycle, the LH levels begin to rise, coinciding with the fall in E_2 and P.

Ovaries

The morphologic events that take place in the ovaries are the result of both gonadotropin stimulation and intraovarian "short-loop" feedback control mechanisms. During the late luteal phase of the preceding cycle and during the early part of the follicular phase, 10 to 15 primordial follicles, composed of a primary oocyte surrounded by a single layer of granulosa cells and a basement membrane, develop into primary follicles with several layers of granulosa cells and a theca interna outside the basement membrane (Fig. 6–4). The events initiating the recruitment and early growth of the follicles are independent of gonadotropins. FSH receptors develop on the granulosa cells, and under the influence of FSH, the primordial follicle grows with an increase in the number of granulosa cells and the accumulation of follicular fluid between granulosa cells, forming an antrum. Concurrently, the theca interna cells grow and develop LH receptors. LH stimulates the theca interna cells to synthesize the androgens, androstenedione and testosterone, which are converted to estrogens by aromatase enzymes present in the theca cells or in the granulosa cells. Estrogen accumulation in the antral fluid further stimulates growth of the follicles. Although several primordial follicles develop in the primary and secondary follicles during each menstrual cycle, usually only one secondary follicle continues to grow and develop into a preovulatory (Graffian) follicle under the influence of FSH and LH. The

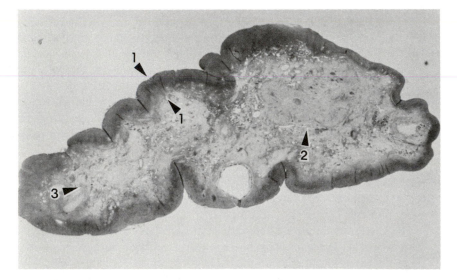

Fig. 6–4. Normal ovary in reproductive years. Section of ovary from a woman during the reproductive period. 1. Ovarian cortex comprised of cortical stroma and scattered primordial and developing follicles. The cortical stroma expands beneath the tunica albuginea that confines the ovary, the outer surface of which is covered by the coelomic or germinal epithelium. 2. Mature corpus luteum with convoluted borders and luteinized follicular cells. 3. Medulla of ovary containing loose connective tissue and blood vessels (×4 magnification).

remainder undergo follicular atresia through mechanisms that are presently unclear. Between 12 and 30 hours following the midcycle LH peak, follicular rupture takes place with the extrusion of the egg. The mechanism responsible for ovulation is unknown but may be related to the rapid increase in intra-follicular fluid accumulation and progesterone-induced synthesis of proteolytic enzymes which weaken the follicular wall. After ovulation, LH induces the transformation of the follicle into a corpus luteum, which secretes P, E_2, and androstenedione. If pregnancy does not occur, the corpus luteum regresses after approximately 14 days of function and is replaced by a scar (corpus albicans).

During the last few days of the luteal phase of the preceding menstrual cycle, the levels of E_2 rapidly decrease and remain low during the early part of the follicular phase. Under the influence of FSH and LH, levels of E_2 rise slowly during the first half of the follicular phase and more rapidly during the second half, peaking approximately 24 hours before the LH peak. Just before ovulation, the E_2 levels decrease, only to rise again when corpus luteum steroidogenesis begins. Progesterone levels continue to decline during the first half of the follicular phase and then rise gradually, reaching a peak during the middle of the luteal phase. The thermogenic effect of P leads to a parallel rise in basal body temperature. Luteal phase E_2 and P secretion are primarily controlled by LH, modulated by intrinsic changes in the sensitivity of the corpus luteum to LH secretion.

Uterus

The uterine endometrium is composed of three layers. The basal layer is not lost during menses and serves to regenerate the other two layers during the cycle. A superficial layer of compact columnar epithelial cells lines the endometrial cavity, with an intermediate layer of spongiosum. These two layers show the principal endometrial changes during the menstrual cycle. Approximately 5 days after the start of the menses under the influence of rising levels of E_2, the denuded endometrium begins to be regenerated from the basal layer. At that time, the surface epithelium is cuboidal with a compact stroma and straight glands. During the proliferative phase, the endometrial lining increases in width, the epithelium becomes more columnar and the glands elongate. After ovulation, the E_2 secreted by the corpus luteum maintains the growth of the endometrium, while P induces the glands to become coiled, sawtoothed, and secretory. As the levels of E_2 and P decline during the late luteal phase, the stroma becomes edematous, endometrial and blood vessel necrosis occurs, and menstrual bleeding ensues. Because the histologic changes during the menstrual cycle are so characteristic, endometrial biopsies may be used to accurately date the stage of the cycle and assess the tissue response to gonadal steroids.

Endocervix

The endocervical glands also undergo cyclic changes in morphology and function. The product of these glands—the cervical mucus—demonstrates a series of characteristic changes. Under the influence of E_2, the quantity, elasticity, water content, and sperm penetrability of the mucus increases, peaking at midcycle, while the viscosity and cell count decrease. The changes in viscosity and elasticity are easily quantitated by measurement of the length that the cervical mucus can be stretched (spinnbarkeit). Ferning, the ability of the sodium chloride present in the cervical mucus to crystallize in an arborized pattern as the mucus dries, is also a manifestation of the estrogen effect and reaches a peak at midcycle. During the luteal phase, P induces a decrease in the quantity, pH, spinnbarkeit, sperm penetrability, and ferning ability of the mucus, with a concomitant increase in the viscosity and cellular content.

Vagina

Four well-defined layers of cells make up the stratified squamous epithelium of the vagina. The basal germinal layer is not desquamated and is responsible for regeneration of the epithelium. The other three layers—the parabasal, the intermediate or precornified squamous, and the cornified squamous epithelium—change during the cycle. In the proliferative phase, the estrogens induce thickening of the vaginal epithelial cell layers and increase the number of cornified cells. After ovulation, stimulation by P results in more precornified cells, an increased number of polymorphonuclear leukocytes, cellular debris, and clumping of the desquamated cells. These changes may be quantitated by a variety of histologic methods and are useful qualitative indices of estrogen stimulation.

Summary of Hormonal Events During the Menstrual Cycle

The low levels of E_2 and P at the end of the preceding cycle induce a rise in the FSH and LH concentrations, which in turn stimulate follicular growth and E_2 production during the early follicular phase. The rise in E_2 suppresses FSH, but not LH, during the last half of the follicular phase. Because of the rapid rate of rise of E_2, the absolute amount of E_2, or synergism of P and E_2, GnRH secretion increases and the sensitivity of the gonadotrope to GnRH increases, resulting in a midcycle LH and FSH secretory discharge. The rapid elevation of gonadotropin concentrations results in further growth of the follicle and secretion of antral fluid, which together with possible weakening of the follicular wall due to enzymes brings about ovulation. The LH-stimulated secretion of E_2 and P by the corpus luteum results in GnRH suppression and, therefore, LH and FSH suppression. The decreased LH levels, together with the inherent decreasing sensitivity of the corpus luteum to LH, leads to a decrement in E_2 and P secretion, which through decreased negative feedback inhibition results in rising levels of FSH and LH and a new cycle.

VARIATIONS OF THE MENSTRUAL CYCLE

The preceding discussion describes the typical, normal, ovulatory menstrual cycle observed in the majority of women between the ages of 20 and 40 years. However, approximately 20% of the cycles in apparently normal women may be abnormal. This percentage of abnormal cycles increases at both ends of the reproductive years. A brief discussion of the hormonal and clinical findings in several varieties of such cycles follows.

Short Luteal Phase

This abnormality is characterized by cycle lengths that are usually short because of a decreased duration of the luteal phase (10 days or less), with an inadequate rise and duration of rise of the basal body temperature, lower-than-normal serum P levels, and endometrial development that does not correspond with the cycle date. This defect appears to be the result of an inadequate early follicular FSH rise and subsequent incomplete maturation of the follicular steroid-producing cells that become luteinized. If this defect persists, it may lead to infertility.

Inadequate Luteal Phase

These cycles are often found in obese, oligomenorrheic women, and during the menopausal transition. The amount of P secreted by the corpus luteum is not great enough to mature the endometrium fully. Hence, the cycle lengths may be short or long, and the endometrial development is always out of phase with the cycle date. The pathogenesis of this defect is similar to that of the short luteal phase.

Long Follicular Phase

Prolonged cycles with delayed, but ultimately normal, follicular maturation and ovulation are commonly found shortly after menarche. The duration of the luteal phase and the hormonal patterns during this phase are completely normal.

Short Follicular Phase

Regularly menstruating, premenopausal women may demonstrate short ovulatory cycles, which are characterized by a short follicular phase, with lower than normal midcycle and luteal E_2 levels. This condition appears to be an age-related decrease in E_2 secretory ability of the follicles and corpus luteum. The endometrial lining and cervical mucus usually do not develop properly during this type of cycle.

Perimenopausal Anovulatory Cycles

Although a variety of pathologic processes may lead to anovulatory cycles, the menopausal transition is often characterized by long cycles with irregular bleeding. During the menopause, which usually takes place between 45 and 55 years, the ovaries undergo an obliterative endarteritis that ultimately leads to a reduction in ovarian size and replacement of the parenchyma with connective tissue (Fig. 6–5). As the E_2 production decreases, the gonadotropins rise and the woman may experience a variety of signs and symptoms of the

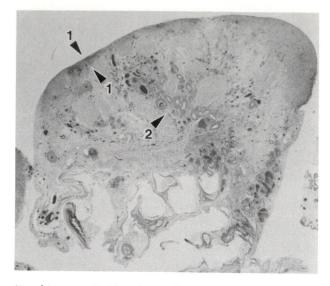

Fig. 6–5. Atrophic ovary. Section of ovary from a woman in post-menopausal years demonstrating ovarian atrophy. 1. Thin, atrophic ovarian cortex depleted of primordial and developing follicles. Scattered corpora albicantia are scarified follicles from previous ovulation. 2. Medulla filled with thickened and sclerotic blood vessels. Adjacent to the medulla is the hilum of the ovary, which contains blood vessels and hilar cells (×9.5 magnification).

menopause, including hot flushes, sweating, and atrophy of the breasts, vagina, and vulva. Prolonged estrogen deficiency is a risk factor for the development of osteoporosis. Early during the menopausal transition, the rising gonadotropin levels may be sufficient to stimulate some follicular estrogen synthesis. If ovulation does not occur and P is not secreted, the endometrium continues to proliferate, eventually resulting in irregular, prolonged shedding. These irregular cycles may persist from months to years before the woman becomes amenorrheic.

FEMALE REPRODUCTIVE DISORDERS

Disorders that affect the glands and organs involved in female reproduction are common. Although such topics as the endocrinology of pregnancy, contraception, and infertility fall into this category of gynecologic endocrinology, they are not discussed here. Rather, this section concentrates on two problems, amenorrhea and hirsutism. These topics were chosen because disorders of virtually all the endocrine glands may result in either one or both of these problems. Therefore, they illustrate the close interaction of the endocrine glands in maintaining normal female reproductive homeostasis.

Amenorrhea

Amenorrhea, or the absence of menses, occurs in every woman surviving to the age of 60. Many women have long lapses between menses during the first 1 or 2 years after menarche, with between 40 and 55% of the cycles being anovulatory. During the active reproductive years, pregnancy is the most common physiologic cause of amenorrhea. Between the extremes of menarche and the menopause, a variety of pathologic processes may produce the symptoms of amenorrhea and oligomenorrhea.

Definitions

Primary amenorrhea is the absence of a menses in a phenotypic female by age 16. Older publications often set the age limit between 18 and 20 years. However, the age of menarche has been decreasing at a rate of 4 months per decade from 1830 until 1968 (secular trend), probably due to improved nutrition. In the United States, the age of menarche at present is approximately 12.8 $\pm$ 1.2 (SD) years. Therefore, the age of 16 is $2\frac{1}{2}$ SD from the mean, justifying the previously cited age limit for defining primary amenorrhea. Since menarche occurs relatively late in the pubertal process (approximately 3 years after the first pubertal change of breast budding), absence of menarche *and* secondary sexual maturation at age 14 should be considered abnormal. *Secondary amenorrhea* is the absence of a menses for a period equal to or greater than 3 times the length of the usual menstrual cycle in a previously menstruating female or 6 months of amenorrhea. *Oligomenorrhea* refers to infrequent, irregular bleeding episodes, at intervals of more than 45 days.

Causes of Primary Amenorrhea. Primary amenorrhea is a symptom of an underlying disorder that may involve the genital tract, ovaries, adrenal, thyroid, pituitary, or hypothalamus. This section lists the causes of primary amenorrhea and then describes some of the clinical and laboratory features associated with these disorders.

Lower Tract Defects
Vaginal aplasia
Imperforate hymen
Congenital vaginal atresia

Uterine Disorders
Congenital absence of the uterus
Endometritis

Ovarian Disorders
XO gonadal dysgenesis and variants
XX gonadal dysgenesis
XY gonadal dysgenesis
Congenital absence of the gonad
Testicular feminization syndrome
17-hydroxylase deficiency of the ovaries and adrenals
Autoimmune oophoritis
Resistant ovary syndrome
Polycystic ovary syndrome

Adrenal Disorders
Congenital adrenal hyperplasia

Thyroid Disorders
Hypothyroidism

Pituitary-Hypothalamic Disorders
Hypopituitarism
Constitutional delay in the onset of menses
Nutritional disorders

Lower Tract Defects. Defects in the uterus and vagina result in amenorrhea, but do not alter the hypothalamic-pituitary-ovarian axis. Therefore, development of the secondary sexual organs occurs normally. In addition, midcycle ovulation pain (mittelschmerz) and cyclic premenstrual tension symptoms such as breast enlargement and tenderness, weight gain, edema, bloating, and behavioral symptoms may be present due to the normal cyclic change in ovarian function.

Vaginal Aplasia. This condition most frequently involves the upper third of the vagina and is often associated with absence of the uterus and fallopian tubes due to defective Müllerian duct development. Anomalies of the urinary tract may also be present.

Imperforate Hymen. At menarche, cyclic monthly lower abdominal pain, often with a palpable lower abdominal mass, occurs without visible menstruation. Pelvic examination usually reveals a bluish hymeneal membrane at the lower part of the vagina, which is distended with menstrual secretions (hematocolpos). This condition is a form of cryptomenorrhea in which menstruation occurs but does not appear externally owing to the obstruction. In some individuals distention of uterus (hematometria) and fallopian tubes (hematosalpinx) also occurs. This distention may lead to retrograde menstruation with hemoperitoneum, resulting in endometriosis. Surgical excision of the hymeneal membrane is curative.

Congenital Vaginal Atresia. Membranous or fibrinous obliteration may occur at any level of the vaginal canal, owing to incomplete fusion of the Müllerian duct structures with the vaginal plate originating from the urogenital sinus. Symptoms are similar to those occurring with an imperforate hymen.

Congenital Absence of the Uterus. This disorder is usually associated with absent or rudimentary fallopian tubes and absence of the upper third of the vagina due to defective development of the Müllerian duct. Congenital anomalies of the urinary tract, vertebral column, and heart may also occur in such patients.

Endometritis. Chronic and acute inflammation and destruction of the endometrium by diseases such as tuberculosis or schistosomiasis may prevent the normal endometrial ripening and shedding during the menstrual cycle.

45,X (XO) Gonadal Dysgenesis (Turner's Syndrome). This syndrome is thought to result either from the fertilization of a hypoploid (lacking a chromosome) gamete, egg, or sperm, by a normal gamete, or from the loss of the second sex chromosome when fertilization has established an XX or XY zygote. These patients are characterized by short stature, streaked gonads, and a variety of somatic abnormalities in a phenotypic female. The prevalence of this syndrome is 1 in 2000 to 3000 female newborns and accounts for approximately 25 to 40% of patients with primary amenorrhea. The short stature is present at birth, with height and weight below the third percentile. The final adult height is almost uniformly below 5 feet and is related in part to the parental height. Growth hormone (GH) secretion is normal, and the response to exogenous GH is poor. Somatomedin levels have been reported to be elevated, implying an end-organ resistance to its effect. The gonads are replaced with bilateral fibrous streaks, which are characterized by sheets and whorls of fibrous tissue with absence of germinal tissue (Fig. 6–6). The uterus, fallopian tubes, and external genitalia are structurally normal, although often hypoplastic. Multiple somatic anomalies have been noted, including triangularly shaped facies, hypoplastic chin, epicanthal folds, abnormally shaped and low-set ears, high-arched palate, strabismus, short and broad neck (often with webbing), low posterior hairline, multiple pigmented nevi, broad shield-like chest with widely spaced nipples, congenital lymphedema of the hands and feet, clinodactyly, short fourth and fifth metacarpals, cubitus valgus, multiple renal malformations, coarctation of the aorta (25 to 30%), and osteopenia. The frequency of diabetes mellitus, red-green color blindness, hypertension, and chronic lymphocytic thyroiditis is increased in these patients. Ovarian estrogen secretion is decreased, and FSH and LH levels are increased due to decreased negative feedback by the gonadal steroids. A buccal smear reveals the absence of the Barr body (inactive X chromosome), and a karyotype establishes the diagnosis. Postzygotic loss of an X chromosome may result in mosaicism. These patients may present with a few or many of the physical stigmata of Turner's syndrome, depending upon what tissues have the deleted X chromosome.

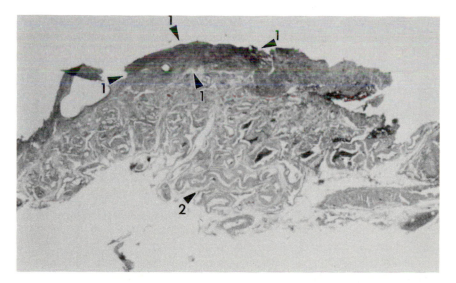

Fig. 6–6. Streak gonad. Section of a rudimentary gonad from a patient with gonadal dysplasia (Turner's syndrome, XO/XY mosaic karyotype). 1. Gonadal tissue comprised of a thin condensed zone of sex mesenchyme. 2. Hilar portion of the gonad containing thick walled vessels (×23 magnification).

XX Gonadal Dysgenesis. These patients are phenotypic females with streaked gonads, eunuchoid habitus, decreased secondary sexual characteristics, primary amenorrhea, and normal female karyotype. Their pituitary gonadotropins are high and ovarian estrogen secretion is low due to fibrous replacement of the ovaries. In essence, they have gonads that are identical to those found in Turner's syndrome, but do not have the somatic features of Turner's syndrome. Since the E_2 levels are not sufficient to close the epiphyses of the long bones, these patients continue to grow, under the influence of GH, and they develop eunuchoid proportions.

XY Gonadal Dysgenesis (Swyer Syndrome). These phenotypic females are similar to the patients with XX gonadal dysgenesis, except that they have a 46 XY karyotype and often develop postpubertal virilization due to androgen secretion from their dysgenetic gonad. Many of these gonads undergo neoplastic transformation to dysgerminomas or gonadoblastomas and, therefore, should be removed.

Congenital Absence of the Gonad. If a gonad is absent after the fifth week of fetal life, both the internal and external genitalia differentiate in a female fashion owing to the lack of testosterone and Müllerian duct inhibitory factor. Many of these patients have an XY karyotype. A few patients have had external female genitalia and absence of the internal genitalia, implying a maldevelopment of the Müllerian duct primordia.

Testicular Feminization Syndrome. These phenotypic females appear normal at birth, although occasionally an inguinal hernia is present. The growth and development of the patient are usually normal, and breast development occurs at the expected time. However, both axillary and pubic hair are deficient, and no menses occur. Pelvic examination reveals a blind vaginal pouch and no cervix or uterus. The gonads are often located in the inguinal hernia and resemble cryptorchid testes. They may undergo malignant transformation (10 to 20%). The karyotype is 46 XY, and the disorder is transmitted as either a sex-linked recessive trait or a sex-limited autosomal dominant disorder. Testosterone secretion from the testes is normal, and testicular estrogen production is often increased. The defect is the result of end-organ insensitivity to testosterone and its active metabolite, dihydrotestosterone, with a normal responsiveness to the estrogen secreted from the testes. Because the fetal testes secrete Müllerian duct inhibitory factor, the Müllerian ducts regress. The resistance to the biologic effects of testosterone leads to regression of the Wolffian duct structures, and formation of external genitalia along female lines. The normal pubertal estrogen secretion results in development of the breasts. Axillary and pubic hair are deficient due to inability of the androgen sensitive pilosebaceous units to respond to androgens. These patients present to their physicians not only with amenorrhea, but also with pain on intercourse (dyspareunia) due to the short vaginal pouch, and infertility.

17-Hydroxylase Deficiency of the Ovaries and Adrenals. Since the 17-hydroxylase enzyme is required in the adrenal for cortisol synthesis and in both the ovary and adrenal for androgen and estrogen synthesis (but not mineralocortical synthesis), these women have primary amenorrhea, hypertension, hypokalemia, and lack secondary sexual characteristics. Plasma cortisol levels are decreased, as are the serum androgen and estrogen levels. ACTH and gonadotropins are elevated, and the mineralocorticoid, corticosterone, is overproduced. Plasma renin levels are depressed. Replacement of the glucocorticoids does not correct the amenorrhea since this does not alter the defect in the ovary.

Autoimmune Oophoritis. This rare disorder may cause primary or secondary amenorrhea and is often associated with autoimmune thyroiditis and adrenalitis. Idiopathic hypoparathyroidism, pernicious anemia, diabetes mellitus, myasthenia gravis, Graves' disease, and vitiligo are also seen in this form of polyhormonal disorder. The ovarian steroid production is low, and gonadotropin levels are elevated. This disorder appears to involve cellular immunity, with round cell infiltration of the affected organs and secondary production of autoantibodies directed toward the involved glands. This syndrome may be familial and has been associated with the HLA-B8 histocompatibility antigen. Primary ovarian failure has also been noted in some patients who have antibodies to ovarian FSH receptors.

Resistant Ovary Syndrome. When first seen, patients with this unusual syndrome may have primary or secondary amenorrhea. The ovaries contain normal-appearing, but unstimulated, primordial follicles. Low or low-normal estrogen and elevated levels of gonadotropins are present in the blood. The ovaries are hyporeactive to exogenous stimulation with human menopausal or pituitary gonadotropins. This syndrome is another example of end-organ refractoriness to a hormone, in this instance both LH and FSH, probably due to absence of gonadotropin receptors in the ovaries.

Polycystic Ovary Syndrome. This condition is most commonly associated with secondary amenorrhea. However, it may occasionally cause primary amenorrhea. It is more fully discussed later in this chapter.

Congenital Adrenal Hyperplasia (CAH). Deficiencies of the 21-hydroxylase or 11-hydroxylase enzymes of the adrenal glands, with resultant overproduction of the adrenal androgens, are manifested clinically by primary amenorrhea, virilization, short stature, and hyperpigmentation in the affected females (see Chap. 4). It has recently been apparent that some patients with 21-OH CAH have an allelic variant that may present with secondary amenorrhea, hirsutism, and acne, or with no clinical manifestations. Basal levels of 17-hydroxyprogesterone may be normal but show an excessive rise following injection of ACTH. The spectrum of clinical manifestations has resulted in this also being referred to as cryptogenic or late-onset CAH. When adequate glucocorticoid replacement therapy is instituted, adrenal androgen levels fall, and ovulatory menstrual cycles may ensue.

Hypothyroidism. Although hypothyroidism in childhood may be associated with isosexual precocious puberty, its occurrence during early adolescence is often accompanied by delayed sexual maturation with low gonadotropin secretion. Growth retardation and other findings of hypothyroidism are usually present.

Hypopituitarism. Partial or panhypopituitarism because of congenital defects or acquired disorders such as tumors, infiltrative diseases, and infection often results in primary amenorrhea due to deficiency of gonadotropins. Some of the inherited and sporadic forms of hypogonadotropic hypogonadism are caused by a hypothalamic disorder with inadequate stimulation of the pituitary by GnRH. When hypopituitarism occurs prepubertally, it results in primary amenorrhea, infertility, lack of secondary sexual development, and an eunuchoid habitus if growth hormone secretion is intact. Agenesis of the olfactory nerves with anosmia or hyposmia may be associated with isolated deficiency of the gonadotropins (Kallman's syndrome). Hyperprolactinemia from a prolactin secreting tumor that has developed in a prepubertal female may prevent normal gonadotropin secretion leading to primary amenorrhea with deficient secondary sexual characteristics.

Constitutional Delay in the Onset of Menses. Approximately 2% of the women begin menstruating after the age of 17 years. These patients often give a history of late onset of menses in their mothers and other female relatives. They can be distinguished from most women with other causes of hypogonadism by the presence of pubertal changes, such as breast buds by age 13, pubic hair, and peak height velocity. This condition is considered to be a delay in the normal maturation of the hypothalamic-pituitary feedback responsiveness to levels of circulating gonadal steroid hormone.

Nutritional Disorders. See discussion later in this chapter.

Diagnostic Evaluation of Primary Amenorrhea

The most important aspects of the evaluation are the history and physical examination. Important background information includes the age of onset of menarche in the patient's mother, grandmothers, and siblings, family history concerning congenital adrenal hyperplasia or congenital hypopituitarism in siblings, symptoms of organic hypothalamic-pituitary disorders, hypothyroidism, and cyclic lower abdominal pain. On physical examination, special attention should be directed toward determining whether the primary amenorrhea is associated with a general lack of secondary sexual maturation or with normal secondary sexual maturation. Lack of secondary sexual maturation is found with hypothyroidism, organic pituitary-hypothalamic disorders, and all the gonadal disorders except testicular feminization. Normal secondary sexual maturation is characteristic of constitutional delay in the onset of menses and local vaginal or endometrial disorders. Pelvic examination is usually sufficient to diagnose the vaginal causes of primary amenorrhea. The presence of a uterus eliminates testicular feminization and congenital absence of the uterus from consideration. The patient's ability to smell should be formally tested in order to determine whether she has Kallmann's syndrome. Both classical congenital adrenal hyperplasia and Turner's syndrome have sufficiently distinctive clinical features to allow an accurate preliminary diagnosis.

Laboratory tests should include serum FSH, LH, and E_2 levels as well as thyroid function tests. Elevated gonadotropins with low E_2 levels (hypergonadotropic hypogonadism) point to an ovarian cause of the primary amenorrhea, and further evaluation should include chromosome analysis with banding and, if necessary, laparoscopy with gonadal biopsy. Persistently low gonadotropins and E_2 levels (hypogonadotropic hypogonadism) in a patient with primary amenorrhea and lack of secondary sexual maturation require a full hypothalamic-pituitary evaluation in order to eliminate serious organic problems in this area. Endometrial biopsy, hystosalpingography, and laparoscopy may be needed to diagnose primary endometrial problems accurately.

Causes of Secondary Amenorrhea

Of the disorders causing secondary amenorrhea (see list), many may also result in oligomenorrhea. Following the list of causes, the prominent clinical pathologic and endocrinologic features of these disorders are discussed. A few have been discussed in the section dealing with primary amenorrhea and are not described further.

Uterine Disorders
Pregnancy
Post-traumatic uterine synechia
Progestational agents

Ovarian Disorders
Polycystic ovary syndrome
Ovarian tumors
Premature menopause
Antimetabolite therapy

Adrenal Disorders
Late onset adrenal hyperplasia
Cushing's syndrome
Virilizing adrenal tumors
Adrenocorticoid insufficiency

Thyroid Disorders
Hypothyroidism
Hyperthyroidism

Pituitary Disorders
Acquired hypopituitarism
Physiologic or pathologic hyperprolactinemia

Hypothalamic Disorders
Tumor and infiltrative diseases
Drug suppression
Nutritional disorders

Extrahypothalamic Nervous System Disorders

Pregnancy. The most frequent cause of secondary amenorrhea is pregnancy, which should be considered despite the most vehement protestations of virginity. A pregnancy test that measures the presence of human chorionic gonadotropin in the serum or urine should be performed on every amenorrheic woman.

Post-traumatic Uterine Synechia (Asherman's Syndrome). Secondary amenorrhea may occur after a uterine curettage, especially in the postpartum or postabortive state, because of formation of adhesions and damage to the basal layer of the endometrium.

Progestational Agents. Prolonged use of progestational agents for contraceptive purposes or for the treatment of endometriosis may induce an irreversible endometrial atrophy.

Polycystic Ovary (Stein-Leventhal) Syndrome. As originally described in 1935, this syndrome is composed of secondary amenorrhea or oligomenorrhea, infertility, obesity, hirsutism, and enlarged, polycystic ovaries. Since the initial description, the criteria for this entity have been reduced. It now includes any clinical picture associated with enlarged ovaries that have a thickened tunica albuginea and numerous cystic and atretic follicles in the cortex (Fig. 6–7). These patients tend to have high-normal or mildly elevated serum levels of the adrenal androgen, dehydroepiandrosterone sulfate (DHEA-S), mildly elevated serum testosterone levels, low or normal FSH levels, and elevated LH levels. These patients are well estrogenized and have high serum levels of estrone and usually normal levels of E_2. Catheterization of the adrenal and ovarian veins has demonstrated that the elevated androgen levels may arise from either or both of these organs. Ovulation and subsequent pregnancies have been achieved by a variety of techniques including unilateral or bilateral ovarian wedge resection, adrenocortical steroid therapy, clomiphene therapy, or human menopausal gonadotropin therapy. The origin of this syndrome has not been established, and some authorities consider it to

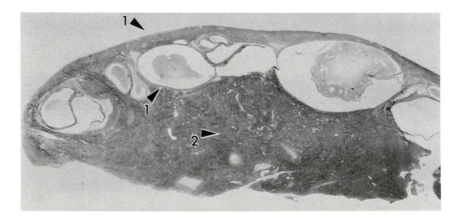

Fig. 6–7. Polycystic ovary. Section of ovary from a woman with polycystic ovary syndrome (Stein-Leventhal syndrome). 1. Ovarian cortex is expanded and occupied by large numbers of cystic follicles exhibiting varying degrees of atresia. The tunica albuginea is slightly thickened. Corpora lutea and albicantia are absent. 2. Dense hyperplastic cortical stroma among and adjacent to cystic follicles (× 4 magnification).

be a primary hypothalamic disease with oversecretion of GnRH leading to increased LH and depressed FSH levels. The elevated LH may stimulate ovarian thecal cell androgen production. The elevated androgens in turn may enhance follicular atresia and stimulate ovarian capsular fibrosis. Peripheral conversion of androgens to estrogens may account for the elevated estrone levels. Alternatively, the defect may lie in the ovaries and/or adrenals with primary oversecretion of androgens leading to increased estrogens, positive feedback on pituitary LH secretion, and negative feedback effect on FSH release. This syndrome can occur sporadically or in a familial setting.

Ovarian Tumors. Ovarian tumors that produce excessive androgens or estrogens cause amenorrhea by suppression of the pituitary-hypothalamic axis. The various types include hilus cell tumors, lipoid cell tumors, arrhenoblastomas, dysgerminomas, gonadoblastomas, and granulosa cell tumors.

Premature Menopause. These patients develop secondary amenorrhea under the age of 40, often preceded by an interval of gradually increasing menstrual irregularities accompanied by menopausal symptoms. The ovaries appear atrophic, with a thickened cortex, interstitial fibrosis, and absent primordial follicles (Fig. 6–5). The E_2 levels are low, and the serum LH and FSH levels are elevated. It is presumed that the original primordial ovarian follicles were deficient in quantity. As previously noted, autoimmune failure of the ovaries may occur as part of the polyglandular autoimmune failure syndrome.

Antimetabolite Therapy. Antimetabolite drugs, such as cyclophosphamide, and irradiation may result in destruction of the primordial follicles and secondary amenorrhea.

Cushing's Syndrome. Cushing's syndrome due to bilateral adrenocortical hyperplasia from excessive pituitary secretion of ACTH or ectopic ACTH production, or due to adrenocortical carcinoma, may be associated with amenorrhea when adrenal androgen secretion is sufficiently elevated to suppress the hypothalamic-pituitary axis. The excessive steroids may also directly interfere with ovarian steroidogenesis. In addition, elevated levels of glucocorticoids may suppress the LH and FSH response to endogenous GnRH.

Virilizing Adrenal Tumors. These uncommon tumors may produce large amounts of adrenal androgens, resulting in a rapid virilization with acne, hirsutism, clitoral enlargement, deepening of the voice, and amenorrhea due to androgen suppression of the pituitary and hypothalamus, and possibly ovarian steroidogenesis. Adrenocortical carcinomas may also secrete glucocorticoids and mineralocorticoids in addition to androgens giving a mixed picture of Cushing's syndrome, hypokalemia, hypertension, and virilization. Virilizing benign adrenocortical adenomas do not generally secrete glucocorticoids and mineralocorticoids concomitantly.

Adrenocortical Insufficiency. Amenorrhea occurs with chronic adrenal insufficiency at a time when weight loss is a prominent feature. The amenorrhea may be due to hypothalamic abnormalities induced by the malnutrition.

Hypothyroidism and Hyperthyroidism. Oligomenorrhea, amenorrhea, and polymenorrhea (frequent menses) may occur with either of these disorders, irrespective of the underlying thyroid pathologic process. Menstrual irregularities may result from changes in the metabolic clearance rate of the gonadal steroids, as well as hypothalamic-pituitary dysfunction.

Acquired Hypopituitarism. Secondary amenorrhea occurs frequently with partial or complete hypopituitarism, whether due to tumors, vascular problems (aneurysms, postpartum necrosis), trauma (stalk section), infection, or infiltrative disorders. Evidence of other trophic hormone deficiency or prolactin hypersecretion may also be present.

Physiologic Prolactin Secretion. Postpartum amenorrhea in lactating mothers may extend to 10 or more months compared to a mean duration of 2 or 3 months for non-nursing postpartum women. Pregnancy rate in the nursing group is approximately 10%, whereas in the non-nursing group the rate is approximately 75%. Recent studies have suggested that the elevated concentrations of prolactin may inhibit the normal secretion of GnRH from the hypothalamus. In addition, hyperprolactinemia inhibits the ovarian response to gonadotropins. Patients with elevated prolactin levels from pathologic processes may also have amenorrhea.

Tumors and Infiltrative Diseases of the Hypothalamus. Craniopharyngiomas, third ventricular ependymomas, optic gliomas, and metastatic tumors to the hypothalamus may lead to deficient GnRH production or release. Through a similar mechanism, infiltrative disorders of the hypothalamus, such as sarcoidosis or histiocytosis X, may lead to secondary amenorrhea.

Drug Suppression of the Hypothalamus. Oral contraceptive agents may induce prolonged suppression of the hypothalamus following discontinuation of the pills. This condition occurs primarily in women whose menstrual cycles were irregular prior to administration of the pills. Although the majority of patients spontaneously regain their menses, a few may remain amenorrheic for several years. An occult pituitary neoplasm must be ruled out in these patients. Psychotropic drugs such as phenothiazines may also suppress gonadotropin secretion, while concurrently promoting prolactin release.

Nutritional Disorders. Rapid weight loss, through voluntary dieting or profound psychologic disturbances (anorexia nervosa), may lead to hypothalamic dysfunction. Patients with anorexia nervosa demonstrate low basal LH and FSH levels, elevated GH levels, abnormalities in the hypothalamic-pituitary-adrenal axis, partial diabetes insipidus, and thermoregulatory deficiencies. Upon refeeding, the patients develop nocturnal LH spikes similar to those found during puberty. The mechanism for the hypothalamic suppression is unknown. Hypothalamic amenorrhea also occurs in ballet dancers and long-distance runners; weight loss, stress, and alterations in lean body mass may be responsible. In this regard, it is of interest that adipose tissue contains an aromatase enzyme system that converts androgens to estrogens. Deficient fat stores seen in these patients may be responsible for the low estrogen levels. Secondary amenorrhea has also been observed with rapid weight gain, although the pathophysiology of this problem has not been elucidated.

Extrahypothalamic Central Nervous System Disorders. The extrahypothalamic central nervous system may profoundly influence the menstrual cycle. Both emotional and physical stress may suppress gonadotropin release, with resulting amenorrhea. This disorder is perhaps best exemplified by the "boarding house amenorrhea" of college girls, who are away from home and develop amenorrhea of varying lengths while under stress. The phenomenon of pseudocyesis (false pregnancy), with the symptoms of pregnancy and weight gain associated with amenorrhea, illustrates that higher cortical areas influence the hypothalamic control of ovulation.

Diagnostic Evaluation of Secondary Amenorrhea

As in the case of primary amenorrhea, the history and physical examination are extremely important in evaluation of patients with secondary amenorrhea. A history should include inquiries about unprotected sexual intercourse, recent curettage or therapeutic abortion, use of progestational agents or oral contraceptives, and recent weight loss or weight gain. These topics help in determining whether the patient's condition is related to pregnancy, post-traumatic uterine synechia, endometrial atrophy, hypothalamic suppression by birth control pills, or hypothalamic dysfunction due to rapid weight changes. Similarly, a history of a traumatic childbirth raises the possibility of postpartum necrosis, and a history of galactorrhea suggests ingestion of drugs such as phenothiazines or the presence of a prolactin-secreting tumor. A history of rapid virilization or symptoms of excessive glucocorticoid production should be sought in order to eliminate the possibility of ovarian tumors, virilizing adrenal tumors, and Cushing's syndrome. Physical examination is often sufficient to diagnose pregnancy, polycystic ovary syndrome, ovarian tumors, Cushing's syndrome, virilizing adrenal tumors, adrenocortical insufficiency, thyroid disorders, and nutritional disorders.

Laboratory studies, which are outlined in Figure 6–8, include an initial pregnancy test. If the test is negative, a progesterone challenge should be performed. If the uterine endometrium is intact and has been exposed to a sufficient amount of estrogen, the administration of progesterone causes sloughing of the endometrium. If no sloughing occurs, either the endometrium is atrophic or the estrogen level is not sufficient to have stimulated the endometrium. If the patient fails to menstruate after withdrawal of progesterone, cyclic estrogen and progesterone may be administered for 1 or 2 months. If no withdrawal bleeding occurs, serum FSH, LH, E_2, testosterone, prolactin, and DHEA-S should be measured. Hypergonadotropic hypogonadism with high FSH, high LH, and low E_2 indicates primary ovarian failure and the need for replacement therapy. Hypogonadotropic hypogonadism with low FSH, LH, and E_2 points to pituitary-hypothalamic dysfunction and needs to be evaluated with neuroradiologic techniques, visual fields, and pituitary function tests. Low or normal levels of FSH and elevated LH, testosterone, or DHEA-S are most compatible with the polycystic ovary syndrome. Severely elevated serum testosterone levels with normal or slightly elevated DHEA-S

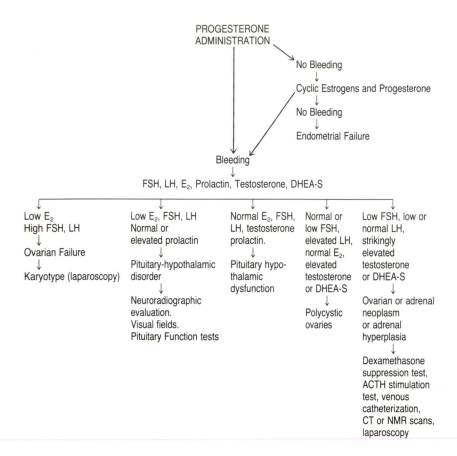

Fig. 6–8.   Flow sheet for evaluation of secondary amenorrhea.

levels suggest an ovarian neoplasm, whereas severely elevated DHEA-S levels with mildly or moderately elevated testosterone concentrations suggest an adrenal neoplasm or acquired adrenal hyperplasia. Normal levels of gonadotropins and E_2 are indicative of a mild pituitary-hypothalamic dysfunction, with absence of the LH and FSH midcycle surges required for ovulation.

HIRSUTISM

Hirsutism may be defined as inappropriately heavy hair growth in the androgen-sensitive areas (such as the beard or mustache region) in a woman. Hirsutism should be differentiated from hypertrichosis, which refers to localized or generalized hair growth not confined to the androgen sensitive hairs. Hypertrichosis may occur due to extrinsic factors such as local trauma. Repeated scratching of an area of the skin may increase the blood supply to that area, resulting in increased stimulation of the pilosebaceous unit (composed of the hair, its follicle, and the sebaceous gland). Certain drugs such as phenytoin (diphenylhydantoin), diazoxide, glucocorticoids, ACTH, and minoxidil may also cause local stimulation of the pilosebaceous unit and increase hair growth. Pigmented nevi often have hair growing from them. Hypertrichosis also accompanies porphyria cutanea tarda, in which repeated irritation of the skin leads to increased blood flow, and thereby stimulation of the hair follicles. Simple hirsutism should also be differentiated from virilization, which includes hirsutism and more pronounced evidence of androgen stimulation, with clitoral hypertrophy, deepening of the voice, temporal hair recession, and male-pattern muscular development. Hirsutism is thus divided into two categories: hirsutism without virilization and hirsutism with virilization.

WITHOUT VIRILIZATION

Normal Individuals
Familial hirsutism
Pregnancy
Menopause
Idiopathic hirsutism
Drugs

Pathologic Conditions
Ovarian Disorders
   Polycystic ovary disease
   Hyperthecosis
Adrenal Disorders
   Bilateral adrenocortical hyperplasia
   Late onset congenital adrenal hyperplasia
Thyroid Disorders
   Hypothyroidism
Pituitary Disorders
   Acromegaly

WITH VIRILIZATION

Normal Individuals
Drugs

Pathologic Conditions
Ovarian Disorders
   Virilizing ovarian tumors
   Polycystic ovary disease
Adrenal Disorders
   Classical congenital adrenal hyperplasia
   Adrenal carcinoma
   Virilizing adrenal adenomas
Male Pseudohermaphroditism
   Incomplete testicular feminization

Without Virilization

Normal women may develop hirsutism due to both intrinsic and extrinsic factors. The amount of hair that grows is related to the potency and concentration of the circulating free androgens, the sensitivity of the hair follicle to these androgens, and the duration of exposure to the androgens. The racial background and familial inheritance of an individual account for the wide range of normalcy in hair growth experienced by females. Women from the Mediterranean area tend to have more hair than those from the northern European countries. When an Italian woman who has a normal amount of hair growth compared to her Italian peers moves to a Scandinavian country, she may be considered to be hirsute by Scandinavian standards. Similarly, Caucasian Americans tend to be more hirsute than American blacks or Spanish-Americans. Many women who have hirsutism on a familial basis will give a history of mothers and female siblings also having excessive hair when compared to the rest of the population. Of importance with this variety of hirsutism is that the patient's menstrual cycle is usually normal. Physiologic hirsutism may also occur during pregnancy, probably because of androgens secreted by the placenta. During the menopause, pre-existing villus hairs may become darkly pigmented, possibly owing to an increase in ovarian androgen secretion under the influence of rising gonadotropin levels. When none of these factors appear to be present in an apparently normal individual, that patient is considered to have idiopathic hirsutism. The pilosebaceous unit in these women may have increased sensitivity to normal circulating levels of androgens.

Multiple pathologic conditions may also give rise to simple hirsutism. The endocrinologic disorders include those of ovarian origin, such as polycystic ovary disease and hyperthecosis, which is clinically similar to the polycystic ovary syndrome with slightly different ovarian pathologic features. Bilateral adrenocortical hyperplasia from pituitary oversecretion of ACTH (Cushing's disease) may lead to hirsutism due to a mild increase of adrenal androgen production. Similarly, late onset CAH may present with simple hirsutism due to the overproduction of adrenal androgens. Acromegaly results in coarsening of pre-existing hairs, as does hypothyroidism.

With Virilization

Women may develop hirsutism with virilization when they receive androgens or some progestational agents that are capable of stimulating the hair follicle and other androgen-sensitive structures. Virilizing ovarian tumors, polycystic ovary disease, congenital adrenal hyperplasia, adrenal carcinomas and adenomas, and incomplete testicular feminization syndrome may also result in hirsutism with virilization. These conditions have been discussed previously.

Clinical Evaluation

One should obtain a history of the age of onset of hair growth as well as the amount, duration, distribution, and rate. Symptoms of virilization such as deepening of the voice, change in libido, and increased odoriferous perspiration should also be sought. The family history, including the racial background and country of origin, is necessary to diagnose the racial and familial forms of this disorder. Menstrual and fertility history, as well as drug history, should also be obtained. Hair growth that begins around the time of puberty and is slowly progressive is most compatible with idiopathic hirsutism, racial and familial hirsutism, late onset CAH, and polycystic ovary disease. The rapid onset of progressive hirsutism and virilization at any age suggests an ovarian or adrenal neoplasm. Normal menstrual function is compatible with the racial and familial varieties, as well as with idiopathic hirsutism, whereas menstrual disturbances are more commonly seen with organic ovarian disorders.

Physical examination should include a measurement of height in order to eliminate classical congenital adrenal hyperplasia as a cause of hirsutism and virilization, a measurement of blood pressure to rule out adrenal 11-hydroxylase deficiency, and assessment of the hair distribution, presence or absence of acne, degree of muscle development, laryngeal development, and female secondary sex characteristics. Abdominal and pelvic masses should be sought, and a measurement of clitoral size obtained (upper limit of normal is 1 cm in diameter). The degree of hirsutism can then be classified as: mild, which includes fine, pigmented hair over the face, extremities, chest, and abdomen; moderate, with coarse pigmented hair over the face (not the complete beard), chest, abdomen, and perineum; severe, with coarse pigmented hair over the face (total beard), ears, nose, and proximal interphalangeal joints; and virilization with temporal hair recession, deepening of the voice, clitoromegaly, and male muscle development.

Laboratory Evaluation

In the normal female, four 17-β-hydroxysteroids present in the blood provide virtually the total androgenic activity. These four are testosterone, dihydrotestosterone, androstenediol, and androstanediol (3-α, 3-β). Of these, testosterone accounts for approximately 50% of the total androgen activity in the blood. Despite variation in testosterone concentrations during the menstrual cycle, approximately one-fourth of the testosterone emanates from the ovary, one-fourth from the adrenal gland, and one-half from the conversion in peripheral tissues, such as the skin and liver, of androgen precursors from the ovaries and adrenals into potent androgens. In all conditions in which the adrenal gland produces excessive testosterone, levels of the adrenal androgen precursors (urine 17-ketosteroids and serum DHEA-sulfate) are elevated. On the other hand, the ovaries are capable of secreting large amounts of testosterone efficiently, and greatly elevated levels of testosterone may be found with little or no elevation of DHEA-sulfate or 17-ketosteroids in ovarian disorders. The activity of the circulating androgen depends on its concentration, potency, and degree of binding to serum proteins. The major protein that binds androgens is testosterone-estradiol binding globulin (TEBG). Because the free androgen is the biologically active material, a situation in which the TEBG level is decreased results in a greater concentration of free androgen, whereas an elevation of TEBG (as seen with estrogen therapy or pregnancy) results in a lowered concentration of free androgen.

The laboratory evaluation of hirsutism should include a measurement of serum testosterone (preferably free testosterone) as well as an assessment of adrenal androgen secretion. The latter may be performed by measuring the plasma DHEA-S level. Because 90 to 96% of DHEA-S arises from the adrenal gland, its level serves as a useful parameter of adrenal androgen secretion. Mildly elevated testosterone or DHEA-S levels are usually of little significance, whereas moderately or severely elevated levels require further studies of ovarian or adrenal function. Measurements of basal and ACTH-stimulated 17-hydroxyprogesterone concentrations should be performed if late onset CAH is considered.

Additional tests include a dexamethasone suppression test (2 mg dexamethasone taken orally each day for 6 days), with testosterone and DHEA-S levels measured before and during the last day of suppression. Inability to suppress is suggestive of an adrenal neoplasm. Severely elevated levels that do suppress with dexamethasone are more compatible with congenital adrenal hyperplasia. Administration of ethinyl estradiol (40 µg/day for 25 days) with medroxyprogesterone acetate (10 mg/day orally during the last 5 days) may be sufficient to suppress serum LH levels; this suppression in turn decreases ovarian androgen secretion. However, because the estrogen may stimulate the liver to produce more globulins, including TEBG, the total serum testosterone level at the end of this suppression may be elevated. A more direct way of determining the androgen production site is by selective ovarian and adrenal venous catheterization with blood sampling for the androgens. Ancillary studies include determination of serum LH and FSH levels when considering the polycystic ovary syndrome, computerized axial tomographic scan or magnetic resonance imaging for adrenal neoplasms, and laparoscopy for suspected ovarian neoplasms.

Approximately 10% of patients with significant hirsutism have normal levels of testosterone, perhaps from an increase in the free fraction of testosterone due to a decrease in TEBG, increased turnover of testosterone, increased levels of other active androgens such as dihydrotestosterone, increased converison of weaker androgens such as DHEA to testosterone, or idiopathic end-organ hypersensitivity to the androgens.

Therapy

Surgical removal of virilizing ovarian or adrenal neoplasms usually causes a prompt regression of hirsutism. Other therapeutic procedures include cosmetic approaches and medical therapy. Excessive hair may be removed by a variety of means including shaving, wax stripping, or chemical depilation. None of these procedures stimulate hair growth, but since they do not destroy the hair follicle, the growth of hair continues. Mild hirsutism may be treated cosmetically by bleaching the hairs, while more severe hirsutism may be treated permanently by electrolysis. During electrolysis the electrologist attempts to destroy the hair follicle, with electrical current. If the hair follicle is destroyed, no further hair grows from that follicle. However, because of the curvature of the hair shaft, it is difficult to successfully eliminate each follicle treated.

Medical therapy includes suppression of adrenal androgen secretion by glucocorticoids, suppression of ovarian androgen secretion by a combination of estrogens and progestogens, and combined adrenal and ovarian suppression. Approximately a third of individuals with familial, idiopathic, or polycystic ovary disease as a cause of hirsutism respond to adrenal suppression, whereas approximately half respond to ovarian suppression. As noted, the prolonged administration of estrogen may increase the TEBG level and may thereby decrease the amount of free androgen available to the hair follicles. Experimental therapies include the use of peripheral antagonists to androgens, such as cyproterone acetate, spironolactone, cimetidine, and medroxyprogesterone acetate. These medical therapies for hirsutism require a minimum of 3 to 6 months of trial before the patient notices a decrease in the rate of hair growth. This long duration of therapy is needed because approximately 10% of the hairs at any one time are in a resting stage, so 3 months pass before the hair falls out and a new hair is formed. Therefore, it takes about 30 months before the androgen-sensitive hairs are turned over.

CLINICAL PROBLEMS

Patient 1. During an evaluation for a heart murmur, a 29-year-old woman confided in her physician that she had never had a menses. She had not spoken to others about this because such subjects were "taboo" in her family. She stated that she had had normal breast development beginning at age 12 and had developed axillary and pubic hair at approximately the same time. She denied hirsutism, galactorrhea, headaches, visual field disturbances, heat or cold intolerance, edema, marked weight changes, excessive exercise, a history of tuberculosis, or intake of oral contraceptives, phenothiazines, or antihypertensive medication. She had not attempted intercourse. She did note occasional lower abdominal discomfort lasting less than a day and also noted at different times breast enlargement, fluid retention, and mild depression lasting 2 to 3 days each month.

On physical examination the patient had a blood pressure of 118/76, pulse 68 and regular, height 5'5" and weight 124 lbs. She was well nourished. There was no webbing of the neck, hypertelorism, cubitus valgus, micrognathia, or lymphedema. Visual fields and extraocular muscle testing was normal. Neck was normal without thyromegaly. Chest was clear to percussion and auscultation. Both breasts were adult in size and configuration and no galactorrhea was demonstrable. Cardiovascular examination revealed a normal sized heart without thrills or rubs. A loud systolic murmur was present over the precordium, with greatest intensity in the 3rd intercostal space at the left sternal border. Abdominal examination was normal. Pubic hair and axillary hair were normal. The labia were well formed and the clitoris was normal in size. The vaginal vault was shallow and ended blindly. No uterus was felt by bimanual examination or upon rectal-vaginal or rectal-abdominal examination. Neurologic examination and musculoskeletal examinations were normal.

QUESTIONS
1. Based upon the history and physical examination what is the most likely diagnosis in this patient?
2. What laboratory tests should be ordered and what results would you anticipate if your diagnosis were correct?
3. What therapy would you recommend for this patient?

Patient 2. A 22-year-old female was brought to the emergency room because of severe weakness. She stated that her weakness had begun approximately 2 months before, but it has become progressively worse. It was associated with a 15 lb. weight loss, orthostatic dizziness, anorexia, and over the preceding 3 days diarrhea. She also noted that she had not had a menses for 2 years and that prior to the cessation of her periods she had been oligomenorrheic for approximately 1 year.

On physical examination, she had a blood pressure of 90/60 right arm supine going to 60/30 when assuming the upright posture. Her pulse rate was 112 supine and rose to 140 when she stood up. She was obviously dehydrated. Hyperpigmentation of the creases of her hands and over her elbows was present. She had an approximately 30 g pebbly firm goiter without discrete nodules. There was no cervical lymphadenopathy. Chest was clear and cardiovascular examination was normal except for soft heart sounds and a tachycardia. Abdominal examination was unremarkable and pelvic examination revealed normal external genitalia, normal vaginal vault, and small but easily palpable uterus. No adnexal masses were present. The rest of her examination was noncontributory.

Initial laboratory studies in the emergency room revealed:

Na = 126
K = 6.4
Cl = 98
HCO_3 = 20 mEq/L
BUN = 48 mg/dl
Creatinine = 1.4 mg/dl
Glucose = 48 mg/dl
Electrocardiogram: Low voltage with nonspecific ST-T wave abnormalities.
Pregnancy Test: Negative

QUESTIONS
1. What is the primary problem that results in the patient being seen in the emergency room? What other abnormalities are present? What is the overall classification of this disorder?
2. What diagnostic tests should be performed to confirm your diagnoses?
3. What treatment should be given?

Patient 3. A 32-year-old woman noted the development of facial hair and abdominal hair growth, acne, and malodorous perspiration approximately 2 months before seeking help. She also noted weakness, polyuria and polydypsia, and headaches. She had also noted some irregular vaginal bleeding. She denied the intake of medications or a known history of diabetes, hypertension, or weight changes. She did admit to easy bruising and some degree of facial plethora and increased facial fullness.

On examination, her blood pressure was found to be 160/106, pulse 88 and regular, height 5'4", and weight 132 lbs. She had some degree of thinning of her skin over the dorsum of her hands and a few scattered ecchymoses. Acne was present over the face, upper chest, and back. Darkly pigmented terminal hairs were present in the chin area, and new hair growth was present from the pubic triangle to the umbilicus. Facial plethora was present. Fundoscopic examination revealed arteriolar spasm, but was otherwise unremarkable. Neck was normal. Pulmonary and cardiovascular examinations were unremarkable. There were no palpable masses on abdominal examination. Pelvic examination was normal with a clitoris that was at the upper limit of normal in size. The rest of the examination was noncontributory.

QUESTIONS
1. What is the likely etiology of this patient's problem?
2. What laboratory tests should be performed?
3. What therapeutic approaches should be considered?

SUGGESTED READING

Biffignandi, P., Massucchetti, C., and Molinatti, G.M.: Female hirsutism: Pathophysiological considerations and therapeutic implications. Endocr Rev, 5:498, 1984.

Coney, P.J.: Polycystic ovary disease: current concepts of pathophysiology and therapy. Fertil Steril, 42:667, 1984.

Friedman, C.I., Barrows, H., and Kim, M.H.: Hypergonadotropic hypogonadism. Am J Obstet Gynecol, 145:360, 1983.

Henley, K.M., and Vaitukaitis, J.L.: Hormonal changes associated with changes in body weight. Clin Obstet Gynecol, 28:615, 1985.

Meldrum, D.R.: The pathophysiology of postmenopausal symptoms. Semin Reprod Endocrinol, 1:11, 1983.

Morris, D.V.: Hirsutism. Clin Obstet Gynecol, 12:649, 1985.

Neinstein, L.S.: Menstrual dysfunction in pathophysiologic states. West J Med, *143*:476, 1985.
Rock, J.A.: Anomalous development of the vagina. Semin Reprod Endocrinol, *4*:13, 1986.
Schlaff, W.D.: Dynamic testing in reproductive endocrinology. Fertil Steril, *45*:589, 1986.
Simpson, J.L.: Genes and chromosomes that cause female infertility. Fertil Steril, *44*:725, 1985.

ACKNOWLEDGMENTS

The photomicrographs were kindly prepared by Dr. Irene Davos and Mr. Robert Heusser, Department of Pathology, Cedars-Sinai Medical Center, Los Angeles, CA.

ANSWERS TO QUESTIONS

Patient 1

1. The most likely diagnosis in this patient is congenital absence of the uterus. The history and physical examinations strongly suggest that she has a normal hypothalamic-pituitary-ovarian axis in that she is of normal height and weight, had normal secondary sexual development at the appropriate age, complaints of lower abdominal pain that suggest ovulation (mittelschmerz), and has the monthly cyclic symptoms of breast enlargement and fluid retention and mood swings that constitute the premenstrual-tension-syndrome. She does not have acne, hirsutism, virilization that would suggest an adrenal disorder, or polycystic ovaries, and no adnexal masses were felt. The lack of a palpable uterus in an otherwise well estrogenized phenotypic female suggests either the congenital absence of a uterus, or the testicular feminization syndrome in which the testicles produce a Müllerian duct inhibitory factor causing regression of the uterus, fallopian tubes, and upper third of the vagina. The fact that this patient has normal axillary and pubic hair rules out classical testicular feminization. Some patients with incomplete forms of androgen insensitivity may have axillary and pubic hair, but generally show some degree of ambiguity of their external genitalia with fusion of the labial-scrotal folds or clitoromegaly. If she had the 5-alpha reductase deficiency syndrome, some degree of virilization at puberty would have been anticipated.

2. The most important initial test to perform would be an ultrasound examination of the pelvic structures. This is an excellent means to diagnose congenital absence of the uterus as well as detecting ovarian structures. One would also expect to find normal serum gonadotropin levels, estrogen levels, and, if blood is sampled during the week to 10 days before the patient's cyclic premenstrual types of symptoms, a luteal phase progesterone concentration would be present. If congenital absence of the uterus is found to be present, the patient should undergo an examination of her urinary tract with an intravenous pyelogram, her vertebral column by appropriate spine films, and her heart. In this case, the patient did have a small ventricular septal defect that was not of any hemodynamic significance.

3. Since the patient has a normal hypothalamic-pituitary-ovarian axis, there is no need for estrogen replacement therapy. The patient is of course infertile. The short vaginal pouch may be elongated manually through the use of progressively larger dilators or surgically. This may be necessary when the patient becomes sexually active in order to avoid dyspareunia. If spinal, urinary tract, or cardiac abnormalities are present they should be treated on their own merits.

Patient 2

1. This patient undoubtedly had primary adrenal cortical insufficiency that has resulted in her weakness, weight loss, anorexia, nausea, vomiting, diarrhea, hyperpigmentation, hyponatremia, hyperkalemia, hypoglycemia, and dehydration. The presence of a firm micronodular goiter in this setting is highly suggestive of the coexistence of Hashimoto's (autoimmune) thyroiditis. Amenorrhea may certainly be associated with long-standing adrenal cortical insufficiency and hypothyroidism. However, the weight loss and other symptoms were not present until 2 years after she became amenorrheic. In the presence of probable autoimmune adrenal insufficiency and autoimmune thyroid disease, the possibility of premature menopause must be considered. Thus, this patient likely suffers from the polyglandular autoimmune failure syndrome. It was appropriate for the emergency

room physician to perform a pregnancy test, since a patient with a history of amenorrhea who enters with shock needs to have the presence of an ectopic pregnancy ruled out.

2. Blood should be obtained for measuring cortisol and ACTH levels and a cortrosyn stimulation test should be performed with measurements of cortisol and aldosterone before and after the injection of the synthetic ACTH. In patients with primary adrenal cortical insufficiency, the basal cortisol and aldosterone are low and the ACTH levels are elevated. Following ACTH administration there is no rise in cortisol or aldosterone. Patients with secondary adrenal cortical insufficiency may not have an appropriate rise in cortisol but generally will show an appropriate rise in aldosterone. Serum T_4, free thyroxine index and TSH should be measured. Serum FSH and estradiol may also be measured to confirm the presence of premature ovarian failure. A variety of autoantibodies, such as antithyroid microsomal antibodies, antithyroglobulin antibodies, antiadrenal antibodies, antiovarian antibodies, and antiparietal cell antibodies may also be measured. A CBC should be performed to rule out the presence of pernicious anemia, and a serum calcium and phosphorus needs to be determined since autoimmune hypoparathyroidism may be present in some patients.

3. The patient should be treated for acute adrenal insufficiency with salt-containing fluids, hydrocortisone, and, if necessary, mineralocorticoid therapy. If the TSH is elevated, then L-thyroxine replacement therapy should be begun. Since patients with premature ovarian failure are at great risk for developing osteopenia, estrogen replacement therapy will be needed. The therapy is best given in a cyclic fashion over approximately 25 days each month and during the last 10 days of estrogen administration concomitant progesterone administration should be given in order to mimic the normal menstrual cycle as closely as possible. This will markedly reduce the risk for the development of endometrial carcinoma from the estrogen replacement therapy.

Patient 3

1. This patient probably has an adrenal cortical carcinoma. She presented with complaints of onset of hirsutism, acne, and malodorous perspiration beginning at the age of 32 with a fairly rapid tempo of progression. Most of the benign causes of hirsutism have their onset in the premenarcheal age range with a slower rate of progression. The presence of thin skin, rounding of the face, some degree of facial plethora, and recent onset of easy bruisability suggests the co-existence of glucocorticoid excess (Cushing's syndrome). In addition, the hypertension, polyuria, polydypsia, and nocturia are compatible with mineralocorticoid excess. Thus, the combination of new onset hirsutism (or virilization), along with features of glucocorticoid and mineralocorticoid excess, point to an adrenal cortical problem. The onset at this age is not compatible with the diagnosis of congenital adrenal hyperplasia and such patients do not have evidence of excessive glucocorticoid. Adrenal cortical adenomas generally overproduce either adrenal androgens, mineralocorticoids (giving the primary aldosteronism syndrome), or glucocorticoids (giving Cushing's syndrome), but do not produce all three of the hormone groups. In contrast, adrenal cortical carcinomas often will produce more than one of the adrenal hormone classes.

2. Serum electrolytes, DHEA-sulfate, and testosterone should be measured. This patient had a hypokalemic alkalosis, markedly elevated DHEA-sulfate and moderately elevated testosterone. A CT scan of the abdomen revealed an 8 cm left adrenal mass that, upon resection, proved to be an adrenal carcinoma.

3. The initial therapeutic approach is to try to surgically remove the tumor. Unfortunately, this is often not successful because such tumors often grow into the vena cava and metastasize. If surgical resection is incomplete or if adrenal cortical carcinoma recurs following such resection (DHEA-sulfate levels may be useful as a tumor marker for picking up recurrence), then adrenolytic agents such as mitotane may be used for palliation. Reduction of the adrenal steroid production may also be achieved through the use of adrenal enzyme inhibitors such as aminoglutethimide (Cytadren).

7

Male Reproductive Abnormalities

Ronald S. Swerdloff and Shalender Bhasin

ABBREVIATIONS

ABP	androgen-binding protein
cAMP	cyclic AMP
DHT	dihydrotestosterone
FSH	follicle-stimulating hormone
GnRH	gonadotropin-releasing hormone
hCG	human chorionic gonadotropin
LH	luteinizing hormone
TEBG	testosterone-estradiol-binding globulin

MALE REPRODUCTIVE PHYSIOLOGY

The reproductive hormonal axis in the adult male consists of four main components: (1) the hypothalamus, (2) the pituitary gland, (3) the testes, and (4) the androgen sensitive end organs (Fig. 7–1). The components of this system function in a closely regulated manner resulting in the concentrations of testosterone required for maintenance of secondary sexual characteristics and male sexual behavior. The reproductive axis also regulates the orderly maturation of sperm necessary for normal fertility.

Gonadotropin Releasing Hormone

The hypothalamus is the site of production of biogenic amines and opioids that regulate the synthesis and secretion of a hypothalamic decapeptide hormone, gonadotropin-releasing hormone (GnRH). GnRH is released into the hypothalamic-pituitary portal circulation in pulses at a frequency of approximately 1 pulse every 70 to 90 minutes. The pulsatile nature of GnRH release appears to be important for optimal synthesis and release of LH and FSH. Although GnRH stimulates the pituitary secretion of both LH and FSH, the frequency of GnRH pulses may be important in determining the relative ratio of LH and FSH secreted into the peripheral circulation. Sex steroids, neu-

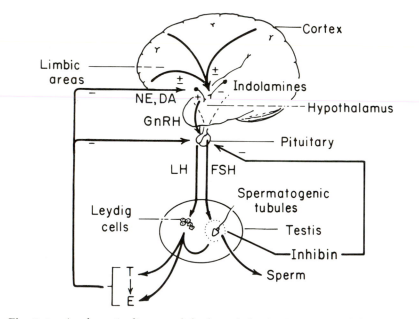

Fig. 7–1. A schematic diagram of the hypothalamic-pituitary gonadal axis in the male. Testicular function is regulated by a series of closed-loop feedback systems. Products of testicular origin, steroid hormones, and inhibin regulate gonadotropin secretion (see text). NE = norepinephrine; DA = dopamine; GnRH = gonadotropin-releasing hormone; LH = luteinizing hormone; FSH = follicle-stimulating hormone; T = testosterone; E = estradiol.

rotransmitters, and pituitary gonadotropins modulate the pulse frequency and amplitude of GnRH secretion. Through an ultrashort feedback loop operating within the pituitary, gonadotropins may also regulate their own secretion.

Gonadotropins

LH is the predominant stimulus for testicular steroidogenesis by the Leydig cell. LH action is mediated by specific, high-affinity receptors in the cell membrane of Leydig cells. Binding of LH to its receptors increases adenylate cyclase activity, which causes a rise in intracellular cyclic AMP (cAMP); cAMP binding to protein kinase leads to dissociation of this holoenzyme, release of its regulatory unit, and RNA and protein synthesis. Both LH and FSH belong to a family of structurally related glycoprotein hormones which also includes TSH and human chorionic gonadotropin (hCG). Each of these glycoproteins consists of two internally linked subunits, alpha and beta. The alpha subunit is common to all 4 glycoprotein hormones, while the beta subunit confers biologic and immunologic specificity. Both alpha and beta subunits contain complex asparagine-linked oligosaccharides that appear essential for transduction of the biologic signal.

LH exerts its stimulatory effect upon steroidogenesis by accelerating the metabolism of cholesterol. Cholesterol entry into the mitochondria is proportionate to the quantity of cholesterol available to the Leydig cells. There, LH also stimulates the conversion of 20- and 22-alpha-hydroxycholesterol to pregnenolone through the action of cholesterol esterase and cholesterol side chain cleavage enzymes. There is no evidence that LH directly affects any of the components of the seminiferous tubules.

FSH receptors are present on Sertoli cell membranes. FSH binds to these receptors, stimulates adenylate-cyclase-mediated production of cAMP, and finally, activates the regulatory subunit of protein kinase.

One of the major actions of FSH is the stimulation of protein synthesis. FSH enhances testicular incorporation of amino acids into protein. FSH promotes the testicular production of at least 5 specific proteins: androgen-binding protein (ABP), inhibin, the plasminogen activator, gamma glutamyl transpeptidase, and a protein kinase inhibitor. The first 3 are secreted into the rete testis fluid.

FSH also stimulates aromatase activity in Sertoli cells. Aromatase is the term for a group of enzymes that convert certain androgens (such as testosterone) to estrogens (such as 17-beta-estradiol). FSH also stimulates a calcium-dependent regulatory protein that influences the distribution of intracellular calcium and the Sertoli cell cytoskeleton by microfilament realignment.

Some FSH effects are age-related. For example, FSH stimulates protein synthesis in the testes of immature rats, but not in the testes of rats older than 25 days. The responsiveness to FSH in mature rats returns following hypophysectomy. The loss of Sertoli cell response to FSH in the adult rat is caused by increased phosphodiesterase activity, which diminishes cAMP production. These age-related effects of FSH cannot be ascribed to changes in FSH receptors since the number of FSH receptors does not decrease with age, but actually increases.

Spermatogenesis and Sperm Transport

Spermatogenesis is the orderly maturation of germinal cells in the spermatogenic tubules from spermatogonia to sperm. Most evidence indicates that FSH and LH are both required for the initiation of this process at puberty. The effect of LH is indirect in that it causes high intratesticular testosterone levels, which in turn act on the spermatogenic tubules to stimulate spermatogenesis. After puberty, spermatogenesis may be maintained by adequate intratesticular testosterone concentration.

The development of germ cells in the seminiferous tubules occurs in 3 phases: spermatogonial multiplication, meiosis, and spermiogenesis. In the seminiferous epithelium, cells in these developmental phases are arranged in defined associations or stages. In most mammals, these stages follow one another in a regular fashion and give rise to a wave of germ cell maturation along the seminiferous epithelium. The time interval between the successive appearance of the same cell association at a given point in the tubule is called the cycle of the seminiferous epithelium. In man, the average length of this cycle is 73 days and includes all 3 phases. Subsequent sperm transport in the epididymis and vas deferens requires an additional 21 days.

FSH and androgens cause changes during different stages in the cycle of the seminiferous epithelium. Maximal binding of FSH in Sertoli cells occurs in those stages of spermatogenesis in which activity of adenylate cyclase in the haploid germ cells is greatest and when the secretion of cAMP by the seminiferous tubules is maximal. The other stages are found when secretion rates of androgen-binding protein and local concentrations of testosterone are highest. The stages of spermatogenesis that appear to be androgen dependent are found when secretion of plasminogen activator and a meiosis-inducing substance is highest.

Testosterone alone will initiate spermatogenesis in hypophysectomized immature rats; FSH is required for maturation of spermatids to form spermatozoa. However, exogenous administration of testosterone to hypogonadotropic men does not induce spermatogenesis. This failure of exogenous testosterone to reinitiate spermatogenesis in the human is most likely attributable to the practical limits of the dose of testosterone that can be administered. Such doses increase circulating testosterone concentrations, but do not provide adequate intratesticular testosterone concentrations. By contrast, hCG administration stimulates an increase in intratesticular testosterone concentrations and promptly initiates spermatogenesis. Furthermore, precocious puberty may occur in boys with localized Leydig cell tumors. The germ cells in tubules adjacent to this androgen-producing tumor undergo maturation, while the germs cells distant from the tumor or in the contralateral testis remain unstimulated, despite virilizing peripheral serum concentrations of testosterone. In hypogonadal men treated with hCG alone, maturation of the seminiferous epithelium does not progress beyond the spermatid stage. FSH alone does not initiate spermatogenesis, but its administration to hCG-primed hypogonadal men results in completion of spermatogenesis and production of an adequate number of sperm to restore fertility. Thus, FSH appears to be essential for spermiogenesis (transformation of spermatids into mature spermatozoa). In hypogonadotropic men primed with hCG and FSH, spermatogenesis can be maintained by hCG alone.

In addition to androgens and FSH, many other proteins are secreted locally in the tubule in a cyclic fashion during the cycle of the seminiferous epithelium. These proteins probably mediate the interaction of Sertoli and germ cells, which is important for the intratesticular control of spermatogenesis.

Sex Steroid Hormones

The secreted gonadal androgens, testosterone and dihydrotestosterone, act on numerous end organs, cause the secondary sexual characteristics of ''maleness,'' and are responsible for male sexual behavior.

Testosterone and Estradiol. Testosterone is the major steroid hormone produced by the testis and cholesterol appears to be the obligatory precursor. The Leydig cells are the main source of the 4 to 7 mg of testosterone produced daily. Cholesterol is converted within the mitochondria of Leydig cells to pregnenolone, which is further metabolized outside the mitochondria to several other steroids, including testosterone. Pregnenolone can be converted to testosterone either via a delta-4 or a delta-5 pathway. During incubation of human testicular tissue in vitro, the delta-5 pathway appears to predominate, while in other species the delta-4 pathway via progesterone predominates.

About 40 μg of estradiol are produced daily in an adult male. Three-fourths of this estradiol is derived from peripheral aromatization of testosterone and androstenedione, while the rest is secreted directly from the testes. Virtually all of the dihydrotestosterone produced (300 μg/day) is derived from peripheral conversion of testosterone, much of it in the prostate gland. Thus, testosterone functions as a prohormone for both 17-beta-estradiol and dihydrotestosterone formation. Sertoli cells appear to be the intratesticular site of estradiol synthesis. The production of estradiol within the human testis may be important in the regulation of Leydig cell function.

The role of dihydrotestosterone in spermatogenesis is probably minimal since little of this androgen is produced within the testes, and it is not required for spermatogenesis. Males with 5-alpha-reductase deficiency cannot produce normal quantities of dihydrotestosterone, yet spermatogenesis occurs.

Most of the circulating testosterone is bound to a high-affinity beta globulin, testosterone-estradiol binding globulin (TEBG), but only free, or unbound testosterone, is available for entry into most testosterone-responsive cells. The hepatic production of TEBG is affected by a number of physiologic and metabolic factors. Estrogen stimulates and testosterone inhibits production of TEBG. Thyroid hormones also influence TEBG levels: TEBG synthesis is reduced in hypothyroidism and increased in hyperthyroidism. TEBG concentrations are low in obese men and in patients with acromegaly.

Androgen Receptors

Androgen-responsive tissues contain a specific receptor protein that binds dihydrotestosterone (DHT) with high affinity. The binding affinity of this intracellular receptor is less for testosterone, and less yet for 3-alpha-androstanediol. Earlier biochemical and autoradiographic studies suggested that the receptor is present in the cytosolic fraction of cells from many androgen-responsive tissues. It was believed that the hormone binding induces receptor transformation and translocation of the hormone receptor complex to the nucleus where the biologic response is initiated (Fig. 7–2). However, recent data have cast some doubt on the belief that androgen receptors are primarily located within the cytoplasm. Emerging data suggest that the receptors for many steroid hormones are located within the nucleus and not within the cytoplasm. Whether the receptors for testosterone also reside within the nucleus remains a matter of some controversy. At any rate, it is clear that steroid binding to the receptor transforms it into a biologically active form. The transformed active receptor then binds to specific nuclear acceptor sites resulting in induction (or occasionally repression) of mRNA transcription, altered protein synthesis and thereby regulation of cell function. Dihydrotestosterone and testosterone are bound to a single androgen receptor protein, although claims of separate receptors for each steroid and distinct receptors in different tissues have been presented. In the majority of androgen-sensitive

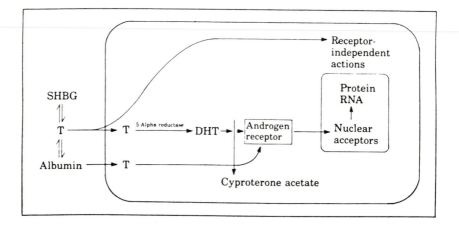

Fig. 7–2. Molecular basis of androgen action. The traditional concept envisions penetration of the plasma membrane by testosterone in androgen-sensitive tissues and its conversion to DHT by 5-alpha reductase. DHT binds to a high affinity receptor. The DHT receptor complex binds to nuclear acceptors, which stimulate androgen-dependent RNA and protein synthesis. Cyproterone acetate is a competitive inhibitor of androgen action. T = testosterone; DHT = dihydrotestosterone; SHBG = sex hormone-binding globulin; RNA = ribonucleic acid.

cells, testosterone readily diffuses through the cell membrane and is converted to DHT by 5-alpha-reductase. In cells in which 5-alpha-reduction of testosterone occurs to a limited extent (e.g., seminiferous tubules), testosterone itself binds to the receptor. The gene for the intracellular androgen receptor protein is located on the X chromosome.

Gonadal Regulation of Gonadotropins

Regulation by Gonadal Steroid. Secretion of LH and FSH is regulated by the negative feedback effects of testicular hormones. Testosterone is believed to be the predominant inhibitor of LH secretion and a major controller of FSH secretion. The role of estrogens in the feedback control of gonadotropin secretion in the male is controversial, but estrogens may be involved in this process. Similarly, the role of 5-alpha-reduction of testosterone in feedback regulation of gonadotropins remains unclear although 5-alpha-reductase activity is widely distributed within the pituitary and other parts of the brain.

Inhibin. An additional peptide hormone, inhibin, produced by the Sertoli cells has been implicated in the selective inhibition of FSH secretion. Support for a physiologic role of inhibin arises from the demonstration that selective damage to the germinal epithelium results in moderate increases in serum FSH without affecting either serum testosterone or LH. Complete nucleotide sequences for the precursors of the two forms of porcine inhibin, human follicular fluid inhibin and a bovine follicular fluid inhibin, have recently been determined. The recent development of a radioimmunoassay for inhibin should provide new insights to its importance as a regulatory hormone.

LABORATORY TESTS

Serum Testosterone

Serum testosterone is now routinely measured by radioimmunoassay. Its level should be determined in all patients with hypogonadism. The measurement of serum testosterone includes both protein-bound and free testosterone. Only the unbound (or free) testosterone is biologically active, and this free testosterone concentration is only about 1% of the total testosterone concentration. Thus, hypogonadism (underandrogenization) may be associated with a lower free testosterone but a normal total plasma testosterone level. Serum testosterone has a circadian rhythm with a peak in the early morning. Normal total serum testosterone values in adult men are 350 to 1050 ng/100 ml.

Table 7–1.   Serum LH, FSH, Testosterone, and Estradiol Levels in Normal Adult Males

Hormone	Level
LH	1–15 mIU/ml
FSH	<1–15 mIU/ml
Testosterone	350–1050 ng/100 ml
Estradiol	<40 pg/ml

Serum LH and FSH

Serum LH is measured by radioimmunoassay; normal values vary from laboratory to laboratory. Elevated levels usually indicate a primary failure of the testis to produce testosterone, while low levels may indicate hypothalamic or pituitary failure. Serum levels of LH fluctuate widely, varying 2- or 3-fold over a 2-hour period. Thus, several samples must be drawn and assayed to give a reasonable measure of the mean level of serum LH. Recent data have demonstrated occasional discrepancies between radioimmunoassayable LH and LH bioactivity. This may occur as the result of the production of an altered LH molecule or due to interference with LH action at the Leydig cell. In vitro bioassays can identify the presence of LH with less biologic activity. While these bioassays are extremely valuable in selected instances, they remain a research tool.

Serum FSH is measured by radioimmunoassay, and is elevated (as is LH) in patients with primary hypogonadism. In addition, serum FSH can be increased selectively in patients with primary damage to the spermatogenic tubules. Since much less variation exists in the plasma levels of FSH than of LH, multiple sampling is not needed. However, in many laboratories some normal men have undetectable serum FSH, making it difficult to separate those with normal FSH from those with low FSH.

Serum Estradiol

Serum estradiol is measured by radioimmunoassay; normal values in men are 40 pg/ml or less. Measurement of serum estradiol is helpful in cases of gynecomastia or feminization.

GnRH Stimulation Test

Synthetic GnRH is now available for testing of pituitary LH and FSH secretory reserve. Administration of 100 µg GnRH intravenously causes tripling of serum LH within an hour in normal men; the rise of serum FSH is inconstant and of smaller magnitude. Patients with hypogonadism secondary to pituitary destruction or tumor generally have no increase in serum LH after administration of GnRH. Patients with hypothalamic disorders resulting in hypogonadism may have normal or impaired LH responses to a single dose of GnRH; a blunted LH response to GnRH may return to normal if GnRH is given in repeated doses in a pulsatile fashion. In primary testicular failure, the loss of the normal inhibitory effect of testosterone results in an exaggerated rise in serum LH after GnRH administration. In practice, testing with a single injection of GnRH has not been a reliable method for separating hypothalamic from pituitary causes of hypogonadism.

Clomiphene

Clomiphene citrate is a compound that stimulates the release of LH and FSH, probably by blocking the inhibitory effect of testosterone and estrogen on the hypothalamus. In normal men, administration of 150 mg clomiphine per day for 10 days causes a doubling of serum LH. A failure to respond to clomiphene coupled with normal pituitary function indicates probable hypothalamic cause of hypogonadism. Since the ability to respond to clomiphene does not develop until stage III of puberty, this test has usually not been helpful in assessing disorders of delayed puberty. It is used primarily as a test of hypothalamic-pituitary function.

hCG Stimulation Test

Administration of human chorionic gonadotropin, which has biologic activity similar to LH, directly stimulates the testes to secrete testosterone. Normal men double their serum testosterone after 2 injections of 2000 IU of hCG; patients with primary testicular failure may have either no response or a blunted response. Patients with pituitary or hypothalamic causes of hypogonadism may have a small rise in serum testosterone after hCG; prolonged administration of hCG may restore this response to normal.

Semen Analysis

Semen analysis (as a test for evaluation of infertility) is performed optimally by examination of a specimen obtained after 48 to 72 hours of abstinence. Normal men have at least 15 million spermatozoa per milliliter with 60% motility and 60% normal forms. Specific abnormalities may be associated with specific disorders; for example, the presence of a large number of tapered forms suggests varicocele. Recent studies have suggested that sperm function can be assessed by: (1) the determination of the ability of sperm from a semen specimen to penetrate hamster eggs that have been chemically treated to remove the zona pellucida (zona free hamster test), and (2) the ability of sperm to move through cervical mucus (cervical mucus penetration test).

Buccal Smear and Karyotype

Examination of epithelial cells from the buccal mucosa (buccal smear) for Barr bodies and karyotyping of peripheral blood lymphocytes enables determination of sex chromosome composition and is indicated when a congenital defect may exist. It is especially indicated when serum FSH or LH are elevated, since the most common cause of hypergonadotropic hypogonadism in adult males is Klinefelter's syndrome.

Microscopic examination of the buccal smear reveals the presence of Barr bodies (dark chromatin clumps) in patients who have more than one X chromosome per cell. The Barr body represents the heterochromatin of the extra X chromosome; the number of Barr bodies per cell is one less than the number of X chromosomes. Normal males have Barr bodies in fewer than 5% of their buccal mucosal cells; in normal females, Barr bodies are present in more than 20% of buccal mucosal cells. A more specific method of determining sex chromosome composition is by karyotyping, that is, the examination of photomicrographs of the metaphase plates of cultured peripheral blood lymphocytes. In these preparations, the Y chromosome can be located by its characteristic fluorescence when exposed to quinacrine. Recently, it has become possible to determine the presence of a Y chromosome without karyotyping by looking for the presence of a specific "Y antigen" on the surface of cells.

MALE REPRODUCTIVE DISORDERS

Hypogonadism

Clinical Manifestations

DEPENDENCE ON AGE OF ONSET. Hypogonadism or impaired testicular function may be reflected clinically as underandrogenization, infertility, or a combination of the two. The clinical features of decreased testosterone secretion depend on the degree of deficiency and the age of onset of the disorder. Deficiencies occurring during early fetal development result in pseudohermaphroditism, and those occurring during late gestation may result in micropenis.

The clinical onset of testosterone deficiency prior to puberty will result in eunuchoid proportions and female hair distribution. Eunuchoid proportions include an arm span 2 inches greater than height and an upper-body-to-lower-body ratio of less than one. (These proportions may be normal for black men from East Africa.) Patients with hypogonadism acquired after puberty have normal body proportions and male temporal hair recession, but show other clinical signs of hypogonadism (Fig. 7–3).

FACIES. The distribution of facial beard in normal males depends on the person's racial background. Deviations from the facially determined norm indicate the presence of hypogonadism. Hair distribution on the cheek, moustache, chin, and neck varies greatly amongst different races; most Caucasian males need to shave daily, while men of black, Oriental, or American Indian extraction may shave normally only once in 2 to 3 days. Detailed questioning of other male family members is helpful in assessing the clinical status of a suspected hypogonadal patient. Hypogonadism is also associated with increased fine wrinkling of the skin around the mouth and eyes.

BODY HAIR DISTRIBUTION. Body hair distribution also varies with racial background. Many normal black, Oriental, and Indian men have body hair limited to the axillary, pubic, and sternal areas, while many Caucasian men have additional pectoral, back, and flank hair. The male pubic hair distribution is diamond-shaped with hair extending up toward the umbilicus. When the pubic hair has an inverted triangle appearance, it is described as a female escutcheon. Severe long-standing hypogonadism results in absence of chest hair and sparseness of pubic hair. Less severe defects produce more subtle changes, which should be evaluated with the patient's racial and family hair patterns as a guide.

TESTICULAR SIZE. Ninety percent of the normal testis volume consists of spermatogenic tubules. The testes should be measured in all patients; testes greater than 4.0 cm in length or greater than 15 ml in volume (measured with

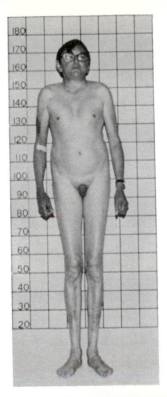

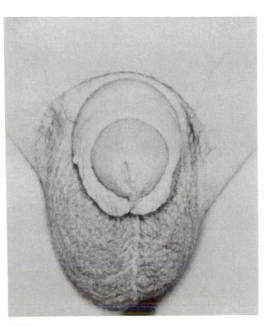

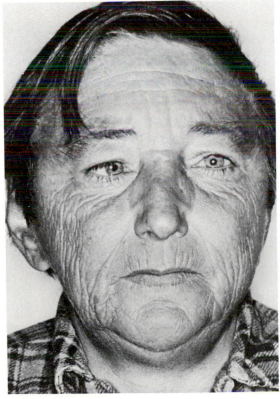

Fig. 7–3. A 43-year-old man with hypogonadotropic hypogonadism due to a chromophobe adenoma. Prepubertal onset is apparent from the eunuchoidal proportions. The sparse pubic hair, absence of beard (never shaved), infantile genitalia, and increased facial wrinkling indicate severe androgen deficiency.

a Prader orchidometer) are normal in size. Most patients with hypogonadism have testes that are smaller than normal. If the onset of the lesion is prepubertal, the testes are often infantile in size. Hypogonadism beginning after puberty results in testicular size varying from small, soft organs to those that are near normal. Severe tubular injury not associated with underandrogenization may result in small testes and normal Leydig cell function.

Causes of Male Hypogonadism. Hypogonadism occurs in three main categories: (1) hypothalamic-pituitary defects (hypogonadotropic), (2) primary gonadal defects (hypergonadotropic), and (3) defective androgen action. Each of these categories consists of multiple subcategories described in Table 7–2. (Some rare disorders have not been included.)

From a clinical standpoint it is important to: (1) define the anatomic site of the defect; (2) determine whether the defect has additional serious consequences to the patient such as would occur in patients with hypothalamic or pituitary tumors, panhypopituitarism, hypothalamic syndromes, and many congenital adrenal and testicular enzymatic defects; (3) determine whether a genetic disorder requires genetic counseling to the family; and (4) characterize the physiologic nature of the hormonal deficiency and its consequences in order to optimize therapy. (Patients with hypogonadotropic hypogonadism could be treated with testosterone to produce virilization, but restoration of fertility would require treatment with gonadotropins.)

Localization of Site of Defect. Evaluation of patients with clinical evidence of underandrogenization should begin with measurements of basal serum testosterone, LH, and FSH levels. In almost all such cases, serum testosterone concentrations are lower than normal, thus confirming the diagnosis of hypogonadism. In such patients, the serum LH and FSH concentrations separate the patients into two main categories: hypergonadotropic (high LH and FSH) or hypogonadotropic (low or inappropriately normal LH and FSH).

HYPOGONADOTROPIC HYPOGONADISM. Hypogonadotropic hypogonadism may be further dissected into the hypothalamic and pituitary abnormalities. Ability to smell should be tested in all hypogonadotropic patients because its absence suggests a congenital hypothalamic cause of hypogonadism (Kallmann's syndrome). CT scans and skull roentgenograms including special views of the sella turcica must be obtained in such patients. These films may detect: (1) enlargement of the sella turcica, suggesting an intrapituitary or suprasellar mass; (2) calcification in or above the sella, suggesting a craniopharyngioma; and (3) evidence of increased intracranial pressure. CT scans are highly efficient means of assessing the above structural defects and can identify pituitary microadenomas.

Additional laboratory tests should be done in hypogonadotropic patients. Serum prolactin measurements are required because a marked elevation suggests a prolactinoma. Lesser elevations of prolactin may occur in many disorders (see Chap. 2). Hyperprolactinemia may suppress LH and FSH secretion in the absence of anatomic damage to the GnRH and gonadotropin-secreting cells. Lowering prolactin levels with a dopamine agonist (bromocriptine) will

Table 7–2. Classification of Hypogonadism

1. Abnormalities in Hypothalamic-Pituitary Function
   a. Panhypopituitarism (congenital or acquired)
   b. Hypothalamic syndromes (acquired or congenital)
      Structural defects (neoplastic, inflammatory infiltrative)
      Prader-Willi syndrome (mental retardation, hypogonadism, hypotonia, and obesity)
      Laurence-Moon-Biedl syndrome (mental retardation, hypogonadism, retinitis pigmentosa, and hand anomalies)
   c. Isolated LH or FSH deficiency (may be associated with anosmia [Kallmann's syndrome])
   d. Hyperprolactinemia (prolactinoma is the most common cause)
   e. Malnutrition and anorexia nervosa
   f. Drug-induced suppression of LH (androgens, estrogens, tranquilizers, antidepressants, antihypertensives, barbiturates, cimetidine, GnRH analogs, and opiates

2. Primary Gonadal Abnormalities
   a. Acquired (irradiation, orchitis, castration, cytotoxic, and other drugs and toxins)
   b. Chromosomal
      Klinefelter's and variants
      Autosomal and sex chromosomal polyploides
      True hermaphroditism
   c. Defective androgen biosynthesis
      20-alpha-hydroxylase (cholesterol 20,22-desmolase) deficiency
      17,20-desmolase deficiency
      3-beta-hydroxysteroid dehydrogenase deficiency
      17-keto-hydroxylase deficiency
      17-keto-reductase (17-beta-hydroxysteroid dehydrogenase) deficiency
      5-alpha-reductase (17-beta-hydroxysteroid dehydrogenase) deficiency
   d. Testicular agenesis
   e. Selective seminiferous tubular disease
   f. Miscellaneous
      Noonan's syndrome (short stature, pulmonary valve stenosis, hyperteloris, and ptosis)
      Streak gonads
      Myotonia dystrophica
      Cystic fibrosis and other syndromes of immotile sperm

3. Defects in Androgen Action (Pseudohermaphroditism)
   a. Complete androgen insensitivity (also called testicular feminization)
   b. Incomplete androgen sensitivity
      Testosterone receptor defect
      Testosterone postreceptor defect
      5-alpha-reductase deficiency

reverse the hypogonadotropic state. All hypogonadotropic patients should have a complete assessment of hypothalamic-pituitary function. Additional tests of reproductive function may be indicated to characterize the lesion. The response to clomiphene is abnormally low in patients with either hypothalamic or pituitary disease. GnRH administration increases LH and FSH levels in most patients with hypothalamic disease and fails to do so in most patients with a pituitary cause of hypogonadism. Unfortunately, the ability of this test to determine the site of the defect is not foolproof. Some patients with pituitary disease respond normally, and others with a hypothalamic problem respond only after prolonged treatment with GnRH.

HYPERGONADOTROPIC HYPOGONADISM. Patients with low serum testosterone and elevated serum LH and FSH have a primary testicular disorder. In some patients with borderline testosterone levels, an hCG test may demonstrate the presence of impaired Leydig cell reserve.

The clinical history frequently indicates whether there has been infection or trauma. Chromosome analysis identifies patients with disorders such as Klinefelter's syndrome and its variants (see next section). Most defects of testosterone biosynthesis result in pseudohermaphroditism (see Chap. 5). Other rare disorders can be identified by their clinical characteristics, such as Noonan's syndrome and myotonia dystrophica.

Klinefelter's Syndrome. Klinefelter's syndrome, the most common cause of male hypogonadism, is a congenital disorder characterized by the presence of XXY sex chromosome composition in the testis. The abnormal testicular function resulting from this genetic defect is responsible for the manifestations of Klinefelter's syndrome seen in the reproductive tissues. In addition, the abnormal sex chromosome composition may also be found in other body tissues (such as buccal mucosa and skin fibroblasts) or may be associated with mosaicism with variable cell sex chromosome composition. These mosaics may show features of Klinefelter's syndrome to a variable degree, but they all possess at least one or more cell lines containing two X chromosomes and one Y chromosome. The incidence of Klinefelter's syndrome is approximately 0.2% of live male births. The cause of the disorder is thought to be nondisjunction, and, like some other chromosomal disorders, it seems to be associated with advanced maternal or paternal age.

The cardinal physical finding in patients with Klinefelter's syndrome is small, firm testes, which on biopsy show germ cell loss, hyalinization of spermatogenic tubules, and Leydig cell clumping and hyperplasia. These abnormalities usually result in azoospermia and infertility, but the temporal pace of germ cell loss and tubular hyalinization allows a broad range in testicular size and consistency on physical examination. Androgen deficiency, manifested by decreased facial and pubic hair growth, reduced muscle mass, small penis size, and impaired sexual potency are usually present in Klinefelter's syndrome, but some patients may appear normally virilized. Gynecomastia, as evidenced microscopically by hyperplasia of the interductal breast tissue, is often present. These individuals tend to have a tall stature and long legs, in association with the typical eunuchoidal proportion of upper-segment-to-lower-segment ratio less than one. In contrast with other disorders resulting in eunuchoidal proportions, Klinefelter's patients may have an arm span less than their height.

Klinefelter's syndrome is also associated with a number of nonreproductive abnormalities, including diabetes, chronic bronchitis, breast cancer, thyroid abnormalities, and mental retardation in as many as 15 to 25% of patients. The association with mental retardation is confirmed by observations that the prevalence of Klinefelter's syndrome in institutions for the mentally retarded is 1%, which is higher than that in the general population.

Laboratory findings in Klinefelter's syndrome reflect both the genetic and hormonal abnormalities. The XXY chromosomal composition may be detected by examining a buccal smear for the presence of Barr bodies. More definitive diagnosis requires complete karyotyping of peripheral blood lymphocytes, and the presence of mosaicism may in some cases be detected only by determining the karyotype of several cell lines. Semen analysis in these patients usually shows azoospermia. Plasma testosterone levels are low-to-normal or reduced, and the loss of inhibitory feedback is reflected by high-normal or frankly elevated serum levels of LH and FSH. Some patients may have selective damage to the germinal elements and come to the clinic with elevated serum levels of FSH and normal testosterone and LH concentrations, but most patients show impaired testicular steroid reserve when challenged with injections of hCG.

Testicular Dysfunction with Aging. Testicular function is often abnormal in an aged male population. This abnormality is usually associated with elevated serum LH and FSH levels, which indicate a primary defect at the level of the testis. Some controversy exists as to whether the testicular failure seen in the aged is a normal consequence of growing older or a result of concomitant disease processes.

End-Organ Resistance. Some patients may have signs of underandrogenization and yet have normal or elevated serum testosterone levels. These patients often come to the clinic with male pseudohermaphroditism manifest by a broad range of physical appearances. In the most severe form (testicular feminization), the phenotypic appearance is female. In less severe forms the patients may have hypospadias and gynecomastia. Even more subtle examples of this disorder may be manifested by isolated decrease in sperm number and function. The several defects described include inability to convert testosterone to dihydrotestosterone (5-alpha-reductase deficiency) and unresponsiveness to testosterone and dihydrotestosterone in androgen-sensitive tissues (androgen receptor defect). In the latter case, estradiol levels are usually above the normal male range, serum testosterone and LH levels are normal or high, and FSH is usually normal or low.

Infertility

The evaluation of an infertile couple requires an assessment of both partners. In the initial evaluation, semen analysis should be performed on the male partner. Patients with decreased sperm counts (less than 15,000,000/ml) should have serum LH, FSH, and testosterone values determined; patients with panhypogonadism have low serum levels of testosterone. Many oligospermic or azoospermic patients do not show evidence of Leydig cell dysfunction. Hormonal parameters are normal, or an isolated increase of FSH is seen. A few patients may have had previous testicular injury, infection, chemotherapy, or irradiation, which would explain the isolated germinal element damage. Some patients have unsuspected sex or autosomal chromosome abnormalities. Significant numbers of patients have obstruction to the ductal system. Obstruction to the semen excretory ductal system is strongly suggested by normal serum FSH levels in a patient with azoospermia. Varicoceles (worm-like dilatation of the spermatic venous system) may be associated with infertility; an increased number of tapered forms on morphologic examination of the sperm suggests such a possibility. The role of autoimmunity, sperm and cervical mucus incompatibility, and female antisperm antibodies is under investigation. In the majority of oligospermic and azoospermic patients, the pathogenic cause of impaired spermatogenesis cannot be determined. Many patients with unexplained infertility may have impaired sperm function without evidence of an abnormal routine semen analysis.

Gynecomastia

Gynecomastia is defined as an increase in the nonfatty tissue of the male breast. This increase may be in either the parenchymal or stromal elements and may be bilateral or unilateral. The incidence of gynecomastia in the general population is an issue of some controversy. Reports vary from 5 to 9% in several autopsy series to 36% in a clinical survey. Breast enlargement in the male is seen in many clinical situations, some of which are:

1. Puberty (seen in 50 to 70% of normal boys)
2. Cirrhosis (especially after recovery from hepatic decompensation)
3. Chronic renal failure with chronic hemodialysis
4. Drugs (estrogens, digitalis, spironolactone, ketoconazole, cyproterone, marijuana, reserpine, and other drugs known to act on the central nervous system)
5. Hyperthyroidism or, rarely, hypothyroidism
6. Rapid weight gain (especially after previous weight loss)
7. Primary testicular failure (including Klinefelter's syndrome)
8. Hypogonadotropic hypogonadism (less common than in primary testicular failure)
9. Cancer
   a. with overproduction of estrogens
   b. with production of an hCG-like peptide hormone

The mechanisms producing gynecomastia are diverse. The relationship between an increase in the estrogen to androgen ratio and breast enlargement is well known, and the mechanism of gynecomastia in men taking estrogens for prostatic carcinoma or those with estrogen-producing adrenal carcinoma is obvious. In hyperthyroidism and cirrhosis, the total plasma levels of estrogens and androgens may be normal, but abnormalities of the globulin that binds them in plasma may lead to an increase in the physiologically active free-estrogen-to-free-androgen ratio and consequent gynecomastia. On the other hand, spironolactone seems to block both the synthesis of testosterone and the attachment of androgens to their receptors on target tissues (including the breast) and leads to an increase in the estrogen to androgen ratio at the cellular level. Similarly, in patients with testicular feminization, these androgen receptors on the target tissues may be entirely absent. The mechanism producing gynecomastia in normal boys during puberty remains controversial; some investigators find elevated plasma estrogen levels and others do not.

When evaluating a patient with gynecomastia, one must keep in mind that most cases are either pubertal or idiopathic. Careful history and physical examination identifies most of the known causes of gynecomastia listed previously. Special attention should be paid to history of sexual functioning and examination for signs of virilization, since most patients with normal libido, potency, and virilization do not have a life-threatening underlying disorder. Normal levels of plasma LH, FSH, testosterone, and estradiol are often found and are typical of the idiopathic cases. Serum LH should be measured in all cases of gynecomastia because high levels may indicate primary hypogonadism (e.g., Klinefelter's syndrome) or hCG production by choriocarcinoma of the testis or other tumor. In the latter case, the presence of beta-hCG in the serum, as determined by specific radioimmunoassay, would confirm the diagnosis of tumor since beta-hCG is not normally present in males. A high level of plasma estradiol may suggest a feminizing adrenal carcinoma. Idiopathic or pubertal gynecomastia usually regresses spontaneously.

CLINICAL PROBLEMS

Patient 1. A 33-year-old male accountant was referred by his general physician for complaints of decreased libido, loss of morning erections, and diminished body and beard hair. He developed in a normal pubertal fashion between ages 14 through 17 with normal sexual drive. He married at age 23 and divorced at the age of 26. His wife had no pregnancies, but used birth control agents. During the past 6 years, he noted progressive loss of facial, chest, and lower abdominal hair. His sexual drive, frequency of morning erections, and frequency of coitus diminished during this period. He complained of recent onset of bifrontal headaches and decrease in lateral vision.

PHYSICAL EXAMINATION. His height was 73 inches (upper segment 37 inches, lower segment 36 inches, arm span 72 inches). A decrease in the lateral visual fields was observed. He had minimal facial hair, no chest hair, and a female pubic hair distribution. Mild gynecomastia without galactorrhea was present. His penis was of normal size without hypospadius; his scrotum, epididymis, and vas were normal. The testes were 13 ml bilaterally and somewhat softer than normal.

LABORATORY DATA. Serum testosterone was 150 ng/dl; serum LH 5 mIU/ml; serum FSH 2 mIU/ml; serum prolactin was 92 ng/ml; serum estradiol was 38 pg/ml.

QUESTIONS
1. Does this patient have hypogonadism?
2. What is the most likely site of his lesion?
3. Is this likely to be an acquired disorder?
4. What is the most likely pathophysiologic cause of his problem?
5. Testing of his visual fields demonstrated a bitemporal hemianopsia (bilateral loss of lateral visual fields). What diagnosis does this suggest?
6. What further tests or x rays should be obtained?
7. Would a single dose GnRH test be likely to demonstrate a normal or diminished response?

Patient 2. The patient is a 23-year-old black male referred for marked gynecomastia, and decreased male secondary sexual characteristics. He had decreased libido and no sexual activity. The patient underwent only partial secondary sexual development during the normal pubertal age. He presently has a sparse beard requiring him to shave only once a week. Breast enlargement began at the age of puberty and has progressively increased to the present time. The patient denies morning erections, has low libido, and denies sexual intercourse or masturbation.

PHYSICAL EXAMINATION. He is obese and has striking gynecomastia. His height is 72 inches with the span 3 inches greater than his height. The lower segment measurements were 38 inches and the upper segment 35 cm. He had 6 cm of non-tender glandular tissue palpable in both breasts. No abdominal masses were present. The penis was 10 cm in length and the testes were 4 ml bilaterally and somewhat firmer than usual.

LABORATORY DATA. The serum LH and FSH concentrations were elevated above the adult normal range (35 and 50 mIU/ml, respectively), serum testosterone was low (100 ng/dl). Serum estradiol was 58 pg/ml.

QUESTIONS
1. What is the anatomic site of the defect?
2. What is the most likely diagnosis?
3. What test will confirm the most likely diagnosis?
4. Why does he have gynecomastia?
5. Is a skull x ray necessary?
6. Will he always be infertile?
7. Can you characterize his response to GnRH?
8. If you should administer hCG what would his response be?

SUGGESTED READING

Reproductive Hormone Physiology

Clermont, Y.: The cycle of the seminiferous epithelium in man. Am J Anat, *112*:35, 1963.

Crowley, W.F., Jr., Filicori, M., Spratt, D.I., and Santoro, N.F.: The physiology of GnRH secretion in men and women. Recent Prog Horm Res, *41*:473, 1985.

Handelsman, D.J., and Swerdloff, R.S.: Pharmacokinetics of gonadotropin-releasing hormones (GnRH) and its analogs. Endocr Rev, *7*:95, 1986.

Parvinen, M.: Regulation of the seminiferous epithelium. Endocr Rev, *3*:404, 1982.

Swerdloff, R.S., and Bhasin, S.: Male reproductive physiology. *In* Infertility—Diagnosis and Management. Edited by E.J. Aimen. New York, Springer/Verlag, 1984, pp. 177–184.

Swerdloff. R.S.: Physiology of male reproduction. Hypothalamic-pituitary function, the hypo-thalamic-pituitary-gonadal axis. *In* Campbell's Urology. 5th Ed. Edited by J. Hartwell Harrison. Philadelphia, W.B. Saunders Co., 1985, pp. 186–200.

Yanaihara, T., and Troen, P.: Studies of the human testis. Biosynthetic pathways for androgen formation in human testicular tissue in vitro. J Clin Endocrinol Metab, *34*:783, 1972.

Hypogonadism

Handelsman, D.J., and Swerdloff, R.S.: Male gonadal dysfunction. Clin Endocr Metab, *14*:89, 1985.

Swerdloff, R.S., and Sokol, R.Z.: Manifestations of androgen deficiency and effects of androgen therapy. *In* Reproductive Medicine. Edited by E. Steinberger, G. Fajese and A. Steinberger. Serono Symposium, Vol. 29, 1986, pp. 39–53.

Spratt, D.I., Hoffman, A.R., and Crowley, Jr., W.F.: Hypogonadotropic hypogonadism and its treatment. *In* Male Reproductive Dysfunction. Edited by R.J. Santen, and R.S. Swerdloff. New York, Marcel Dekker, 1986, pp. 227–249.

Aging and Reproductive Function

Harman, S.M., and Tsitouras, P.D.: Reproductive hormones in aging men. J. Clin Endocrinol Metab, *51*:35, 1980.

Nieschlag, E.: Testicular function in senescence. *In* Male Reproductive Dysfunction. Edited by R.S. Santen, and R.S. Swerdloff. New York, Marcel Dekker, 1986, pp 199–209.

Sparrow, D.R., Bosse, R., and Rowe, J.W.: The influence of age, alcohol consumption, and body build on gonadal function in men. J Clin Endocrinol Metab, *51*:508, 1980.

Infertility

Sherins, R.J., and Howards, S.S.: Male infertility. *In* Campbell's Urology. 5th Ed. Edited by Hartwell Harrison. Philadelphia, W.B. Saunders Co., 1985, pp. 640–697.

Swerdloff, R.S., Overstreet, J.W., Sokol, R.Z., and Rajfer, J.: Infertility in the male. Ann Intern Med, *103*:906, 1985.

Gynecomastia

Carlson, H.E.: Gynecomastia. N Engl J Med, *303*:795, 1980.

Frantz, A.G., and Wilson, J.D.: Endocrine disorders of the breast. *In* Williams' Textbook of Endocrinology. 7th Ed. Edited by J.W. Wilson and D.W. Foster. Philadelphia, W.B. Saunders Co., 1985, pp. 402–421.

Knorr, D., and Bidlingmaier, F.: Gynecomastia in male adolescents. Clin Endocrinol Metab *4*:157, 1975.

Nuttal, F.Q.: Gynecomastia as a physical finding in normal men. J Clin Endocrinol Metab *48*:338, 1979.

ANSWERS TO QUESTIONS

Patient 1.

1. Yes. Symptoms of decreased libido, loss of morning erections, and regression of secondary sexual characteristics along with low serum testosterone concentrations clearly demonstrated that the patient is hypogonadal.

2. The patient has hypogonadotropic hypogonadism since serum LH and FSH concentrations are low normal and are not elevated in the face of decreased serum testosterone concentrations. Thus, the site of lesion is likely to be either at the hypothalamus or the pituitary gland. Decreased lateral visual fields also suggest that the lesion is in the hypothalamic pituitary area and compressing the optic chiasm.

3. Yes. Normal development of the genitalia and normal upper and lower body proportions suggest that the disease process causing hypogonadism started after puberty.

4. The most likely cause of patient's hypogonadism is hyperprolactinemia. In the absence of drugs, renal or hepatic failure, and hypothyroidism, prolactin secreting pituitary adenomas are the most likely cause of increased serum prolactin. Prolactin secreting pituitary adenomas may cause hypogonadotropic hypogonadism in two ways; increased prolactin concentrations may inhibit LH and FSH secretion or the tumor may itself compress the normal pituitary, thus compromising hormonal function.

5. The presence of bitemporal hemianopsia suggests that the tumor is suprasellar in location and is compressing the midline decussation of the optic chiasm. Tumors compressing the optic chiasm from below often initially present with loss of the upper outer quadrant of the visual fields. The most common cause of optic chiasm compression is a suprasellar tumor; most often this represents a pituitary adenoma with suprasellar extension. In young adults or children, a craniopharyngioma is a likely diagnosis.

6. A CT scan of the hypothalamic-pituitary area is indicated to characterize the anatomic location of the tumor.

7. A single GnRH test is likely to show a diminished response since the lesion is at the pituitary site. Some patients with hyperprolactinemia and hypogonadotropic hypogonadism may overcome their block of LH secretion with a high dose of GnRH.

Patient 2

1. The patient has hypergonadotropic hypogonadism (high LH and FSH). Therefore, the lesion is at the testicular level.

2. The most common cause of hypergonadotropic hypogonadism in a phenotypic male is Klinefelter's syndrome.

3. The demonstration of a XXY karyotype on chromosome analysis will confirm the diagnosis.

4. Increased serum estradiol to testosterone ratio is the most likely cause of gynecomastia.

5. No. A skull x ray is unlikely to provide any useful information.

6. Yes. Patients with primary testicular failure rarely respond to fertility therapy.

7. He is likely to have an exaggerated LH response to GnRH.

8. Since he has primary testicular failure, he will either fail to increase his testosterone level after hCG or have a blunted response.

8

Diabetes Mellitus and Hypoglycemia

Mayer B. Davidson

ABBREVIATIONS

CoA	coenzyme A
DKA	diabetic ketoacidosis
HNKC	hyperosmolar nonketotic coma
IDDM	insulin-dependent diabetes mellitus
IGF-1	insulin-like growth factor-1 (somatomedin C)
IGT	impaired glucose tolerance
MODY	maturity-onset diabetes of youth
NDDG	National Diabetes Data Group
NIDDM	noninsulin-dependent diabetes mellitus
NSILA	nonsuppressible insulin-like activity
OGTT	oral glucose tolerance test
SSPG	steady state plasma glucose
SSPI	steady state plasma insulin
WHO	World Health Organization

This chapter describes the pathophysiology, diagnosis, and treatment of adult hypoglycemia and diabetes mellitus. The metabolic pathways that characterize the fasting and fed states are reviewed, so that hypoglycemia and hyperglycemia (diabetes mellitus) can be discussed in terms of specific departures from these normal homeostatic mechanisms.

It is important to have a solid understanding of the disorders of carbohydrate metabolism. No matter which area of medicine students choose to enter, they will encounter some aspect of the many problems presented by the diabetic patient. On the other hand, some practitioners contend that hypoglycemia is responsible for many modern ills, such as alcoholism, sexual inadequacy, allergies, drug addiction, depression, learning disorders, and behavior problems. Clearly, hypoglycemia is not the problem in these situations; however, it is important for any physician who cares for patients to know how to make a bona fide diagnosis of hypoglycemia and to determine which of many conditions may be responsible for it.

NORMAL METABOLISM

The metabolic machinery of mammals is geared to handle a wide variety of metabolic situations. For instance, a Peruvian miner working at high altitude may ingest 5000 calories a day and maintain a stable normal weight. A neurotic individual living at sea level with no unusual caloric expenditure eating 5000 calories a day may gain 50 kg in a year. An extremely obese individual undergoing a protein-sparing diet may lose 50 kg in one year. The Eskimo eating approximately 2000 calories a day, 80% of which is in the form of fat, has a normal body composition. All these individuals are able to function normally, a testimony to our amazing versatility in adjusting to various metabolic conditions.

Fasting State

Metabolic homeostasis after an overnight fast is depicted in Figure 8–1. During a short fast, only a few tissues require glucose. The most important obligate glucose consumer is the brain that uses most of the available glucose (125 to 150 g/day). In vitro studies suggest that the red blood cells are the next most avid glucose consumer but use a much smaller amount (35 to 50 g/day) than does the central nervous system. Platelets, leukocytes, peripheral nerves, and the renal medulla also require glucose during a short fast; as a group, however, these tissues consume only half as much as the red blood cells. All other tissues use predominantly free fatty acids (FFA) that are produced by the breakdown of adipose tissue triglycerides. A small amount of the energy required by these tissues is provided by ketone bodies which are produced from the hepatic catabolism of FFA (see below). Recent data obtained by catheters placed in the artery and vein across a leg suggest that muscle tissue may also use a small amount of glucose after an overnight fast.

The liver is the sole source of glucose production during short fasts. Glucose is produced through two separate pathways: glycogenolysis and gluconeogenesis. Glycogenolysis is the breakdown of glycogen, the storage form of glucose. Approximately 30% of the carbohydrates contained in meals is stored directly as hepatic glycogen. A large proportion of the remainder is broken down by either muscle or splanchnic tissue to gluconeogenic precursors, alanine and lactate (see below), recycled to the liver, and then converted into glycogen. Hepatic glycogen is slowly hydrolyzed and released as glucose in order to maintain stable plasma levels of glucose during periods when an individual is not eating. After an overnight fast, approximately 75% of hepatic glucose is produced by glycogenolysis.

PRECURSORS   GENERATOR   CONSUMERS

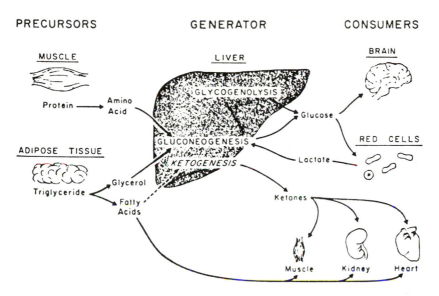

Fig. 8–1. Fasting homeostasis. (From Arky, R.A.: Pathophysiology and therapy of the fasting hypoglycemias. Edited by Harry F. Dowling: DM. Chicago, Year Book Medical Publishers, Inc. 1968. Reproduced with permission.)

Gluconeogenesis is the synthesis of new glucose from noncarbohydrate precursors. There are three major gluconeogenic substrates (Fig. 8–1). One is lactate, an end product of the glucose used by the peripheral tissues. The second category of substrate is composed of the amino acids supplied by muscle tissue. The most important of the gluconeogenic amino acids is alanine. A transamination pathway in muscle facilitates the conversion of pyruvate, another product of glucose metabolism, to alanine, which is released and delivered to the liver. The final substrate for gluconeogenesis is glycerol, the other product (along with FFA) of triglyceride hydrolysis. Thus, gluconeogenic precursors are derived from the catabolism of glucose (lactate and pyruvate), protein (glucogenic amino acids other than alanine), and fat (glycerol). The rate-determining step for gluconeogenesis seems to be the amount of substrate presented to the liver. Although only 25% of hepatic glucose production derives from gluconeogenesis after an overnight fast, the contribution from glycogen decreases considerably soon thereafter, and gluconeogenesis becomes dominant as the period of fasting lengthens.

Most stored energy is contained in adipose tissue triglycerides. The breakdown of triglyceride yields FFA and glycerol. As stated earlier, glycerol is a gluconeogenic precursor, whereas FFA are the main source of energy for most tissues in the fasting state. The FFA delivered to the liver have three metabolic fates. First, they can be re-esterfied back into triglycerides. Second, they can be used as an energy source for the liver through β-oxidation to acetyl-coenzyme A (CoA) with subsequent metabolism through the Krebs cycle. Third, the acetyl-CoA can be channeled into ketone bodies, acetoacetate and β-hydroxybutyrate.

Although the molar ratio of insulin to glucagon in the portal vein influences ketogenesis, the most important control of hepatic ketone body formation is the amount of FFA delivered to the liver. After synthesis, the ketone bodies are released into the general circulation where they can be used to some extent by the peripheral tissues. The amount that can be taken up by peripheral tissues is limited, however, and after 12 to 24 hours without food, the ketone bodies spill over into the urine (ketonuria). This condition is known as starvation ketosis and must be carefully distinguished from diabetic ketosis described later. Ketosis can also be seen in subjects ingesting low carbohydrate diets. When dietary carbohydrate is limited (fewer than approximately 50 to 80 g/day), lipolysis increases, enhancing FFA delivery to the liver and thus increasing ketone body formation. The body has powerful homeostatic mechanisms to maintain glucose concentrations during total starvation so that the tissues that are obligate glucose consumers can continue to function normally. When calories are totally withheld, an initial drop of glucose concentration by 15 to 20 mg/100 ml usually stabilizes after approximately 3 days. Some individuals of normal weight undergoing total caloric deprivation (especially women) may have glucose levels as low as 30 to 35 mg/100 ml but remain asymptomatic. During the next several weeks, hepatic glucose production is equal to glucose utilization by the brain and red blood cells; therefore, glucose concentrations remain stable. Insulin levels uniformly decrease and glucagon concentrations increase. FFA concentrations are approximately double while ketone body concentrations rise some 200-fold (Fig. 8–2). Glucogenic amino acid levels (especially alanine levels) decrease to approximately one-third of their prefast value with a concomitant increase in hepatic extraction of these precursors. Plasma lactate and pyruvate concentrations show no change.

After 3 to 4 weeks of starvation, the body makes certain alterations in an attempt to conserve the protein stores. If continued breakdown of muscle protein were to occur in order to supply the glucogenic amino acids, a severe depletion would ensue. To counteract this continued drain, the brain adapts so that ketone bodies can be used for energy. Thus, less glucose is required for the most important (and avid) obligate consumer with consequent sparing of protein. At this point, the kidney (the other tissue capable of gluconeogenesis) begins to contribute glucose to the general circulation. Prior to this time, glucose synthesized by renal gluconeogenesis was used locally by the renal tissue itself, and the kidney did not supply glucose for other tissues. With regard to the work-up of a patient with hypoglycemia that occurs in the fasting state (after an overnight fast or when a meal is missed), the important point is that when normal subjects

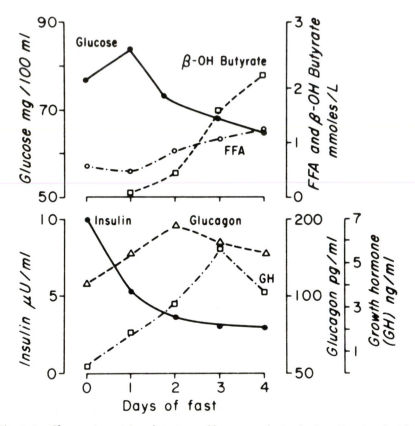

Fig. 8–2. Changes in certain substrates and hormones during fasting. (Reprinted with permission from Ensinck, J.W., Williams, R.H.: Disorders causing hypoglycemia. *In* Textbook of Endocrinology. 5th Ed. Edited by R.H. Williams. Philadelphia, W.B. Saunders Co., 1974.)

starve, the fall in glucose concentrations is associated with a much greater proportional decrease in insulin levels (Fig. 8–2).

Fed State

A normal diet includes both simple (mono- and disaccharides) and complex (polysaccharides) carbohydrate. The simple form, which constitutes approximately half of the total carbohydrate in the typical American diet, is quickly absorbed either directly or after rapid hydrolysis to glucose and the other constituent sugar in the small intestine. The complex form, composed mainly of large polymers of glucose, is also hydrolyzed and absorbed. The rising concentration of glucose in the blood stream stimulates insulin secretion by the β-cell of the pancreas into the portal vein. The newly released insulin traverses the liver first, where approximately 50% is degraded on each passage. The remainder escapes into the general circulation in which its half-life is approximately 5 minutes. The hormone binds to specific receptors in the three insulin-sensitive tissues—liver, muscle and adipose tissue; there, it may exert an effect for 1 to 2 hours after the initial binding.

Approximately 30% of dietary carbohydrate is taken up directly by the liver. The remaining 70% is used by the other tissues. The rise in glucose and insulin concentrations following a meal shuts off hepatic glucose production. Thus, some of the meal-derived glucose is used by the obligate glucose consumers, mainly brain and red blood cells. The remainder is metabolized, mostly by muscle with a few percent stored in fat. As mentioned above, some of the glucose is converted to alanine and lactate and recycled back to liver glycogen. The remainder is either stored as muscle glycogen or oxidized (following a meal, glucose oxidation replaces lipid oxidation to produce energy).

Normal postprandial changes in concentrations of glucose and insulin are shown in Figure 8–3. Blood samples were taken each hour from subjects fed three meals at the indicated times. Each meal consisted of 600 calories, of which 40% were carbohydrate, 20% protein, and 40%

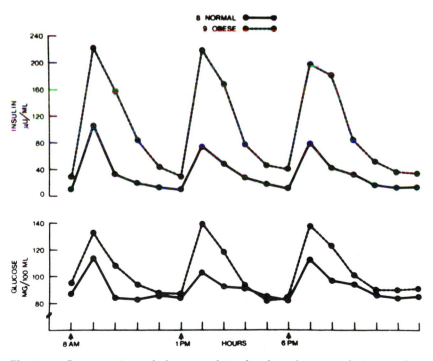

Fig. 8–3. Concentrations of glucose and insulin throughout a 16-hour period in subjects who had normal carbohydrate tolerance and ate three identical meals. (Reprinted with permission from Genuth, S.M.: Ann Intern Med, *79*:812–822, 1973.)

fat. Approximately half of the carbohydrate was in the simple form. All subjects were considered to have normal carbohydrate metabolism, but glucose concentrations were higher in the obese individuals whose weights ranged from 169 to 315% of their ideal body weight. Glucose values peaked 1 hour after a meal and had returned to basal levels 3 to 4 hours later. The glucose elevations were modest, especially in lean subjects. Insulin concentrations followed a similar pattern, peaking 1 hour after a meal and returning to baseline levels by 3 to 4 hours. The hyperinsulinemia, which is a result of the insulin antagonism caused by obesity, is well demonstrated in these overweight subjects.

HYPOGLYCEMIA

Definition

Hypoglycemia is a biochemical abnormality that has many causes. First, one has to document the low glucose concentration. Then, one systematically determines which condition is responsible for it.

The glucose concentration measured in whole blood is approximately 15% lower than that measured in plasma or serum because approximately 30% of the red cell is composed of solid material that is not capable of dissolving glucose. Thus, when whole blood is used, glucose is distributed in only 85% of the volume tested (assuming a hematocrit of 50%). Since this result is expressed per milliliter, the value for whole blood is actually 15% (not 15 mg/100 ml) less than that for plasma or serum. In adults, plasma or serum glucose concentrations of less than 50 mg/100 ml (and of whole blood less than 40 mg/100 ml) are abnormally low following oral glucose. In the fasting state, plasma glucose concentrations of less than 60 mg/100 ml (50 mg/100 ml for whole blood) signify hypoglycemia.

Hormonal Responses to Hypoglycemia

Glucoreceptors in the hypothalamus initiate certain hormonal responses (catecholamines, glucagon, growth hormone, cortisol) to low concentrations of glucose or to rapidly falling concentrations that are not yet in the hypoglycemic range. (Glucagon secretion from the α-cell located in the pancreatic islets of Langerhans may also be stimulated directly by glucose deprivation itself.) The released hormones stimulate potent metabolic mechanisms that prevent glucose concentrations from dropping to dangerously low levels. The four hormones secreted in response to hypoglycemia are depicted in Figure 8–4; in the study illustrated, hypoglycemia was induced by an I.V. insulin tolerance test. The nadir of glucose concentrations is reached 20 minutes after injection of insulin. Secretion of epinephrine, norepinephrine, and glucagon quickly increases, whereas that of cortisol and growth hormone increases more slowly. Secretion of the latter two hormones is sustained, whereas concentrations of the catecholamines and glucagon return almost to basal levels 2 hours after the administration of insulin.

In response to hypoglycemia, glucose concentrations are increased by the following mechanisms. A signal emanating from the hypothalamus increases the activity of the sympathetic nervous system; this increase is reflected by increased levels of norepinephrine and epinephrine in plasma. The sympathetic nerve endings in the liver and pancreas stimulate directly hepatic glycogenolysis and glucagon secretion, respectively. Epinephrine secretion by the adrenal medulla stimulated by the sympathetic nervous system increases blood sugar levels by: (a) stimulating hepatic glycogenolysis; (b) inhibiting muscle utilization of glucose; (c) stimulating glucagon secretion; and (d) inhibiting insulin secretion. Glucagon stimulates both hepatic glycogenolysis and gluconeogenesis but has no effect on the utilization of glucose by peripheral tissues. Cortisol increases hepatic gluconeogenesis. The major effect of growth hormone is to block peripheral glucose utilization. This hormone may also increase hepatic gluconeogenesis. There is a 1- to 2-hour lag period before growth hormone and cortisol begin to act, and their effects may last for 4 to 6 hours.

Thus, the response to hypoglycemia is finely orchestrated (Table 8–1). The activation of the

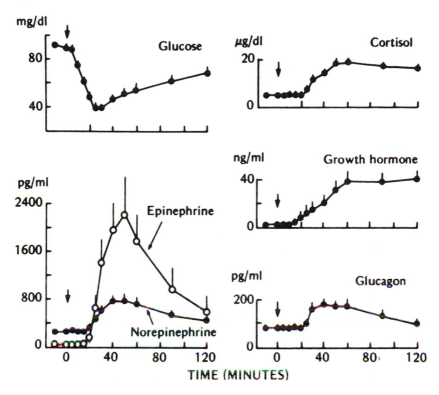

Fig. 8–4. Hormonal responses to hypoglycemia induced by insulin (0.15 U/kg) in six normal subjects. (Reprinted with permission from Cryer, P.E.: Diagnostic Endocrinology. London, Oxford University Press, 1976.

autonomic nervous system and of epinephrine and glucagon secretion is quick and has a rapid effect that is soon dissipated. The secretion of cortisol and growth hormone is somewhat delayed, and their effects are further delayed and last for many hours. Therefore, antihypoglycemic factors (termed counterregulatory hormones) start to exert their effects almost immediately after hypothalamic recognition of a low or rapidly falling glucose concentration and continue to operate for 4 to 6 hours.

Although it is not germane to the diagnosis and treatment of hypoglycemia, it is important to realize that these hormonal responses to hypoglycemia are altered in Type 1 diabetic patients. (See below for discussion of Type 1 and Type 2 diabetes.) Selective blockade of each of these hormones during insulin-induced hypoglycemia revealed that: (a) as long as glucagon was secreted, glucose levels were restored normally; (b) if glucagon was absent but the catecholamines were present, restoration was delayed but eventually occurred; (c) growth hormone and cortisol secretion was unnecessary for return of glucose levels to normal, at least in the short term; and (d) if both glucagon and catecholamines were absent, glucose concentrations remained at the nadir levels. This latter observation becomes extremely important in type 1 diabetic patients because within a year or two of diagnosis, the glucagon response to hypoglycemia is impaired even though glucagon is hypersecreted in these patients under other circumstances. By 4 years after the diagnosis, the glucagon response is minimal. Furthermore, the catecholamine response to hypoglycemia may become blunted after 5 years of type 1 diabetes. Thus, in type 1 patients who have had their diabetes for more than 5 years, there is a good chance that secretion of both of the critical hormones necessary to respond to hypoglycemia is either absent or markedly impaired. This has important ramifications for treating these insulin-requiring patients. Secretion of the counterregulatory hormones remains either intact, or nearly so, in type 2 diabetic patients.

Table 8–1. Hormonal Responses to Hypoglycemia

Hormone	Onset of Secretion	Action	Effects
Epinephrine	Rapid	Rapid	Inhibits glucose utilization by muscle; increases hepatic glycogenolysis and gluconeogenesis; stimulates glucagon secretion; inhibits insulin secretion
Glucagon	Rapid	Rapid	Increases hepatic glycogenolysis; increases hepatic gluconeogenesis
Cortisol	Delayed	Delayed	Increases hepatic gluconeogenesis
Growth hormone	Delayed	Delayed	Inhibits glucose utilization by muscle; increases hepatic gluconeogenesis (?)

Table 8–2. Signs and Symptoms of Hypoglycemia

Adrenergic[a]	Neuroglucopenic[b]
Weakness	Headache
Sweating	Hypothermia
Tachycardia	Visual disturbances
Palpitations	Mental dullness
Tremor	Confusion
Nervousness	Amnesia
Irritability	Seizures
Tingling of mouth and fingers	Coma
Hunger	
Nausea[c]	
Vomiting[c]	

[a]caused by increased activity of the autonomic nervous system; may be triggered by a rapid fall in the glucose concentration.
[b]caused by decreased activity of the central nervous system; require an absolutely low level of glucose.
[c]unusual

Signs and Symptoms

The signs and symptoms of hypoglycemia (Table 8–2) fall into two categories: adrenergic (those caused by increased activity of the automatic nervous system) and neuroglucopenic (those caused by depressed activity of the central nervous system). Since the hypothalamic glucoreceptors can sense a rapid fall in glucose concentrations, a subject may show adrenergic signs and symptoms at a time when glucose levels are only mildly decreased, normal, or even high (i.e., if the patient is a diabetic who has recently taken regular insulin). If glucose concentrations fall slowly enough, however, the autonomic nervous system may not be activated, and only the neuroglucopenic signs and symptoms will appear. Many of the latter are similar to some of the signs and symptoms of cerebral hypoxia. They develop only in the presence of low glucose levels, and not simply with rapidly changing concentrations. Although the signs and symptoms of hypoglycemia vary widely among subjects, the pattern in an individual patient tends to be similar during each episode. It cannot be emphasized too strongly that hypoglycemia does not cause allergies, alcoholism, drug addiction, depression, sexual dysfunction, chronic fatigue, poor concentration, behavioral problems, and other such maladies.

Although mental deterioration and even schizophrenia have been reported to be possible permanent sequelae of hypoglycemia, such an association is extremely rare and is found only after repeated and profound hypoglycemic episodes.

Classification

A functional classification of most causes of adult hypoglycemia is given in Table 8–3. This classification separates the causes into fasting and fed hypoglycemias, a useful approach in the work-up of individual patients. It is extremely important to ascertain whether the hypoglycemia occurs in the fasting state (i.e., after an overnight fast or when a meal is missed) or only after eating. Because the onset of fasting hypoglycemia is often gradual, the adrenergic component of the signs and symptoms is minimal or absent in many cases. Fasting hypoglycemia is usually persistent and requires glucose administration for reversal. The fasting hypoglycemias are potentially much more serious than the fed hypoglycemias.

Table 8–3.   Differential Diagnosis of Hypoglycemia in Adults

Fasting	Fed (Reactive)
Drugs[a]	Hyperalimentation
Ethanol	Impaired glucose tolerance
Non-β-cell tumors	Idiopathic reactive
Hepatic failure	Adrenal insufficiency[b]
Adrenal insufficiency	β-cell tumors (insulinomas)[b]
Renal failure	Insulin autoantibodies[c]
β-cell tumors (insulinomas)	
Insulin autoantibodies	
Insulin receptor autoantibodies	
Sepsis	

[a]includes factitious hypoglycemia
[b]although fed hypoglycemia occasionally occurs, fasting hypoglycemia predominates
[c]experience is too limited to determine which form of hypoglycemia predominates

Hypoglycemia can occur both in the fasting state and after meals in three situations: adrenal insufficiency, the presence of insulinomas, and the presence of autoantibodies to insulin. All of the other factors and conditions listed in Table 8–3 cause either fasting *or* postprandial hypoglycemia. This fact underscores the importance of determining whether the signs and symptoms occur in the fasted state or after a meal in a patient with suspected hypoglycemia. This distinction is also helpful in cases involving adrenal insufficiency or insulinomas, because in these instances fasting hypoglycemia is much more prominent than postprandial hypoglycemia, which is usually not evident. Whether fasting hypoglycemia predominates in patients with autoantibodies to insulin cannot be determined because the number of reported cases are small.

Fasting Hypoglycemias

Drugs. The most common form of fasting hypoglycemia is drug ingestion (Table 8–4). Drug-induced hypoglycemia is often associated with restricted food intake, hepatic or renal disease, ethanol intake (see below), old age, or a combination of these factors. Insulin is the drug most commonly associated with hypoglycemia, and the sulfonylurea agents are the next most common. Almost all hypoglycemia due to these 2 agents occurs in diabetic patients. In a few instances, emotionally disturbed nondiabetic patients take these drugs to induce hypoglycemia for secondary gain. The diagnosis of this factitious hypoglycemia will be discussed under β-cell tumors, a condition that is easy to confuse with surreptitious drug ingestion. Although the other drugs listed in Table 8–4 can cause hypoglycemia by potentiating the effects of insulin and sulfonylurea agents, they can also induce hypoglycemia by themselves. Salicylates, monoamine oxidase inhibitors, pentamidine, and quinine lower glucose concentrations by increasing insulin secretion. Although quinine-induced hypoglycemia is much more likely to occur in patients with severe Falciparum malaria, especially if they are pregnant, it can also be seen in patients without malaria. Although specific evidence is lacking, the other drugs must decrease hepatic glucose production directly since a normal fasting glucose concentration cannot be maintained in their presence.

Table 8–4.   Drugs Associated with Hypoglycemia

Common	Uncommon
Insulin	Salicylates
Sulfonylurea Agents	Propranolol (β-adrenergic antagonist)
	Monoamine oxidase inhibitors
	Disopyramide (Norpace)
	Pentamidine
	Quinine
	Oxytetracycline

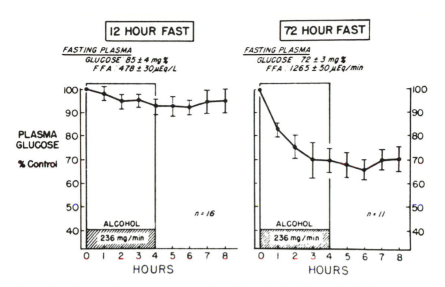

Fig. 8–5. Plasma glucose response to ethanol in fasted healthy subjects. The response is expressed as a percentage of the glucose concentration before infusion, which was set at 100%. FFA, free fatty acids. (Reprinted with permission from Arky, R.A., and Freinkel, N.V.: N Engl J Med, *274*:426–433, 1966.)

Ethanol. Ingestion of ethanol is associated with hypoglycemia much more frequently than the relatively small number of reports in the literature would suggest. Concomitant intake of ethanol has been noted in many of the reported cases of drug-induced hypoglycemia. Studies with normal volunteers suggest that ethanol causes hypoglycemia by interfering with gluconeogenesis (Fig. 8–5). After an overnight fast, a 4-hour infusion of ethanol has little effect on glucose concentrations. In fact, little effect would be expected, since, as discussed earlier, approximately 75% of hepatic glucose production at this time results from glycogenolysis. After 72 hours of fasting, when gluconeogenesis is the sole source of circulating glucose, the same infusion lowers glucose levels by 30%. The mechanism is related to the oxidation of ethanol to acetaldehyde and subsequently to acetate. Both reactions involve the reduction of diphosphopyridine nucleotide (NAD), and the resultant increase in the ratio of NADH (the reduced form) to NAD provides an unfavorable intracellular environment for gluconeogenesis. Therefore, alcoholic hypoglycemia is more likely under circumstances of restricted food intake. This condition often occurs in malnourished chronic alcoholics, but may also develop in heavy weekend drinkers or even in social drinkers who miss meals. It should be stressed that ethanol decreases glucose concentrations in patients with normal liver function. Children are particularly sensitive to this effect of alcohol. Clinically, the neuroglucopenic signs and symptoms predominate in alcoholic hypoglycemia. The adrenergic response is often diminished or absent, possibly because of the gradual decrease in glucose levels. Prompt diagnosis and treatment are important. The failure to recognize this syndrome may be responsible for the high mortality: estimated at approximately 25% in children and 10% in adults.

Non-β-Cell Tumors. A number of non-β-cell tumors are associated with hypoglycemia. Large, relatively rare, mesenchymal tumors account for approximately one-half to two-thirds of the cases reported. The tumors weigh at least 1 kg and are located in the thorax, retroperitoneal space, or pelvic area. These mesenchymal tumors, many of which are benign, include mesotheliomas, fibrosarcomas, neurofibromas, neurofibrosarcomas, spindle cell sarcomas, leiomyosarcomas, and rhabdomyosarcomas. The next most common cause of tumor hypoglycemia is the hepatocellular carcinoma (hepatoma), which accounts for approximately 20 to 25% of cases of hypoglycemia associated with tumors. Adrenal carcinomas, gastrointestinal tumors, and lymphomas account for 5 to 10% each. Most other tumors have occasionally been associated with hypoglycemia. Of these remaining types, kidney tumors, lung tumors, anaplastic carcinomas, and carcinoid tumors are most commonly associated with hypoglycemia.

The mechanism whereby any of these non-β-cell tumors causes hypoglycemia is not clear. Although it is commonly held that glucose requirements of the large mesenchymal tumors eventually exceed the ability of the liver to produce glucose and thereby lead to hypoglycemia, good evidence for this sequence of events is lacking. Indeed, in a few studies in which glucose kinetics were evaluated under such circumstances, hepatic glucose production was found to be decreased. Immunoreactive insulin has been extracted from a few of the involved tumors. However, in view of: (a) evidence that extracts of most normal tissues contain immunoreactive insulin; (b) normal or low concentrations of insulin in the plasma of these patients; and (c) failure to demonstrate the actual release of insulin (by arteriovenous differences across the tumor at surgery), it can be asserted that few, if any, of these cases of hypoglycemia are caused by tumor secretion of the same hormone (i.e., insulin) contained in the pancreatic β-cell.

A likely explanation for many cases of tumor hypoglycemia is the synthesis and release of certain polypeptide growth factors that also have hypoglycemic properties. It has been known for many years that most of the insulin-like activity of plasma measured in vitro was not attributable to insulin, since very little of this activity was neutralized or suppressed by antibodies to the hormone. The material responsible for these findings was termed nonsuppressible insulin-like activity, or NSILA. Further work has identified two compounds of relatively small molecular weight that are soluble in ethanol and are designated NSILA-S. A compound of greater molecular weight that precipitates in alcohol has been isolated and is designated NSILA-P. NSILA-S has been shown to be composed of two separate insulin-like growth factors, IGF-1 and IGF-2. An older term for IGF-1 was somatomedin C. These peptides promote growth of tissues as well as stimulation of carbohydrate metabolism.

All three hypoglycemic growth factors, IGF-1, IGF-2, and NSILA-P, have been found to be elevated in the circulation of some (but not all) patients with non-β-cell tumor hypoglycemia. A refinement of assay techniques and a much clearer understanding of these polypeptides will be required to substantiate this hypothesis.

Hepatic Failure. Death from hepatic failure is common, but associated hypoglycemia is distinctly unusual. This is because the liver has a tremendous capacity to produce glucose, and hypoglycemia ensues only when the liver is severely compromised. The diagnosis is obvious since the patient has all of the clinical and laboratory stigmata of hepatic failure. Although treatment is simple (i.e., support of the glucose concentration with I.V., dextrose until the liver regenerates the capacity to maintain appropriate levels itself), hypoglycemia in this situation is a serious prognostic sign, indicating that there is little functioning hepatic tissue left. Indeed, the capacity of the liver to produce glucose may be restored and the patient may still succumb to the other complications of hepatic failure.

Adrenal Insufficiency. An important cause of fasting hypoglycemia is adrenal insufficiency. The mechanism by which this hormonal deficiency causes hypoglycemia is decreased hepatic gluconeogenesis. A high index of suspicion is often necessary for consideration of the diagnosis that is made by appropriate testing of the pituitary-adrenal axis. Replacement with glucocorticoids is an effective treatment. Because patients with pituitary insufficiency who are treated with glucocorticoids do not have difficulties with hypoglycemia, growth hormone deficiency does not cause hypoglycemia in the adult (although it may in small children).

Renal Failure. Hypoglycemia accompanying renal failure is being increasingly recognized. A clear-cut picture of the setting in which this syndrome is most likely to occur has not yet emerged. Insulin requirements have long been known to decrease in diabetic patients with progressive uremia and this decrement can happen rapidly in patients with acute renal failure. However, fasting hypoglycemia occurs in uremic diabetic patients who either are taking sulfonylurea agents or are controlled with dietary therapy alone; it has also been reported in uremic nondiabetic individuals. The relation of the hypoglycemic episodes to dialysis is variable. Although poor dietary intake has been associated with many of the reported cases, some patients are clearly well fed. Most authors suggest that impairment of hepatic gluconeogenesis underlies the hypoglycemia. On the other hand, some patients remain hypoglycemic despite the I.V. administration of large amounts of glucose. This latter finding points toward enhanced glucose use in this situation.

Insulinomas (β-Cell Tumors). Although insulinomas (β-cell tumors) are rare, they are an important cause of fasting hypoglycemia. They are usually curable but may have permanent neuropsychiatric effects on the patient if the diagnosis is missed. Of these patients, 80 to 90% have single tumors while 10 to 20% have multiple tumors. Approximately 90% of these tumors are benign and 10% are malignant although histologically this distinction can be difficult. Hyperplasia of the β-cell, as part of the multiple endocrine adenomatosis type 1 syndrome, is rare. The mechanism of the hypoglycemia is uncontrolled secretion of insulin.

Insulinomas are small tumors (usually <2 cm in diameter) located with equal frequency in the tail, body, and head of the pancreas. Women develop insulinomas more commonly than do men. These tumors usually become manifest between the ages of 30 and 50 years; patients almost invariably present clinically with fasting hypoglycemia. Since the glucose level often drifts down slowly in affected patients, adrenergic signs and symptoms (Table 8–2) are often lacking and the presence of hypoglycemia may thus be obscured. Patients with insulinomas tend to present with the more confusing neuroglucopenic signs and symptoms that can include visual difficulties, transient neurologic syndromes, mental confusion, convulsions, and personality changes. Weight gain is common in these patients because chronic hyperinsulinemia and hypoglycemia lead to excessive caloric intake and subsequent fat deposition.

The diagnosis of a β-cell tumor is usually not difficult once it is considered. The cardinal rule in the evaluation of glandular function is to stimulate the gland if hypofunction is suspected and to suppress it if hyperfunction is suspected. The most physiologic test to suppress insulin secretion is fasting. Characteristic changes in the relation between glucose and insulin concentrations during total caloric deprivation are the most reliable diagnostic criteria for insulinomas and will be found in almost every patient who is tested appropriately. Levels of both glucose and insulin fall during starvation (Fig. 8–2). As mentioned earlier, in some individuals, especially women, plasma glucose concentrations commonly decrease asymptomatically to values as low as 30 to 35 mg/100 ml after 24 to 72 hours without food. However, insulin levels fall disproportionally more than the glucose concentrations. Therefore, the most reliable way to diagnose a β-cell tumor is simply to extend an overnight fast until the patient becomes symptomatic. Blood samples for glucose and insulin determinations are drawn after the overnight fast and then every 4 hours. Approximately two-thirds of the patients will experience hypoglycemic symptoms within the first 24 hours of food deprivation. Another one-quarter or so will become symptomatic during the second 24 hours of starvation. A third day of fasting is required in fewer than 5% of patients who harbor insulinomas. The response to fasting is evaluated by calculating the insulin (μU/ml) to glucose ratio. Values >0.3 are abnormal. This is illustrated in Figure 8–6. The 12 control subjects were women whose glucose concentrations fell to <35 mg/100 ml during 72 hours of fasting. Nevertheless, their insulin-to-glucose ratios all decreased, and in 11 of the 12 this value fell considerably. In contrast, the insulin-to-glucose ratios increased in 6 patients with verified insulinomas during the 10 to 36 hours in which they were able to fast. The fasting data, shown in Figure 8–6 in the normal women, are for the times at which the glucose concentration was lowest.

One specialized test can be helpful in confirming or occasionally even establishing the diagnosis of an insulinoma. Insulin is synthesized via a single-chain precursor called proinsulin. Enzymes cleave the proinsulin molecule into insulin and a connecting (C-) peptide, both of which remain stored in the granules of the normal β-cell (Fig. 8–7). At the time of secretion, both insulin and the C-peptide are released along with a small amount of intact

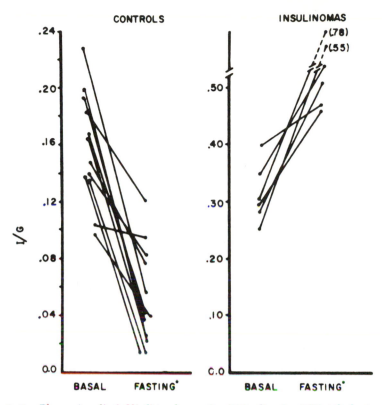

Fig. 8-6. Plasma insulin (μU/ml)-to-glucose (mg/100 ml) ratios (I/G) at the beginning of a fast (basal) and at the nadir of the glucose concentration. (Reprinted with permission from Merimee, T.J., and Tyson, J.E.: Diabetes, *26*:161, 1977.)

proinsulin. The antibodies used to measure plasma insulin also react with proinsulin (but not with C-peptide). Therefore, the insulin concentration that is measured is really the sum of the concentrations of insulin and proinsulin. Under normal circumstances, proinsulin constitutes <20% of the fasting insulin concentration. In patients with an insulinoma, the percentage of proinsulin in fasting serum samples is almost always elevated.

An occasional patient with an insulinoma does not manifest hypoglycemia after 72 hours of fasting. In this situation, the diagnosis can be established by the high proportion of proinsulin in a sample obtained after an overnight fast.

No stimulatory tests are recommended for the diagnosis of an insulinoma. In the past, stimulation of insulin secretion by administration of tolbutamide, glucagon, calcium, or leucine was suggested for this purpose. However, many false-negative results and even some false-positive results occur in these tests. There is no rationale for an oral glucose tolerance test in a patient in whom an insulinoma is suspected. Because normal, impaired, and flat oral glucose tolerance test results are all seen in patients with β-cell tumors, this test is

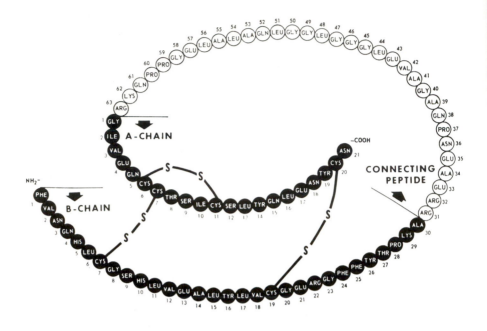

Fig. 8–7. Structure of porcine proinsulin. Cleavage occurs at the straight lines, yielding equimolar amounts of the connecting C-peptide and insulin. (From Chance, R.E.: Diabetes, *21* (Suppl. 2):461, 1972. Reproduced with permission.)

distinctly unrewarding in this situation (as well as in all other conditions of fasting hypoglycemia) and should be avoided.

Once the presence of an insulinoma is established biochemically, localization of the tumor is extremely helpful to the surgeon because of the small size of this type of lesion. This can be accomplished by arteriography (successful in approximately 50% of patients) and computed tomographic (CT) scanning with enhancement by contrast material (successful in the majority of patients although experience is still too limited to be certain what percentage). It should be emphasized, that once the insulin-to-glucose ratios establish the diagnosis, the surgeon should proceed even if the lesion has not been pinpointed preoperatively. The tumor is often identified only under the scrutiny of a skilled surgeon.

Factitious. In many cases, once the biochemical hallmarks of an insulinoma are found, factitious hypoglycemia must be considered. In this unusual form of drug-induced hypoglycemia, emotionally disturbed patients surreptitiously take insulin or sulfonylurea agents. These individuals are usually women in health-related occupations or relatives of diabetic patients who are legitimately taking these drugs. Patients with factitious hypoglycemia often undergo extensive medical testing, and even repeated laparotomies with eventually total pancreatectomy, without divulging the true nature of their hypoglycemia. The major diagnostic problem is to distinguish factitious hypoglycemia from β-cell tumors of the pancreas, since the biochemical hallmark of both conditions are a low glucose concentration with a relatively high insulin concentration. Because administration of insulin and sulfonylurea agents also cause this combination of low glucose and high insulin levels, differentiation between the two conditions may seem difficult at first glance. Fortunately, new techniques for measuring insulin antibodies, C-peptide, and metabolites of the sulfonylurea agents permit the identification of patients with factitious hypoglycemia once the proper diagnosis is suspected.

Daily administration of insulin to diabetic patients over a period of several months causes the production of IgG insulin-binding antibodies. Therefore, the presence of these antibodies in a patient in whom factitious hypoglycemia is suspected (and who is not an insulin-dependent diabetic) provides fairly good evidence for the diagnosis if insulin administration has occurred frequently. The measurement of C-peptide (Fig. 8–7) should reliably distinguish between factitious hypoglycemia and β-cell tumors. Insulin and C-peptide are secreted from the pancreatic β-cell in equimolar amounts. However, because C-peptide is only minimally degraded by the liver, its half-life is much longer than that of insulin. Consequently, C-peptide concentrations are proportionately higher than insulin levels after secretion. On the other hand, commercial insulin preparations do not contain C-peptide. Therefore, a combination of low concentrations of glucose and C-peptide with high concentrations of insulin assures the diagnosis of factitious hypoglycemia secondary to administration of exogenous insulin, whereas a combination of low glucose concentration with high insulin and C-peptide levels usually indicates secretion of endogenous insulin. Since surreptitious administration of sulfonylurea agents also results in the latter combination, measurement of the appropriate compounds in serum or urine is necessary in order to rule out this cause of factitious hypoglycemia.

Autoantibodies to the Insulin Molecule. In recent years, the spontaneous development of hypoglycemia for no apparent reason has been described in a few patients. During their evaluations, extremely elevated "insulin" concentrations were noted. Upon further testing, autoantibodies to the insulin molecule were measured in the plasma of these patients. These autoantibodies caused the spuriously high values for insulin allegedly found in the radioimmunoassay. None of these patients had ever received exogenous insulin. Hypoglycemia associated with autoantibodies to insulin has been reported in patients with Graves' disease, rheumatoid arthritis and lupus erythematosus. These cases suggest that the formation of autoantibodies to insulin may be associated with the general syndromes of autoimmunity. The mechanism involved in the hypoglycemia is probably related to the binding of large amounts of endogenous insulin with the subsequent release of free insulin at inappropriate times. Although most of the patients had both fasting and postprandial hypoglycemia, a few seemed to experience postprandial episodes only.

Autoantibodies to the Insulin Receptor. An occasional patient (usually female) has a syndrome of insulin resistance and acanthosis nigricans associated with the following conditions in various combinations: obesity, hirsutism, amenorrhea, polycystic ovaries, and certain immunologic features, such as elevated erythrocyte sedimentation rates, high titers of antinuclear and anti-DNA antibodies, and decreased complement levels. Affected patients also have autoantibodies to the insulin receptor (not to the insulin molecule). The presence of these antibodies accounts for insulin resistance in these patients since insulin is unable to exert its action at the critical initial step of binding. A few of these patients inexplicably manifest recurrent hypoglycemia. One patient with an autoantibody to the insulin receptor had only hypoglycemia and no evidence of insulin resistance. The hypoglycemia in these cases is probably due to an insulin-like effect of the antibody after binding to the receptor, a sequence of events for which there is good evidence.

Sepsis. Hypoglycemia is not clinically associated with infection. In fact, insulin antagonism and hyperglycemia have been described in conjunction with infection. However, a few patients have been described in whom hypoglycemia was associated with overwhelming sepsis and no other cause for hypoglycemia could be found. With regard to possible mechanisms, the administration of endotoxin (produced by gram-negative organisms) to animals causes hypoglycemia, probably through an inhibition of hepatic gluconeogenesis, but some of the patients described were infected with gram-positive organisms.

Miscellaneous. There are also some other rare causes of fasting hypoglycemia. A few patients with *congestive heart failure* have developed fasting hypoglycemia. Common features have included weight loss, anorexia, low cardiac output, and only mild hepatic dysfunction. In such instances, hypoglycemia is postulated to be secondary to decreased delivery of gluconeogenic substrates to the liver as a result of poor appetite and diminished hepatic blood flow. In view of the extremely high prevalence of congestive heart failure and the mere handful of reported cases of hypoglycemia, this association is probably quite rare.

Eating *unripe fruit from the akee tree,* which is found in West Africa and Jamaica, is associated with vomiting and hypoglycemia. The toxic ingredient, called hypoglycin, causes the accumulation of medium-chain dicarboxylic acids. This indicates that hypoglycin interferes with the normal sequence of β-oxidation of long-chain fatty acids in the liver that is necessary for gluconeogenesis. Once the akee fruit ripens, it no longer produces hypoglycin.

Moderate hypoglycemia often occurs in *protein-calorie malnutrition* (kwashiorkor). Severe hypoglycemia is rare and is usually fatal when it does occur. Although involuntary protein-calorie malnutrition to this degree would be quite rare in a developed country, voluntary *inanition* of this magnitude occasionally occurs in patients with marked anorexia nervosa. Curiously, the resulting hypoglycemia seems refractory to infusions of large amounts of glucose.

Inborn errors of metabolism in both the carbohydrate and lipid pathways may also occasionally lead to fasting hypoglycemia in adults. Examples of the former are deficiencies of glucose-6-phosphatase, amylo-1,6-glucosidase (debrancher enzyme), fructose-1, 6-diphosphatase, and fructose-1-phosphate aldolase (hereditary fructose intolerance). Examples of the latter are systemic carnitine deficiency and glutaric aciduria, type 2. Finally, there are rare patients in whom the cause of well-documented, recurrent fasting hypoglycemia is unclear with our present state of knowledge.

Fed (Reactive) Hypoglycemias

In contrast to the signs and symptoms of fasting hypoglycemia, those of fed (reactive) hypoglycemia are predominantly adrenergic. Their onset is characteristically rapid. The neuroglucopenic component is unusual in reactive hypoglycemia. This type of hypoglycemia is transient and is usually reversed by normal hormonal responses (Table 8–1). Administration of exogenous glucose will hasten, but is not necessary for, the abatement of the adrenergic signs and symptoms.

The differential diagnosis of fed hypoglycemia is described in Table 8–3. As discussed earlier, two of the six causes listed (adrenal insufficiency and insulinomas) cause predominantly fasting hypoglycemia. This may be true also for a third cause, the presence of autoantibodies to insulin, although there are too few reported cases on which to base a firm conclusion. The remaining three diagnoses listed must be considered when a patient gives a history suggestive of postprandial hypoglycemia only: hyperalimentation, impaired glucose tolerance, and idiopathic reactive hypoglycemia.

Hyperalimentation

The normal responses to an oral glucose challenge are peak glucose and insulin concentrations at ½ to 1 hour, with a subsequent return toward fasting levels (Fig. 8–8). In the fed hypoglycemic seen after gastrectomy or a drainage procedure on the stomach (labeled in Fig. 8–9 as alimentary hyperglycemia), the mechanism appears to be the rapid absorption of glucose from the small intestine. This rapid absorption of glucose leads to an excessive insulin response and subsequent hypoglycemia occurring usually within two hours. The initial glucose levels are often high, sometimes exceeding 300 mg/100 ml. A diagnosis is easily made by taking a careful history.

Impaired Glucose Tolerance (IGT)

The second cause of fed hypoglycemia is IGT (formerly called latent or chemical diabetes mellitus, and labeled in Fig. 8–9 as diabetes). The mechanism seems to be a delayed rise of insulin that peaks late (Fig. 8–9). This delayed peak drives down the glucose concentration between 3 and 5 hours

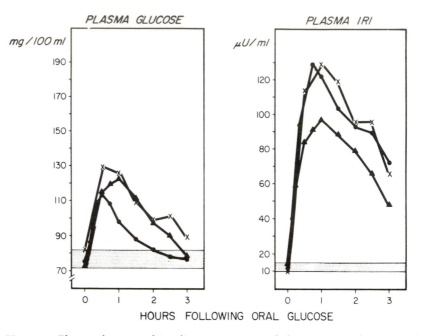

Fig. 8–8. Plasma glucose and insulin responses to oral glucose in nonobese normal subjects. ●=●, n = 21; ▲=▲, n = 9; x=x, n = 17. (Results of three separate studies reviewed by Freinkel, N., and Metzger, B.F.: Reprinted, by permission, from N Engl J Med, *280*:820, 1969.)

after carbohydrate ingestion. That the early glucose concentrations are higher than normal suggests the diagnosis of impaired glucose tolerance.

Idiopathic

The third cause of reactive hypoglycemia is the most controversial. Formerly called functional hypoglycemia, it is often the subject of much publicity in the press. A better term is idiopathic reactive hypoglycemia. The pattern is one of normal glucose concentrations early in the glucose tolerance test with later hypoglycemia occurring 3 to 5 hours after oral administration of glucose (Fig. 8–9). The mechanism is uncertain. Excessive insulin secretion can be shown in some patients and increased intestinal absorption of glucose in a few others. However, in most patients, the mechanism remains unknown. Idiopathic reactive hypoglycemia is uncommon. Overdiagnosis is due to the fact that low glucose levels 3 to 5 hours after oral glucose are a normal occurrence in the healthy population. Up to one-third of normal subjects, especially if they are young and overweight, have plasma glucose levels below 60 mg/100 ml after an oral glucose load. The prevalence of "hypoglycemia" was almost 1 in 3 among young obese women; approximately 1 in 5 among young, relatively thin females; 1 in 10 among older obese subjects; but only 1 in 50 among older thin individuals. A high prevalence of low glucose levels during an oral glucose tolerance test is not limited to females. The results of

LATE HYPOGLYCEMIA FOLLOWING ORAL GLUCOSE LOAD (100 gm)

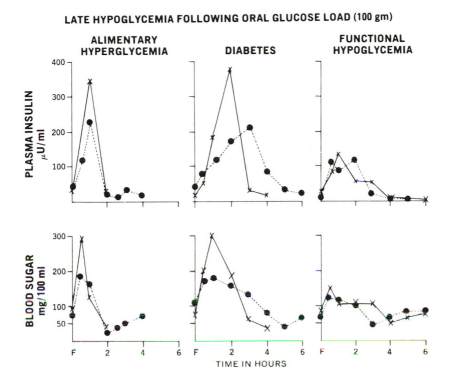

Fig. 8–9. Glucose and insulin responses in reactive hypoglycemia. Each curve represents an individual patient. (From Conn, J.W., and Pek, S.: Current concepts: on spontaneous hypoglycemia. Scope monograph published by the Upjohn Co., Kalamazoo, Mich., 1970. Reproduced with permission.)

measuring glucose concentrations 2 hours after the ingestion of 100 g of dextrose in almost 5,000 inductees into the U.S. Army are shown in Figure 8–10. Approximately 2% had plasma glucose concentrations below 40 mg/ 100 ml. Plasma glucose levels were between 40 and 49 mg/100 ml in another 7% and between 50 and 59 mg/100 ml in 16%. Thus, one-quarter of healthy young men had plasma glucose concentrations below 60 mg/100 ml 2 hours after oral glucose challenge! The prevalence of low glucose values would certainly have been much higher if values at later times had also been included. Two other large series comprising both men and women have been reported. In one, 24% of 147 subjects had nadir plasma glucose levels <50 mg/100 ml. In the other in which 650 oral glucose tolerance tests were evaluated, 2.5% of the nadir glucose concentrations were <39 mg/100 ml, 5% were <43 mg/100 ml, 10% were <47 mg/100 ml, and 25% were <54 mg/100 ml.

Therefore, since relatively low glucose concentrations after an oral dextrose

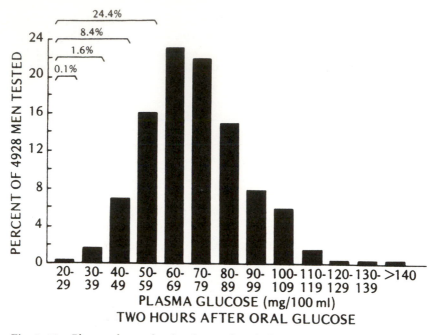

Fig. 8–10. Plasma glucose levels 2 hours after challenge with a 100-g oral glucose load in overtly healthy, young adult men. The results are expressed as the percentage falling into each glucose range listed on the horizontal axis. The cumulative frequency of the lower values is shown in the upper left part of the figure. (Reprinted with permission from Cryer, P.E.: Diagnostic Endocrinology. London, Oxford University Press, 1976.)

challenge are so common, *an oral glucose tolerance test (OGTT) is inappropriate to diagnose reactive hypoglycemia.* Seventy-five to 100 g of simple carbohydrate is hardly a physiologic stimulus. A low blood sugar must occur after the patient eats his or her usual diet, that is, in an environment in which their symptoms are taking place. Thus, to make a valid diagnosis of idiopathic reactive hypoglycemia, four criteria have to be met:

1. Hypoglycemia has to be documented (a plasma glucose level below 50 mg/100 ml or a whole blood glucose level below 40 mg/100 ml).
2. Symptoms of which the patient complains must occur at this time.
3. These symptoms have to be relieved quickly (within 10 to 20 minutes, not 1 to 2 hours) by eating.
4. This pattern (symptoms of hypoglycemia after meals, relieved quickly by eating) must be regular, rather than an isolated occurrence.

In my experience, only a few individuals meet this criteria. Usually, a patient gives a vague history that includes some of the following: tiredness, lethargy, anxiety, weakness, depression, mental dullness, headache, paresthesia, loss of vitality, irritability, and a "trembly" feeling inside. It is usually difficult to obtain a clear description of these symptoms; rather, the history is characterized by its vagueness. There is no clear relation between food intake and either the onset or the relief of symptoms. Patients often wake up with symptoms, many of which improve only slowly (several hours) after eating. Other patients complain of the onset of symptoms within 30 to 60 minutes of eating. Unfortunately, these individuals are usually convinced they are "hypoglycemic" and that they will improve if only the correct diet, vitamin or mineral, or other nostrum is prescribed.

The reason for the overdiagnosis is that the signs and symptoms of anxiety and hypoglycemia are similar since they are both due, in large part, to excessive epinephrine secretion. Both patient and doctor, in seeking an organic cause for the various symptoms of psychoneurosis, have equated the commonly occurring low plasma glucose concentrations during an oral glucose tolerance test with the many psychogenic symptoms that unfortunately are also common in our population. Indeed, many patients with alleged symptoms of hypoglycemia have personality disorders as judged by both psychiatric interviews and Minnesota Multiphasic Personality Inventory testing. There are no correlations among their glucose tolerance, their alleged symptoms, and the severity of their personality disorder.

One other situation should be mentioned with regard to the diagnosis of idiopathic reactive hypoglycemia. Patients whose oral glucose tolerance tests give "flat" results are sometimes considered to have fed hypoglycemia. However, a flat glucose tolerance test result is seen in approximately 20% of the normal population (especially younger subjects) and simply reflects the efficiency of normal homeostatic mechanisms in disposing of an oral glucose load.

The treatment for all forms of reactive hypoglycemia is primarily dietary. Avoiding simple carbohydrates is usually all that is needed. If that does not suffice, a high protein, low carbohydrate diet (35% of calories derived from carbohydrate) should be tried. Multiple feedings (5 to 6 times a day) are sometimes necessary, especially after a gastrectomy. Weight loss in obese patients with impaired glucose tolerance is important. If these dietary measures fail, several drugs have been successful. Anticholinergic agents (which inhibit gastric emptying) can be helpful, but their unpleasant side effects limit their use. Propranolol (a β-adrenergic antagonist) has been found to be effective for unknown reasons. Diazoxide and phenytoin (Dilantin), both of which directly inhibit insulin secretion, have occasionally been used.

DIABETES MELLITUS

Diabetes mellitus has a tremendous impact, not only on the health of individuals, but also on the health care system in the United States. According to the National Commission on Diabetes, this disease now affects 5% of the population of this country (approximately 11 million people), and it is estimated that a similar number of patients remain undiagnosed. Because the incidence of diabetes is increasing by 6% per year, the size of the diabetic population will double in 15 years. Diabetes and its associated vascular complications are the third leading cause of death in this country. Diabetes is the leading cause of new cases of blindness in this country in individuals under 65 years of age. Compared with nondiabetics, diabetic patients are 25 times more likely to develop blindness, 17 times more likely to develop renal disease, 20 times more likely to develop gangrene, 30 to 40 times more likely to undergo a major amputation, and twice as likely to develop heart disease or suffer a stroke. Fourteen percent of diabetic patients (usually the elderly) are bedridden for an average of 6 weeks per year. The total annual economic impact of diabetes mellitus was estimated at more than 5 billion dollars in 1974, approximately 8 billion dollars in 1979 and 14 billion dollars in 1985.

Definition

Diabetes mellitus is a syndrome with both metabolic and vascular components that are probably interrelated. The metabolic syndrome is characterized by an inappropriate elevation of blood glucose concentrations associated with alterations in lipid and protein metabolism. The vascular syndrome consists of a nonspecific macroangiopathy (atherosclerosis which is no different pathologically than that which occurs in nondiabetic patients but appears earlier and often runs a more severe course) and a more specific microangiopathy, particularly affecting the eye and the kidney. The peripheral and autonomic nervous systems are also affected in a great many patients, secondary to hyperglycemia in most instances.

To appreciate the pathophysiology of the signs and symptoms of the metabolic syndrome of diabetes mellitus, it is helpful to describe a gradual worsening of glucose tolerance: from normalcy through mild to moderate glucose intolerance, progressing to fasting hyperglycemia, ketosis, and finally ketoacidosis. Most patients do not show this sort of progression. Many patients have impaired glucose tolerance (IGT) and are asymptomatic. Others manifest fasting hyperglycemia but only a minority are symptomatic. Most of these patients never become ketotic. A smaller number have ketosis, which may progress to frank ketoacidosis if not treated with insulin.

Carbohydrate Abnormality

Figure 8–11 depicts a series of oral glucose tolerance tests. For the sake of this discussion, imagine that these results are occurring after eating. The heavily shaded line between 1 and 2 hours represents the expected upper limits of glucose concentrations following a meal. The bottom two curves depicted in solid lines are examples of a mild carbohydrate abnormality that is certainly not diabetes mellitus but might fulfill the criteria of IGT on more formal testing (see below). These subjects have no signs or symptoms related directly to their abnormality in carbohydrate metabolism but may suffer from atherosclerosis.

The patients whose glucose tolerance curves are depicted by dashed lines in Fig. 8–11 have a more marked abnormality and would fulfill the criteria for diabetes mellitus (see below). These patients may complain of fatigue. If their postprandial glucose concentration exceeds the renal tubular threshold (T_m) for glucose (approximately 180 mg/100 ml in the presence of a normal

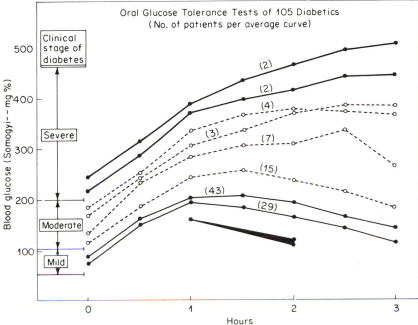

Correlation of Fasting Glucose Level with Severity of Diabetes

Fig. 8–11. Oral glucose tolerance tests in 105 diabetics with varying degrees of carbohydrate abnormality. (The numbers in parentheses on each curve represent the numbers of patients per average curve.) (From Seltzer, H.S.: Diagnosis of diabetes. *In* Diabetes Mellitus: Theory and Practice. Edited by M. Ellenberg and H. Rifkin. New York, McGraw-Hill Book Co., 1970. Used with permission.)

glomerular filtration rate), they show glucosuria at that time. On the other hand, if patients have more marked fasting hyperglycemia (upper two dashed curves in Fig. 8–11), their glucose concentrations throughout the day often exceed their T_m. Consequently, glucosuria may be a chronic condition and may lead to presence of glucose in the renal tubules that causes an osmotic diuresis. This mechanism accounts for a prevalent symptom in uncontrolled diabetes, *polyuria* (increased urination). The resultant fluid loss through the kidneys leads to a mild state of dehydration that the patient tries to correct by increasing water intake. This causes the second prevalent symptom of uncontrolled diabetes, *polydipsia* (increased thirst). If the glucose concentrations exceed the T_m overnight, the patient will experience *nocturia* (urination at night). Because of the decreased amount of effective insulin, the body is not able to use sufficient calories; this leads to the third prevalent symptom of uncontrolled diabetes, *polyphagia* (increased appetite) in the face of persistent weight loss. At this point, patients may show increased susceptibility to certain infections. Especially prominent are fungus *infections,* usually moniliasis, which appear as candidiasis of the vagina, nails, or occasionally the mouth (oral thrush) and infections due to Staphylococcus aureus, which are marked by recurrent furuncles or carbuncles. Patients may also have *blurring of vision* due to alterations in the shape of the lens that occur because of osmotic changes secondary to the hyperglycemia.

Ketosis

As the metabolic syndrome worsens because of less and less effective insulin, ketosis appears. Its mechanism is depicted in Figure 8–12. Insulin stimulates glucose uptake and utilization by muscle, liver, and adipose tissue. In muscle and adipose tissue, insulin stimulates glucose transport into the cells. The situation in the liver is more complex. Insulin increases the phos-

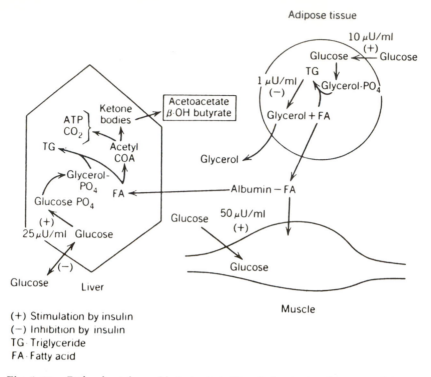

Fig. 8–12. Pathophysiology of ketosis. (+), Stimulation by insulin; (−), inhibition by insulin; TG, triglyceride; FA, fatty acid. See text for discussion.

phorylation of glucose rather than its transport. In addition, through mechanisms that are not entirely clear, insulin also inhibits hepatic glucose production. In vitro studies have shown that concentrations of insulin that increase glucose utilization by tissues range from 10 to 50 μU/ml.

Insulin also plays a critical role in controlling lipolysis of adipose tissue triglyceride. This reaction is sensitive to insulin; an effective insulin concentration of <5 μU/ml is sufficient to inhibit lipolysis. As discussed previously, the controlling factor for the production of ketone bodies is the amount of FFA delivered to the liver. Therefore, only when almost no effective insulin is left does uncontrolled lipolysis occur, flooding the liver with FFA and leading to an overproduction of ketone bodies. Put another way, as the amount of effective insulin becomes less and less, postprandial hyperglycemia supervenes because of the failure of glucose utilization by the tissues. Fasting hyperglycemia occurs when the amount of effective insulin remaining is unable to control hepatic glucose production overnight. As long as some effective insulin is left, however, lipolysis is controlled and ketone body production remains normal. When overproduction of ketone bodies occurs, effective insulin is essentially absent.

As more and more ketone bodies are produced, the peripheral tissues that use them soon become overwhelmed. They begin to accumulate and the patient then becomes ketotic. The only change in the signs and symptoms at this point is that polyphagia is no longer present because ketone bodies cause *anorexia* and mild *nausea*. Ketone bodies are acidic and therefore have to be buffered. If the body bases become depleted, the patient becomes acidotic. The acidosis due to an accumulation of ketone bodies is termed ketoacidosis which is almost invariably due to diabetes mellitus. The only other cause of ketoacidosis is in patients who are drinking heavily (alcoholic ketoacidosis).

Ketoacidosis

Pathophysiology. Although diabetic ketoacidosis (DKA) is caused by a profound lack of effective insulin, published studies routinely report some measurable insulin concentrations. However, these low levels (usually <10 µU/ml) are clearly inadequate in the metabolic milieu of marked hyperglycemia, ketosis, and acidosis. Although levels of the counterregulatory hormones (catecholamines, glucagon, growth hormone, and cortisol) are elevated as the result of stress, such elevations do not *cause* the metabolic derangements that lead to DKA. Elevated levels of these hormones potentiate the effect of a lack of insulin but patients can become at least mildly ketoacidotic in the absence of high levels of these hormones.

The clinical hallmarks of DKA are acidosis, dehydration, and electrolyte depletion. The mechanisms behind these conditions are outlined in Figure 8–13. The effect of a lack of insulin on all three general areas of metabolism—carbohydrate, protein, and fat—figures prominently in the pathophysiology of DKA. In the absence of effective insulin, ingested carbohydrate is not utilized by the three insulin-sensitive tissues (liver, muscle, and adipose tissues). This impairment of glucose uptake causes hyperglycemia. Not shown directly in Figure 8–13 is the effect of a lack of insulin on glucose production by the liver. In the late postprandial state, after the carbohydrate content of the diet has been stored, insulin is critically important in the modulation of glucose production by the liver. In the absence of insulin, unchecked hepatic glucose production further increases the already elevated glucose concentrations. Hyperglycemia, in turn, causes an osmotic diuresis that results in water and electrolyte depletion. The water and electrolyte losses cause dehydration, which is clinically manifest as intravascular volume depletion. The fluid losses are hypotonic to plasma and a hyperosmolar state therefore develops.

In protein metabolism, a lack of insulin reinforces fluid and electrolyte depletion. In the absence of effective insulin, the transport of amino acids into cells and the incorporation of these intracellular amino acids into protein are decreased. In addition, the normal inhibition of protein degradation by insulin is reversed. Therefore, the effects of a lack of insulin on amino acid transport, protein synthesis, and protein degradation all cause protein catabolism that results in increased release of amino acids from muscle tissue. Some of these amino acids are gluconeogenic precursors and are converted to glucose by the liver. The rate of gluconeogenesis is controlled by the amount of appropriate substrates delivered to the liver. Therefore, the increased flux of amino acids from muscle contributes significantly to hyperglycemia with its attendant fluid and electrolyte losses. The amino acids used for gluconeogenesis are metabolized in order to fulfill

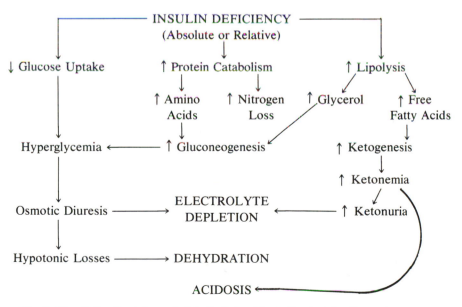

Fig. 8–13. Pathophysiology of diabetic ketoacidosis. See text for discussion.

energy demands. This increased nitrogen loss leads to a depletion of lean body mass, which is an important component of the weight loss suffered by the affected patients.

In the case of fat metabolism, the lack of effective insulin also contributes to fluid and electrolyte depletion. However, ketosis and eventual acidosis are solely attributable to the lack of an insulin effect on adipose tissue. A critical aspect of insulin action on the tissue is an inhibition of the breakdown of triglycerides, a pathway termed lipolysis. Increased lipolysis results in elevated concentrations of glycerol and FFA in plasma. Because glycerol is a gluconeogenic precursor, its increased flux from adipose tissue enhances gluconeogenesis even further. This enhancement, of course, leads to more pronounced hyperglycemia and greater fluid and electrolyte losses. Some of the FFA can be used by tissues for energy or reconstituted as hepatic triglycerides. However, as discussed above, the most important determinant of ketone body formation (ketogenesis) is the amount of FFA delivered to the liver. The ketogenic pathway is further activated by the presence of the low insulin and high glucagon concentrations that characterize DKA. The ketone bodies (acetoacetate and β-hydroxybutyrate) are weak acids that must be buffered upon release by the liver into the circulation *(ketonemia)*. As more and more ketone bodies are produced, the body bases become depleted and acidosis ensues. In addition to causing acidosis, the ketone bodies also contribute to the loss of electrolytes. Although they can be utilized to some extent by various body tissues, the capacity to metabolize ketone bodies is soon exceeded and they are excreted into the urine *(ketonuria)*. This event exacerbates electrolyte depletion as cations must be excreted with the ketone bodies.

Symptoms. The symptoms of DKA are listed in Table 8–5. Polyuria and polydipsia are simply manifestations of the osmotic diuresis secondary to hyperglycemia. Weakness, lethargy, headache, and myalgia are relatively nonspecific symptoms. The gastrointestinal and respiratory symptoms, however, are specifically related to DKA. Although documentation is difficult, ketosis is probably responsible for many of the gastrointestinal symptoms, (ketosis secondary to a low carbohydrate intake—i.e., starvation ketosis—is associated with anorexia, nausea, and occasional vomiting). In any event, nausea, vomiting and abdominal pain are often noted in patients with DKA. The abdominal pain can be quite severe and may even suggest an intra-abdominal process requiring surgery. When questioned more closely, patients who complain of "dyspnea" (shortness of breath on exertion) are found actually to be having difficulty in catching their breath even while sitting or lying quietly. This symptom, of course, represents hyperventilation, which is the ventilatory response to metabolic acidosis originally described by the German physician Kussmaul.

Table 8–5.   Symptoms and Signs of DKA

Symptoms		Signs	
Polyuria	Anorexia	Hypothermia	"Acute abdomen"
Polydipsia	Nausea	Hyperpnea (Kussmaul respirations)	Stupor (coma)
Weakness	Vomiting	Acetone breath	Hypotonia
Lethargy	Abdominal pain	"Dehydration" (intravascular volume depletion)	Uncoordinated movements
Myalgia	"Dyspnea"	Hyporeflexia	Fixed, dilated pupils
Headache			

Signs. The signs of DKA are listed in Table 8–5. It is not generally recognized that low body temperatures are characteristic of patients experiencing DKA. A fever usually denotes an accompanying infection. The depth of respiration (hyperpnea), not the rate (tachypnea), characterizes Kussmaul respirations. Often patients have a normal respiratory rate but on closer inspection are noted to be breathing very deeply. The signal for this hyperventilation is acidosis which stimulates the respiratory center in the brain. The resulting respiratory alkalosis offsets the metabolic acidosis to some extent but cannot compensate for it entirely in the absence of treatment. The structure of and relation among the ketone bodies are depicted in Figure 8–14. Acetoacetate is irreversibly converted to acetone that is excreted by the lungs. Acetone has a fruity odor that is often apparent on the patient's breath although not all observers can distinguish this odor.

Although the term *dehydration* is often used to describe patients experiencing DKA, the signs really result from intravascular volume depletion. In adults, the most sensitive sign of intravascular volume depletion is a change in the way in which the neck veins fill. When normally hydrated subjects lie entirely horizontally (without a pillow), the neck veins fill *from below* to one-half to two-thirds the way up to the angle of the jaw. The neck veins in dehydrated patients will not fill much, if at all, above the clavicles.

The only other reliable sign of intravascular depletion in adults is a fall of systolic blood pressure by 20 mm Hg or greater when the patient moves from a lying to a sitting or standing position. This orthostatic change in systolic blood pressure is a less sensitive measurement than decreased filling of the neck veins from below and thus represents a more marked deficit in intravascular volume. (It must be kept in mind, however, that diabetic patients with dysfunction of the autonomic nervous system may manifest orthostatic changes in blood pressure in the absence of any fluid loss.) The other signs often considered in the determination of dehydration are really not helpful. Dry mucous membranes are noted in patients who breathe with their mouths open. Soft eyeballs and poor skin turgor are seen, at least in adults, only with profound dehydration.

Hyporeflexia may be noted in patients experiencing DKA. If not present

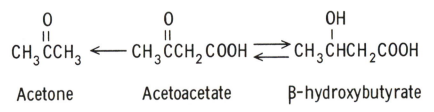

Fig. 8–14. Structure of and relation among the ketone bodies. (Reprinted with permission from Davidson, M.B.: Diabetes Mellitus: Diagnosis and Treatment. 2nd Ed. New York, John Wiley & Sons, 1986.)

initially, it often develops during treatment if the potassium concentration is allowed to fall to low levels.

An abdominal examination of patients experiencing DKA can yield striking results. Abdominal tenderness to palpation and muscle guarding are usual. Bowel sounds may be diminished or even absent. Rebound tenderness is often noted. In an occasional patient, a board-like abdomen with no bowel sounds and rebound tenderness may suggest a catastrophic intra-abdominal process requiring immediate surgical procedure. However, all of these signs can be caused by DKA, although the mechanisms behind them are unknown. Except for the rare patient in whom DKA may be precipitated by such an event, these signs will clear as the patient's biochemical status improves. In any event, since surgical procedure is contraindicated in patients with DKA because of the extremely high mortality, treatment of DKA must precede surgical intervention and signs suggesting the need for surgery almost invariably disappear with treatment.

The mental status of patients experiencing DKA ranges from completely alert to comatose and is not related to the degree of ketosis or acidosis. In fact, the patient's mental status seems best correlated with plasma osmolality. Various degrees of lethargy, stupor, and coma are seen in most patients and altered mental status is an important sign of DKA. Hypotonia, uncoordinated ocular movements, and fixed, dilated pupils are (fortunately) unusual symptoms that are associated with a poor prognosis (as is deep coma).

Fluid and Electrolyte Losses. The magnitude of urinary loss in a diabetic totally without insulin for 24 hours is considerable. Two kinds of experiments have been performed to assess this loss. In one, the amounts of fluid and electrolytes to replenish patients in diabetic ketoacidosis were measured. In the other, insulin therapy was discontinued temporarily in ketosis-prone diabetic patients and the actual losses were measured. The approximate amounts within 24 hours were: water-6.5 L, sodium-500 mEq, potassium-400 mEq, chloride-400 mEq, magnesium-50 mEq, and phosphorus-70 mM.

Laboratory Results. Laboratory findings in patients with ketoacidosis are: increased glucose concentrations (usually between 300 and 800 mg/100 ml), ketonemia, decreased bicarbonate concentrations and pH, increased blood urea nitrogen (BUN), and creatinine (which may be prerenal, reflecting intravascular volume depletion), leukocytosis (even in the absence of infection), increased amylase (in the absence of documented pancreatitis), and increased plasma osmolality (up to 350 mOsm/kg). Potassium and sodium concentrations are variable. They may be low, normal, or high even though total body sodium and potassium stores are severely depleted.

Treatment. The detailed treatment for this condition is beyond the scope of this chapter but includes insulin, fluids (saline solution), and potassium. The need to administer a base (bicarbonate) remains controversial but is usually not necessary. The prognosis for patients in diabetic ketoacidosis is good. The mortality rate is approximately 5 to 10%, and a poor outcome is usually due to a complication rather than to the ketoacidosis itself. The prognosis is not correlated with the degree of acidosis, level of glucose, or any other biochemical parameter. It seems to correlate best with the age of the patient and the level of consciousness at the time of examination, that is, the older the patient and the deeper the coma, the worse the prognosis.

Patients who are in diabetic ketoacidosis need insulin therapy permanently. However, some patients who are initially in ketoacidosis may go through a "honeymoon" period. On recovery from the initial episode, their insulin requirements gradually decrease and some are able to discontinue insulin entirely. During this period, the pancreatic β-cell partially recovers its ability to secrete insulin. This recovery is only temporary and virtually all patients require insulin again, usually within 3 to 6 months.

Hyperosmolar Nonketotic Coma

Some patients may develop hyperosmolar nonketotic coma (HNKC) rather than diabetic ketoacidosis. The pathophysiology for this condition is also shown in Figure 8–13. If enough insulin is present to regulate lipolysis, the chain of events shown on the right side of the figure (i.e., increased lipolysis leading to ketogenesis and ketonuria with subsequent development of acidosis) does not occur. Insulin lack would affect carbohydrate and protein metabolism and would lead only to electrolyte depletion and dehydration. In the absence of the gastrointestinal symptoms caused by ketosis and ketoacidosis, patients may not seek medical attention. Then this sequence of events (hyperglycemia leading to dehydration and electrolyte depletion) occurs over a much longer period of time and leads to severe dehydration which eventually impairs renal plasma flow. Less glucose is presented to the kidney and renal losses of glucose do not keep pace with hepatic overproduction. Glucose concentrations may become extremely high, sometimes exceeding 2000 mg/100 ml.

The signs and symptoms of hyperosmolar, nonketotic coma are marked polyuria, polydipsia, and lethargy. Most of these patients have an altered state of consciousness. In addition, many of them have *focal* neurologic findings; in fact, many are diagnosed as having had a cerebrovascular accident. All have severe dehydration and some may have abdominal tenderness.

The laboratory results are similar to diabetic ketoacidosis except that the glucose levels are usually higher and serum osmolalities are also more elevated (up to 450 mOsm/kg). The contribution of circulating glucose to serum osmolality can be calculated by dividing the glucose concentration by 18 (the molecular weight of glucose is 180). Bicarbonate concentrations and pH are often normal, but there may be a mild decrease in pH and bicarbonate levels because classic HNKC and DKA simply represent two ends of a spectrum. Some patients may have a mild ketoacidosis, but severe hyperglycemia. Evidence suggests that increased osmolality inhibits fat cell lipolysis independent of insulin. Therefore, the high plasma osmolalities attained probably also contribute to the lower FFA levels and the lack of ketosis and acidosis in the syndrome of HNKC.

The prognosis in HNKC is usually not as good as in DKA because many of these patients are older and have other complicating diseases. Thrombosis with resultant emboli is an important complication. Of those patients who survive, a large percentage can be treated eventually with either oral hypoglycemic agents or diet alone. The treatment reflects that these patients are able to secrete some endogenous insulin and that, with proper attention to diet, their glucose levels can be controlled without exogenous insulin. Some salient features of DKA and HNKC are compared in Table 8–6.

Table 8–6.   Comparison of Some Salient Features of DKA and HNKC

| Feature | Conditions | |
	DKA	HNKC
Age of patient	Usually <40 years	Usually >40 years
Duration of symptoms	Usually <2 days	Usually >5 days
[Glucose]	Usually <800 mg/100 ml	Usually >800 mg/100 ml
[Na]	More likely to be normal or low	More likely to be normal or high
[K]	High, normal, or low	High, normal, or low
[HCO₃]	Low	Normal
Ketone bodies	At least 4+ in 1:1 dilution	<2+ in 1:1 dilution
pH	Low	Normal
Serum osmolality	Usually <350 mOsm/kg	Usually >350 mOsm/kg
Prognosis	5 to 10% mortality	30 to 50% mortality
Subsequent course	Insulin therapy required in virtually all cases	Insulin therapy not required in many cases

Abbreviations: [Glucose], serum concentration of glucose; [Na], serum concentration of sodium; [HCO₃], serum concentration of bicarbonate; [K], serum concentration of potassium.

Classification. This classification of diabetes mellitus and other categories of glucose intolerance (Table 8–7) was developed by the National Diabetes Data Group (NDDG) of the National Institutes of Health and amended by the World Health Organization (WHO). It is based on abnormalities of carbohydrate and fat metabolism and does not consider the presence or absence of vascular disease. Diabetes mellitus can be divided into five types.

Table 8–7.   Classification of Disorders of Carbohydrate Metabolism

A. Diabetes Mellitus
  1. Insulin dependent type (IDDM), type 1
  2. Noninsulin dependent type (NIDDM), type 2
  3. Other types
  4. Gestational
  5. Malnutrition-related

B. Impaired glucose tolerance

C. Increased statistical risk for diabetes mellitus
  1. Previous abnormality of glucose tolerance
  2. Potential abnormality of glucose tolerance

Type 1. Insulin-dependent diabetes mellitus (IDDM) was formerly called juvenile-onset diabetes, ketosis-prone diabetes, or unstable diabetes. The currently accepted name is type 1 diabetes mellitus. The important metabolic characteristics of this type of diabetes is the presence of ketosis in the absence of treatment which indicates little effective insulin. Although the onset of type 1 diabetes is more frequent in childhood, adolescence, and young adulthood, it can also occur in the older patient. The signs and symptoms of uncontrolled diabetes can progress rapidly to ketosis and even ketoacidosis, often within a week or two, especially in younger patients.

Type 2. Former terminology for noninsulin dependent diabetes mellitus (NIDDM) included adult-onset diabetes, maturity-onset diabetes, ketosis-resistant diabetes, and stable diabetes. When the disorder occurred in childhood and adolescence, it was termed maturity-onset diabetes of youth (MODY) or, more recently, NIDDMY. The current name is type 2 diabetes mellitus. The important metabolic characteristic of this type of diabetes is the absence of ketosis. Although type 2 diabetes mellitus is much more common in individuals over the age of 40 years, it does occur in younger subjects. Most (80 to 90%) ketosis-resistant diabetic patients are obese. An occasional type 2 diabetic patient may temporarily become ketotic under great stress (trauma, infection, myocardial infarction), but this phenomenon is distinctly unusual. Since approximately three-quarters of these patients have no symptoms of diabetes when the diagnosis is made while they are being evaluated for other reasons, it is estimated that these patients may have had diabetes for years without anyone being aware of it.

Other Types. The third kind of diabetes is now termed other types. It was formerly called secondary diabetes and included: (a) diseases of the pancreas that destroyed the β-cells (e.g., hemochromatosis, pancreatitis, cystic fibrosis); (b) hormonal syndromes (e.g., acromegaly, Cushing's syndrome, pheochromocytoma) that interfere with insulin secretion and/or inhibit insulin action; (c) drugs that may interfere with insulin secretion (e.g., phenytoin) or may inhibit insulin action (e.g., glucocorticoids, estrogens); (d) rare conditions involving abnormalities of the insulin receptor; (e) a variety of rare genetic syndromes in which diabetes mellitus inexplicably occurs more frequently than in healthy persons; and (f) several recently described families in which point mutations in the insulin gene caused amino acid substitution at sites in the insulin structure necessary for hormonal binding to its receptor leading to an ineffective molecule and diabetes mellitus.

Gestational Diabetes. The term gestational diabetes is reserved for women with the onset or the initial recognition of diabetes during pregnancy. Thus, diabetic patients who subsequently become pregnant are not included in this class. In normal pregnancy, insulin antagonistic hormones are produced by the placenta. In approximately 2% of pregnant women, the increased demands on the pancreatic β-cell to produce more insulin cannot be met and abnormal carbohydrate metabolism ensues. Gestational diabetes is associated with increased perinatal risks to the offspring and an increased risk to the mother for progression to diabetes mellitus within the next 10 to 15 years. When the pregnancy ends, these patients require reclassification into previous abnormality of glucose tolerance, impaired glucose tolerance, or diabetes mellitus, depending on the results of their postpartum evaluation.

The WHO has added another category of diabetes that is noted in underdeveloped countries, diabetes mellitus associated with malnutrition. The afflicted individuals are usually young, between 10 and 40 years, at onset. They are symptomatic with marked polyuria, polydipsia, and weight loss. Insulin is usually required to control their hyperglycemia, although they remain ketosis-resistant even when insulin is withdrawn. Some of these patients experience antecedent abdominal pain radiating to the back suggesting pancreatitis. Indeed, many of them show pancreatic calcifications on x-ray and exocrine and endocrine destruction and fibrosis as well as calcium stones in the exocrine ducts at autopsy. Chronic pancreatitis does not account for their diabetes since insulin requirements are high (patients with diabetes secondary to pancreatic inflammation are usually sensitive to insulin) and many of these patients have no evidence of pancreatitis. The role of malnutrition in causing this kind of diabetes is unknown.

Impaired Glucose Tolerance (IGT). The result of oral glucose tolerance tests in patients with IGT are higher than normal, but fail to meet the criteria for diabetes mellitus. Former terminology included chemical, latent, subclinical, borderline, and asymptomatic diabetes. When the subjects are retested with an oral glucose challenge, even after many years, approximately 30% will have reverted to normal, 50% will continue to show IGT and the remaining 20% will be diabetic. Progression to overt diabetes in this latter population occurs at a low rate, 1 to 5% per year. Recent evidence suggests that patients with IGT are unlikely to develop the microangiopathic complications of diabetes, retinopathy, and nephropathy. However, these patients are especially prone to macroangiopathic complications: coronary artery, peripheral vascular, and cerebrovascular disease.

Previous Abnormality of Glucose Tolerance. The classification of previous abnormality of glucose tolerance is restricted to persons whose glucose tolerance test at one time fulfilled the criteria for IGT or diabetes mellitus, either spontaneously or in response to an identifiable stress, but who are currently normal. This group was formerly termed latent diabetes or prediabetes. Gestational diabetic patients are an obvious source for this class, as are formerly obese patients who have lost weight. Subjects undergoing acute stress due to trauma or illness may experience transient hyperglycemia and would fit into this category as well. With the exception of gestational diabetic patients, there has been little systematic study of the propensity of these subjects to subsequently develop diabetes mellitus. It is likely that the risk is increased, and these individuals should be monitored closely when they are in stressful situations.

Potential Abnormality in Glucose Tolerance. The classification of potential abnormality of glucose tolerance is reserved for individuals who have never exhibited abnormal glucose tolerance, but who have a substantially increased risk for the development of diabetes mellitus. The former term for this class was prediabetes or potential diabetes. Subjects who are at increased risk for type 1 diabetes include (in decreasing order of risk): persons with islet-cell antibodies; the monozygotic twin of a type 1 diabetic patient; the sibling of a type 1 diabetic patient, especially one with an identical HLA genotype; and the offspring of a type 1 diabetic patient. The reasons for the increased risk in these individuals will be discussed below.

Individuals who are at increased risk for type 2 diabetes include (in decreasing order of risk): monozygotic twin of a type 2 diabetic patient; first-degree relative (sibling, parent, or offspring) of a type 2 diabetic patient; mother of a baby weighing more than 9 pounds at birth; obese subjects; and members of racial or ethnic groups with a high prevalence of type 2 diabetes (such as certain Indian tribes). The actual degree of risk for any of these circumstances is not well established at the present time, except for the monozygotic twins who are virtually certain to develop diabetes.

Diagnosis

It is important for physicians to be familiar with the site of sampling, the methods of measuring glucose used by the laboratory and the nutritional and clinical status of the patient, such as the presence or absence of stress. Whether plasma (or serum) or whole blood is used for the measurement of glucose is important for a valid interpretation of a glucose tolerance test. The glucose oxidase method, which depends on an enzymatic degradation of glucose, is specific. Other methods give higher values (5 to 10 mg/100 ml) because certain circulating constituents (uric acid, creatinine, glutathione if the red blood cells are hemolyzed, fructose, and galactose) influence the results. However, this slight increase is not clinically important. Capillary blood obtained by finger or ear lobe puncture often gives higher values than those measured in venous samples because capillary samples consist, in large part, of arterial blood, and the peripheral tissues have not had a chance to extract the glucose. The difference between capillary and venous glucose levels is usually small in the fasting state, but may range up to 60 mg/100 ml (average 25 mg/100 ml) for several hours after a glucose challenge.

Two similar sets of criteria for making the diagnosis of diabetes mellitus and IGT have been promulgated by the NDDG and the WHO. The diagnosis of diabetes mellitus in nonpregnant adults can be made by any one of the three sets of criteria [fasting, oral glucose tolerance test (OGTT), random] listed in Table 8–8. To avoid misdiagnosis resulting from laboratory error, it is necessary to document the abnormal values(s) at least twice.

Subjects with less abnormality in their carbohydrate metabolism (who were formerly designated as having asymptomatic, chemical, latent, borderline, or subclinical diabetes) are now categorized as showing IGT. The criteria for making this diagnosis are listed in Table 8–9. The criteria for normal glucose tolerance are listed in Table 8–10.

Table 8—8. Criteria for the Diagnosis of Diabetes Mellitus in Nonpregnant Adults

	NDDG			WHO		
	Venous Plasma Glucose[a]	Venous Whole Blood Glucose[a]	Capillary Blood Glucose[a]	Venous Plasma Glucose[a]	Venous Whole Blood Glucose[a]	Capillary Whole Blood Glucose[a]
Fasting	>140 (7.8)	>120 (6.7)	>120 (6.7)	>140 (7.8)	>120 (6.7)	>120 (6.7)
		or			or	
OGTT[b] (2 hrs)	>200 (11.1)	>180 (10.0)	>200 (11.1)	>200 (11.1)	>180 (10.0)	>200 (11.1)
OGTT (½, 1 or 1½ hrs)	>200 (11.1)	>180 (10.0)	>200 (11.1)	(not part of criteria)		
		or			or	
Random	"gross and unequivocal elevation" of glucose levels with classic symptoms of uncontrolled diabetes			>200 (11.1)	>180 (10.0)	>200 (11.1)

[a] mg/100 ml (mmol/L).
[b] oral glucose tolerance test.

Table 8–9. Criteria for the Diagnosis of Impaired Glucose Tolerance in Nonpregnant Adults

	NDDG			WHO		
	Venous Plasma Glucose[a]	Venous Whole Blood Glucose[a]	Capillary Blood Glucose[a]	Venous Plasma Glucose[a]	Venous Whole Blood Glucose[a]	Capillary Whole Blood Glucose[a]
Fasting	<140 (7.8)	<120 (6.7)	<120 (6.7)	<140 (7.8)	<120 (6.7)	<120 (6.7)
		and			and	
OGTT[b] (2 hrs)	140–199 (7.8–11.1)	120–179 (6.7–10.0)	140–199 (7.8–11.1)	140–199 (7.8–11.1)	120–179 (6.7–10.0)	140–199 (7.8–11.1)
		and				
OGTT (½, 1 or 1½ hrs)	>200 (11.1)	>180 (10.0)	>200 (11.1)	(not part of criteria)		

[a] mg/100 ml (mmol/L).
[b] oral glucose tolerance test.

Table 8–10. Criteria for Normal Glucose Tolerance in Nonpregnant Adults

	NDDG			WHO		
	Venous Plasma Glucose[a]	*Venous Whole Blood Glucose[a]*	*Capillary Blood Glucose[a]*	*Venous Plasma Glucose[a]*	*Venous Whole Blood Glucose[a]*	*Capillary Whole Blood Glucose[a]*
Fasting	<115 (6.4)	<100 (5.6)	<100 (5.6)	<115 (6.4)	<100 (5.6)	<100 (5.6)
OGTT[b] (2 hrs)	<140 (7.8)	<120 (6.7)	<140 (7.8)	<140 (7.8)	<120 (6.7)	<140 (7.8)
OGTT (½, 1, or 1½ hrs)	<200 (11.1)	<180 (10.0)	<200 (11.1)	(not part of criteria)		

[a] mg/100 ml (mmol/L).
[b] oral glucose tolerance test.

Both the NDDG and the WHO committees agree that a 75 g load of glucose or its equivalent should be the oral challenge in nonpregnant adults. The test should be performed after a 10- to 16-hour overnight fast. Water is permitted during this period. The subject should be active and have ingested at least 150 g of carbohydrate daily during the 3 days before the test. The subject should remain seated during the OGTT, and no smoking is allowed.

The interpretation of the results is as follows. According to the NDDG criteria, OGTT results that do not fit into the categories of diabetes mellitus, IGT, or normal are labeled as nondiagnostic and these subjects require a closer follow-up. On the other hand, according to the WHO criteria, the 2-hour OGTT value characterizes the subject. If the value is greater than the equivalent of a plasma value of 200 mg/100 ml, the patient has diabetes mellitus; if it is between 140 and 199 mg/199 ml, the patient has IGT; if it is <140 mg/100 ml, the subject is normal. When both the NDDG and WHO criteria were compared in a large population undergoing OGTT, one-third of the subjects were unclassifiable by the NDDG criteria. The majority of these nondiagnostic OGTT showed IGT by the WHO criteria while the remainder were normal. None of the unclassified subjects by the NDDG criteria was reclassified as a diabetic using the WHO criteria.

If an OGTT is performed, there are two reasons (in my view) to use the WHO rather than the NDDG criteria to interpret it. First, the confusing category of ''nondiagnostic'' is eliminated. Second, only a 2-hour blood sample is required after ingestion of the glucose challenge rather than samples at 30-minute intervals. However, in nonpregnant individuals, OGTT are not usually used for diagnosis. Most commonly, diabetes is diagnosed by either the fasting or random criteria. Pregnancy is an exception to both the dictum that OGTT are usually unnecessary and the recently promulgated less sensitive criteria of the NDDG and WHO. Because even minor abnormalities of glucose tolerance in pregnant women can be associated with increased risk to the fetus at delivery or in the neonatal period, it is recommended that screening with a 50 g glucose load be carried out in all pregnant women, approximately 2% of whom will have gestational diabetes. If the 1-hour plasma value exceeds 150 mg/100 ml, the patient is referred for a formal 3-hour OGTT. This OGTT differs from the OGTT discussed above in three respects. First, the recommended oral glucose load is 100 g. Second, samples are collected before, 1, 2, and 3 hours following the oral challenge. Third, and most importantly, the criteria for making the diagnosis of diabetes in pregnancy are much more sensitive than in the nonpregnant state (Table 8–11).

Several other situations deserve special mention. The criteria for the diagnosis of diabetes mellitus and IGT are the same in children. However, the upper limit of normal for fasting glucose concentrations is 15 mg/100 ml higher in children than in adults (see Table 8–10). Persons who have undergone gastric operations have elevated glucose levels following an oral challenge (see Fig. 8–9). Therefore, an OGTT cannot be used to diagnose diabetes mellitus in these patients and the fasting glucose concentration is the only

Table 8–11. Criteria[a] for the Diagnosis of Diabetes Mellitus in Pregnancy

	Venous Plasma Glucose[b]		Venous Whole Blood Glucose[b]		Capillary Whole Blood Glucose	
Fasting	105	(5.8)	90	(5.0)	90	(5.0)
1 hour	190	(10.6)	170	(9.5)	190	(10.6)
2 hours	165	(9.2)	145	(8.1)	165	(9.2)
3 hours	145	(8.1)	125	(7.0)	145	(8.1)

[a]two or more of the following values after a 100-g glucose challenge must be met or exceeded to make the diagnosis.
[b]mg/100 ml (mmol/L).

criterion. Glucose tolerance deteriorates as individuals age. There is an approximate 10 mg/100 ml increase per decade 1 hour after a glucose challenge in adults. Many former criteria included a 10 mg/100 ml increase per decade in the upper limits of normal after the age of 50 years. The NDDG and WHO did not make such a recommendation, probably because their criteria are much less sensitive (i.e., the glucose values are much higher) than previous ones. Fortunately, the fasting plasma glucose concentration rises only 1 to 2 mg/100 ml per decade. Therefore, as a diagnostic criterion for diabetes mellitus, it is virtually independent of age.

Pathogenesis—Type 1 Diabetes

Genetic Susceptibility. Type 1 diabetes is due to a profound impairment or an absence of insulin secretion secondary to β-cell destruction. Genetic, immunologic, and possibly viral influences are involved. The major risk factor for the development of type 1 diabetes is the human leukocyte antigen (HLA) genes located on the short arm of the sixth chromosome. Their identification requires testing of white blood cells, which accounts for their name. These genes determine which surface antigens are produced by nucleated cells. The surface antigens are involved in a host of cell to cell interactions, one of which includes the rejection process (i.e. the reaction when tissue from one host is transplanted into another). Since many different surface antigens are possible in a population, a large number of separate genes are responsible for them. Two HLA types, DR3 and DR4, are common in Caucasian patients with type 1 diabetes. This means that certain genes, the ones whose expression produces these HLA types, are also common in these patients and provide a marker for the genetic background that increases susceptibility to type 1 diabetes.

Each parent furnishes a gene that codes for different DR antigens. If an offspring should be so unfortunate to have a genotype of DR3/DR4, such as a DR3 from one parent and a DR4 from the other, the lifetime risk for developing type 1 diabetes in that individual is 1:45. If the genotype is DR3/DR3 or DR4/DR4, the lifetime risk is reduced to 1:125 to 150. If the haplotype of an individual contains just one HLA type that confirms susceptibility for type 1 diabetes, that is, DR3 *or* DR4, the lifetime risk is 1:500. If neither DR3 or DR4 is present, there is only a 1:5000 chance of getting type 1 diabetes. However, it is unlikely that the HLA antigens themselves confer the susceptibility. Rather, they either act as inert "markers" for the existence of disease susceptibility or immune response genes (see discussion following) that are in linkage disequilibrium with the HLA system, or more specific subtypes of the DR alleles are responsible. (Linkage disequilibrium is the tendency in a population for some alleles at closely linked loci to occur together in the same haplotype, that is, on the same chromosome, more often than expected by chance.)

Immune Dysfunction. The HLA system in humans is the analog of the major histocompatibility system that occurs in all animals. This chromosomal region consists of loci that not only control the synthesis of transplantation (surface) antigens, but also have fundamental roles in the immune process. Indeed, good evidence suggests that an immune process is active at the onset of type 1 diabetes. Lymphocytic infiltrates are seen in the islets of Langerhans of patients on whom an autopsy is performed soon after the diagnosis. Antibodies against islet cells are present in the sera of over 80% of type 1 patients if they are tested near the onset of their disease; a gradual reduction in antibody titers occurs over the ensuing year in most patients. In addition, islet cell antibodies have now been shown to precede the clinical appearance of type 1 diabetes, sometimes for a period of years. During this time, glucose tolerance is often normal and insulin secretion is either also normal or only subtle changes can be detected.

Viral Influence. The evidence for a viral influence on the onset of type 1 diabetes is indirect and weaker than the case for genetic and immunologic factors. First, there are a number of isolated case reports of different viral syndromes preceding the onset of ketosis-prone diabetes by several weeks. Second, direct epidemiologic data relate the prevalence of new cases of type 1 diabetes in the winter months to seasonal changes of viral illnesses. Third, a similar direct relation exists between antibody titers to Coxsackie B virus (after viral infections, titers rise acutely and then fall) and the onset of new cases of type 1 diabetes. Fourth, certain strains of mice develop diabetes after infection with several different viruses.

The following hypothesis is currently being considered. When susceptible individuals contract a particular viral infection, their β-cells are damaged. Because β-cells do not have the capacity to regenerate, diabetes can result. In some people, repeated viral infections may be necessary. The insult to the β-cells could be due to the virus itself secondary to a compromised immune response. Alternatively, in the process of neutralizing the virus, the altered immune response could damage the β-cells. It is uncertain at present whether the islet-cell antibodies simply reflect damage to the β-cells or cause their destruction. It seems certain that whatever initiates the chronic autoimmune process, be it viral agent, toxin, or random immunologic event, it occurs because of genetic susceptibility. At the present time, the HLA alleles DR3 and DR4 are the best identifying characteristics of these individuals in the population at large.

Pathogenesis—Type 2 Diabetes

The pathogenesis of type 2 diabetes mellitus remains controversial. Some investigators believe that abnormalities of insulin secretion are the primary cause. Others hold that impairment of insulin action is responsible. The true pathogenesis probably involves both possibilities.

Insulin Secretion. Insulin is a polypeptide hormone with a molecular weight

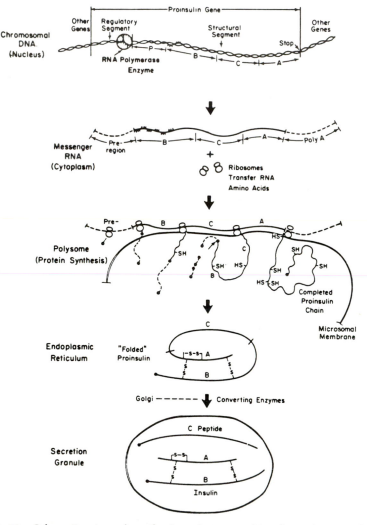

Fig. 8–15. Schematic view of synthesis and storage of insulin and C-peptide in pancreatic β-cell. (Reprinted with permission from Steiner, D.F.: Diabetes, *26*:322, 1977.)

of approximately 6000 (dark structure in Fig. 8–7). It consists of an A and a B chain connected by 2 disulfide bridges. In addition, a disulfide bridge within the A chain connects amino acids 6 and 11. The synthesis of insulin by the β-cell of the pancreas is shown in Figure 8–15. Insulin is first synthesized as a single-chain polypeptide such that the resultant A and B chains of insulin come into opposition to each other and the disulfide bridges between the 2 chains are formed. This molecule, known as proinsulin (entire structure in Fig. 8–7), has a molecular weight of approximately 9000 and consists of the final insulin molecule connected by an amino acid chain termed the C-peptide. Proinsulin is hydrolyzed by trypsin and carboxypeptidase in the Golgi apparatus. The resulting 2 molecules, insulin and the C-peptide (light structure is Fig. 8–7), are packaged into secretory granules that are stored in the cytoplasm of the cell. When insulin secretion is stimulated, the secretory granules are transferred to the plasma membrane of the cell through micro-tubules and insulin and the C-peptide (with a small amount of intact proinsulin) are extruded from the cell via the process of emiocytosis.

Proinsulin cross-reacts with insulin antibodies and is measured in the insulin immunoassay. It has only 10 to 20% of the biologic effectiveness of insulin. No evidence exists for increased secretion of proinsulin in diabetes mellitus. The C-peptide has no known biologic activity, but does serve as a marker for insulin secretion because equimolar amounts of each are secreted by the β-cell. Insulin-treated diabetic patients usually develop insulin-binding anti-bodies that interfere with the immunoassay of insulin. Measurement of C-peptide is useful for assessing insulin secretion in these patients.

Response to Oral Glucose. Since the introduction of the radioimmunoassay for insulin, numerous investigators have measured the insulin response to oral glucose in subjects with abnormal carbohydrate metabolism. The results were initially confusing until two variables were taken into account. First, weight-matched controls were necessary because of the hyperinsulinemia associated with obesity independent of prevailing glucose levels. Second, the insulin response to oral glucose depended on the degree of carbohydrate abnormality. With use of weight-matched controls and a strict definition of the groups under study, a reproducible pattern can be discerned. Patients with IGT, according to the criteria of the NDDG and WHO, have increased secretion of insulin following oral glucose. Patients with type 2 diabetes, according to the criteria of the NDDG and WHO, show blunted insulin response to oral glucose. These relationships are depicted in Figure 8–16, in which the 2-hour plasma glucose and insulin concentrations during an oral glucose tolerance test in nearly 400 Pima Indians are plotted against each other. None of these subjects had been treated for diabetes. As the 2-hour glucose value increases up to about 200 mg/100 ml, the insulin level is greater than normal. Further increases in the 2-hour glucose value over 200 mg/100 ml (above which the criteria for diabetes is met) are associated with a decreasing insulin level that soon falls to below normal. Note that although insulin concentrations are increased in obese subjects compared with lean ones, the same general pattern

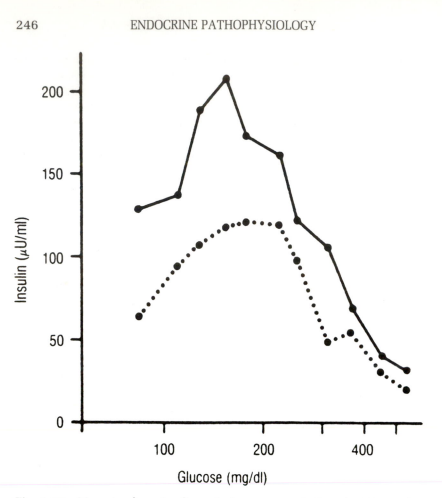

Fig. 8–16. Mean two-hour insulin and glucose concentrations in 396 nonobese (●---●) and obese (●—●) Pima Indians. (Reprinted with permission from Savage, R.J., et al., Diabetes, *24*:362, 1975.)

exists within each group. This pattern of insulin secretion was also noted in large American Caucasian and Scandinavian populations as well.

Response to Meals. On the other hand, both the insulin response to meals and urinary C-peptide levels (which are a measure of insulin secretion during the period in which the urine is formed) are similar in normal subjects and patients with type 2 diabetes. Insulin responses in hyperglycemic patients that are no different than those in euglycemic individuals suggest two things. First, pancreatic β-cell reserve must be impaired because normally one would expect a greater insulin response to these higher glucose levels. Second, the secreted insulin must not be completely effective since nondiabetics with these insulin concentrations are euglycemic.

Response to Intravenous Glucose and Other Secretagogues. Abnormalities in the insulin response to intravenous administration of glucose occur in patients with both IGT and type 2 diabetes mellitus though how they may be related to the altered carbohydrate metabolism in these disorders is not clear. The normal insulin response to intravenous glucose is shown in Figure 8–17. There is an initial rapid response with peak insulin concentrations reached within the first few minutes. This is called the first-phase or "acute" insulin response. A more delayed gradual increase (termed the second-phase response) occurs if large amounts of glucose are administered or if the glucose is given continuously. A small pulse of glucose elicits only the first-phase response. Some other agents given intravenously will also stimulate a first-phase response. These include isoproterenol, which is a β-adrenegic agonist, glucagon, tolbutamide, certain amino acids (e.g. arginine), and secretin.

Persons with fasting glucose concentrations exceeding 115 mg/100 ml have an absent first-phase response to intravenous glucose. This obviously includes patients with IGT as well as those with type 2 diabetes. However, the second-phase response to glucose given intravenously remains generally intact until the fasting plasma glucose level exceeds 200 mg/100 ml. In contrast to the absent first-phase response to intravenous administration of glucose, patients with both IGT and type 2 diabetes retain their acute insulin response to the other intravenously given secretagogues (isoproterenol, arginine, glucagon, secretin, and tolbutamide). Figure 8–18 depicts the acute responses to glucose and isoproterenol in normal persons and type 2 diabetic patients. No acute phase response occurs to intravenous glucose although a nearly normal one does after isoproterenol. Insulin responses to non-glucose secretagogues are dependent on ambient glucose levels; that is, the higher the glucose concen-

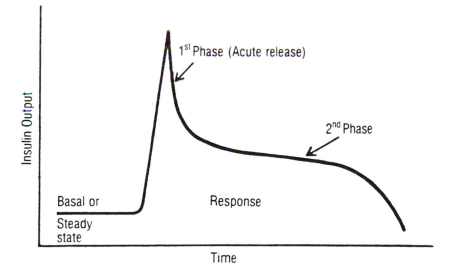

Fig. 8–17. Schematic representation of an normal insulin response to intravenous administration of glucose. (Reprinted with permission from Pfeifer, M.A., Halter, J.B., and Porte, D. Jr.: Am J Med, 70:579, 1981.)

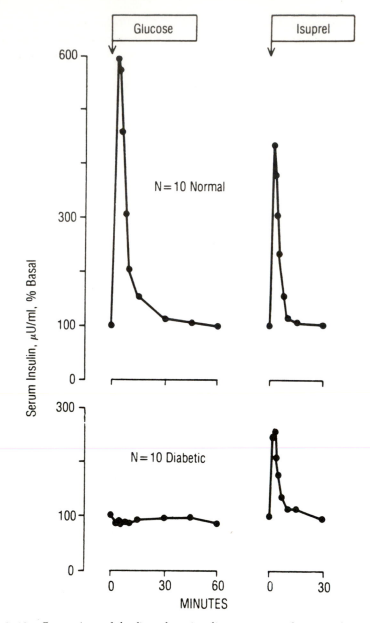

Fig. 8–18. Comparison of the first-phase insulin response to glucose and isoproterenol hydrochloride given intravenously in type 2 diabetic patients and controls. (Reprinted with permission from Robertson, R.P., and Porte, D. Jr.: J Clin Invest, *52*:870, 1973.)

tration, the greater the insulin response. When comparisons between type 2 diabetic patients and normal individuals are carried out at comparable glucose levels (by raising glucose values in normal subjects or lowering them in the diabetic patients), insulin responses to non-glucose stimuli are impaired in persons with type 2 diabetes. Thus, it seems as if recognition of intravenously administered glucose by the pancreatic β-cell is somehow inhibited in patients with IGT and type 2 diabetes.

However, several lines of evidence raise questions whether an absent acute phase response to intravenous glucose *causes* the altered carbohydrate metabolism in patients with IGT and type 2 diabetes. First, as mentioned above, individuals with IGT have an increased insulin response to oral glucose in the presence of an absent first-phase response to intravenous glucose. Second, this absent response is reversible in patients with type 2 diabetes by restoring euglycemia (as well as other manipulations such as inhibiting prostaglandin synthesis and both β-adrenergic and dopaminergic blockade). Third, an absent acute phase insulin response to intravenous glucose with preservation of a normal repsonse to isoproterenol can be induced in normal subjects by 46 hours of hyperglycemia (secondary to an infusion of glucagon and somatostatin). This suggests that this pattern of insulin release may be secondary to the hyperglycemia rather than be a cause of it in patients with IGT and type 2 diabetes. Thus, although the failure to respond to intravenous glucose characterizes these patients with altered carbohydrate metabolism, it is difficult to discern how this β-cell lesion is causally related.

Insulin Antagonism. Two techniques, developed to measure insulin action in human subjects, have revealed insulin antagonism in patients with both IGT and type 2 diabetes. In the steady state plasma glucose (SSPG) method, a solution containing glucose, insulin, epinephrine, and propranolol (a β-adrenergic antagonist) is infused intravenously. The α-adrenergic effect of epinephrine and propranolol inhibits endogenous insulin secretion. Similar steady state plasma insulin (SSPI) concentrations are attained in all subjects because the rate of exogenous insulin infusion is the same. The level at which the glucose concentrations reach a plateau is a measure of the effectiveness of the exogenous insulin. Thus, lower glucose levels signal sensitivity to insulin, whereas higher glucose levels denote an impaired response to insulin. In the second method, the euglycemic clamp technique, insulin is infused at a specified rate and glucose concentrations are measured frequently. This information is used to adjust the rate of a glucose infusion to maintain the plasma glucose concentration at its basal level. Because the glucose concentrations do not change, the amount of glucose infused must equal the amount of glucose disposed of by the tissues. The more glucose deposited into the tissues, the more sensitive the subject is to the infused insulin; the less glucose, the more insensitive to insulin. The results of both the SSPG method (Fig. 8–19) and the euglycemic clamp technique (Fig. 8–20) demonstrate the presence of insulin antagonism in patients with IGT and type 2 diabetes. This

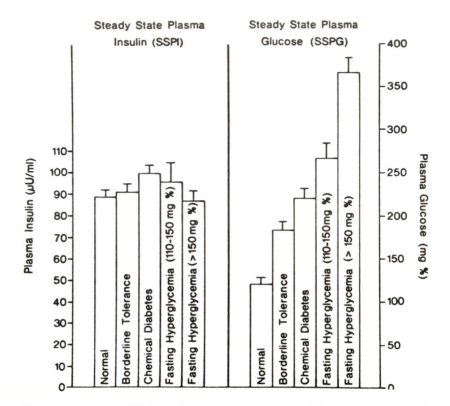

Fig. 8–19. Mean (±SEM) steady-state plasma insulin and glucose levels during the infusion of epinephrine (6 µg/min), propranolol (0.08 mg/kg/min), insulin (80 µU/min), and glucose (6 mg/kg/min) in 5 groups of patients. Chemical diabetes-impaired glucose tolerance. (Reprinted with permission from Reaven, G.M., et al.: Am J Med, 60:80, 1976.)

insensitivity to insulin is above and beyond that due to the obesity that is often present.

Binding of insulin to its receptors located on the plasma membrane of cells is the critical first step of hormonal action. Insulin binding has been measured in a large number of patients with IGT and type 2 diabetes. In general, individuals with IGT have decreased insulin binding a (receptor defect) while patients with fasting hyperglycemia of >180 mg/100 ml have normal binding. Thus, these latter patients have a post-receptor defect. Patients with less severe type 2 diabetes may also show decreased insulin binding. Since insulin antagonism increases as the carbohydrate decompensation worsens (Figs. 8–19 and 8–20), it is unlikely that decreased insulin binding causes the insulin antagonism in type 2 diabetes. Although theoretically a receptor defect could cause the resistance to insulin in IGT, in approximately 20% of these individuals, carbohydrate metabolism will deteriorate to the point where the cri-

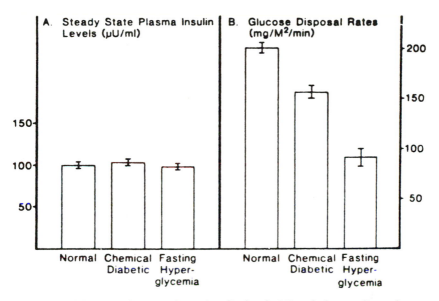

Fig. 8–20. Mean steady-state plasma insulin levels (A) and glucose disposal rates (B) in normal subjects, patients with impaired glucose tolerance (chemical diabetics) and type 2 diabetics. Values obtained from euglycemic clamp studies. (From Olefsky, J.M.: Diabetes, *30*:148, 1981. Reproduced with permission from the American Diabetes Association, Inc.)

teria for diabetes will be met. It is unlikely that there would be separate reasons for insulin antagonism in the two situations.

Patients with IGT and possibly mild type 2 diabetes have hyperinsulinemia (Fig. 8–16). Thus, the decreased insulin binding in these individuals is probably due to *down regulation* of the insulin receptor. After insulin is bound, the insulin-receptor complex is internalized into the cell where the insulin is mostly degraded and the receptor is mostly recycled back to the plasma membrane. In states of hyperinsulinemia, the rate of binding and internalization is more rapid than recycling of the receptor plus de novo receptor synthesis so that the number of insulin receptors remaining on the surface of the cell is diminished. Consequently, when insulin binding to the available receptors on the plasma membrane is measured, it is decreased. (Conversely, when insulin concentrations are chronically low, there is *up regulation* of the surface receptors and measured insulin binding is increased).

How is one to reconcile the following information concerning the pathogenesis of type 2 diabetes? The insulin response to oral glucose is increased in patients with IGT but decreased in those with type 2 diabetes. The insulin response to meals is normal, or nearly so, in type 2 diabetic patients albeit in the presence of hyperglycemia. The acute insulin response to intravenous glucose is markedly impaired in both IGT and type 2 diabetes but is restored toward normal by tight diabetic control. Insulin antagonism characterizes both

IGT and type 2 diabetes and is proportional to the degree of abnormality in carbohydrate metabolism.

Two other facts should be mentioned before attempting to integrate these data into an hypothesis. Insulin antagonism also characterizes two other situations, obesity and aging. Both of these are risk factors for type 2 diabetes. It is estimated that at least 20% of individuals over the age of 65 years will develop type 2 diabetes before they die. Thus, the following (tentative) conclusions seem warranted from the information currently available. Persons destined to have IGT and type 2 diabetes develop insulin antagonism. Those whose pancreatic β-cells can meet this challenge by secreting increased amounts of insulin continue to have normal glucose concentrations or IGT at the expense of hyperinsulinemia. Only in those with a genetic predisposition will type 2 diabetes develop. This predisposition involves a limited ability of the β-cells to continue to synthesize and secrete the extra insulin demanded of them. Therefore, type 2 diabetes ensues when the β-cells can no longer respond well enough to prevent fasting hyperglycemia.

It must be emphasized that this speculation is only that. Its validation requires more experimentation. Furthermore, type 2 diabetes is undoubtedly not one disease. This heterogeneity must be taken into account as we attempt to unravel the pathogenesis.

Glucagon. The α-cells in the islets of Langerhans secrete glucagon, a hormone whose major function is to promote hepatic glucose production by both glycogenolysis and gluconeogenesis. Glucagon secretion is normally suppressed by glucose. In many diabetic patients, especially type 1 patients, basal glucagon levels are higher, and suppression of glucagon by glucose is impaired; that is, the concentration of glucagon does not decrease normally after glucose. Although it has been postulated that one of the primary abnormalities in diabetes may be an inability of the α-cell to respond normally to glucose, the evidence suggests that the abnormality in glucagon secretion is secondary to the uncontrolled carbohydrate metabolism in diabetes. When animal and human diabetes is tightly controlled with insulin, glucagon levels and suppressibility return to normal. This finding suggests that the abnormality of glucagon homeostasis is simply secondary to the altered metabolism and does not constitute a primary lesion of diabetes mellitus. However, increased hepatic glucose production, which causes the fasting hyperglycemia, is due in large part to hyperglucagonemia in concert with low (Type 1 diabetes) or ineffective (Type 2 diabetes) insulin.

Genetics

The inheritance of diabetes mellitus is probably the most controversial of all the many uncertainties surrounding this enigmatic syndrome. Indeed, it has been termed the "geneticist's nightmare." Familial aggregation (the tendency for diabetes to run in families) was first recorded in 1628. Modern studies have shown that overall the prevalence of diabetes is approximately fourfold higher in the parents and ninefold higher in the siblings of diabetic patients as compared to nondiabetics. However, the inheritance of type 1 and type 2 diabetes is clearly different.

Monozygotic twins are genetically identical, whereas the genetic constitution of dizygotic twins is like that of any two siblings. A number of twinships have been identified in which one member has diabetes. If the other twin also has the disease, they are concordant for diabetes; if diabetes is not present, they are discordant for the trait. Monozygotic twins have a much higher concordance for diabetes than dizygotic twins. However, concordance is much different in identical twinships with type 1 and type 2 diabetes. In type 1 twinships, concordance is no more than 50%. Many of the nondiabetic twins have remained normal for 20 to 30 years suggesting that most of these twins will never develop diabetes. It seems probable that in type 1 diabetes, there is a genetic predisposition related to the HLA locus as discussed previously. However, in order for diabetes to occur, an outside cause is required. In recent years, family studies have provided some information concerning the probabilities of developing type 1 diabetes. Offspring of a type 1 diabetic patient have a 5% chance of developing the disease, while the siblings of such patients have a 5 to 10% chance. These statistics can be refined in the siblings if the HLA haplotypes are known. Those siblings who do not share either of the HLA haplotypes of the type 1 diabetic patient have only a 1% chance; if one HLA haplotype is common to both of them, there is a 5 to 7% chance; and if both HLA haplotypes are similar, there is a 20% chance of developing type 1 diabetes at some time in the future.

In regards to type 2 diabetes, concordance in identical twinships approaches 100% with the second twin developing diabetes shortly after the first one. As these twins are usually living apart for many years before the onset of type 2 diabetes, genetic, rather than environmental, factors must play the predominant role. Except for the unusual patient who inherits type 2 diabetes as an autosomal dominant trait (see below), the empiric risk for a first-degree relative (i.e., sibling, parent, offspring) of a ketosis-resistant diabetic patient to develop diabetes is 10 to 15%. There is a 20 to 30% risk for first degree relatives to develop IGT. Avoidance of obesity will prevent the abnormal carbohydrate metabolism in many of these individuals at risk.

Thus, although the evidence is overwhelming that diabetes mellitus is "inherited," the heterogeneous nature of this disorder prevents a clearer understanding of its mode of transmission. Progress will only be made when homogeneous subsets of this syndrome can be identified and studied. This type of study was possible with young type 2 diabetic patients in whom ketosis-resistant diabetes could be traced back through 3 generations. This finding indicates an autosomal dominant inheritance in this small group of type 2 patients. In addition to heterogeneity complicating the genetic analysis of the remaining type 2 patients, certain environmental "stresses" (e.g., obesity, age, pregnancy, infection) seem to be important in the phenotypic expression of the genetic trait. This environmental influence could prevent the identification of all patients who may carry the gene(s). Until these problems can be resolved, diabetes mellitus will remain the "geneticist's night-mare."

Therapeutic Principles

Although the treatment of diabetes mellitus is beyond the scope of this chapter, a general approach can be described to guide the student during the clinical years. Distinguishing features between ketosis-prone and ketosis-resistant diabetes are summarized in Table 8–12. These differences have important implications for therapy. Since ketosis-prone diabetic patients have virtually no effective endogenous insulin, they require exogenous insulin. Although the need for insulin is not as imperative in ketosis-resistant diabetic

Table 8–12.   Metabolic and Clinical Characteristics of the Two Major Types of Diabetes Mellitus

Characteristics	Ketosis-Prone (type 1)	Ketosis-Resistant (type 2)
Synonyms	Juvenile-onset diabetes, growth-onset diabetes, IDDM[a]	Adult-onset diabetes, maturity-onset diabetes, NIDDM[b]
Age of onset	Usually during growth but sometimes occurs in adults	Usually during maturity but occasionally diagnosed in children and adolescents
Precipitating factors	Altered immune response	Age, obesity, pregnancy
Pancreatic insulin	Very low to absent	Present
Insulin response to glucose	Little or none	Decreased
Insulin response to meals	Little or none	Normal in absolute terms, but nondiabetics with this degree of hyperglycemia would have higher levels
Insulin antagonism	Present only when patient out of control	Present (independent of obesity and control)
Response to prolonged fast	Hyperglycemia, ketoacidosis	Normal adjustment established
Response to stress	Ketoacidosis	Hyperglycemia without ketosis
Associated obesity	Absent	Commonly present (~80%)
Sensitivity to insulin	Usually sensitive	Relatively resistant
Response to diet alone	Negligible	Always present to some degree
Response to sulfonylurea agent	Absent	Present

[a]Insulin Dependent Diabetes Mellitus.
[b]Non-insulin Dependent Diabetes Mellitus.

patients (because without insulin they do not become ketotic and slip into acidosis), these patients may require insulin when diet and sulfonylurea agents fail to control their hyperglycemia. Approximately one-quarter of ketosis-resistant diabetic patients take insulin, one-half use sulfonylurea agents, and the remaining quarter are treated by diet alone (Fig. 8–21). The general approach to type 2 (ketosis-resistant) patients is to use diet first, sulfonylurea agents should diet alone fail, and finally insulin if maximal doses of one of the most effective sulfonylurea agents does not control the patient satisfactorily.

What should be the goals of therapy? Although evidence that strict diabetic control benefits large vessel disease is currently lacking, recently acquired data strongly point toward a beneficial effect of near euglycemia on the retinal, renal and neuropathic complications of diabetes. The evidence is as follows:

1. In animals rendered diabetic by agents that destroy the β-cells of the pancreas, retinal, renal, and neuropathic changes consistent with the abnormalities observed in human diabetes were seen.

2. Renal, retinal, and neuropathic abnormalities disappear in diabetic rats whose diabetes was either cured by pancreatic transplantation or controlled tightly with insulin.

3. Diabetic dogs, whose glucose levels were well controlled for 5 years through multiple injections of regular insulin throughout the day, had only mild cataracts and vascular changes in the eye, kidney, and muscle, whereas their counterparts treated with suboptimal daily injections of

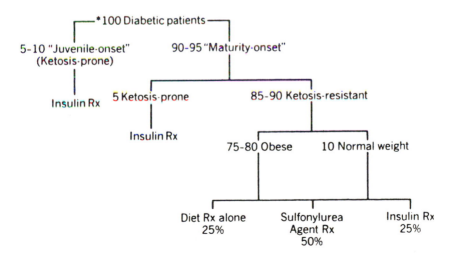

Fig. 8–21. Distribution of ketosis-prone versus ketosis-resistant diabetes in a hypothetical population of 100 diabetic patients. Asterisk indicates that it has recently been recognized that ketosis-resistant diabetes occurs in older children and adolescents; the prevalence of this phenomenon is unknown at present. (Reprinted with permission from Davidson, M.B.: Diabetes Mellitus: Diagnosis and Treatment. 2nd Ed. New York, John Wiley & Sons, 1986.)

intermediate-acting insulin and with poorly controlled diabetes had severe changes.

4. Normal rat kidneys transplanted into inbred diabetic rats developed the vascular changes of diabetes.

5. Vascular abnormalities in kidneys of diabetic rats improved after transplantation into normal inbred rats.

6. In patients with diabetes secondary to pancreatitis or hemochromatosis, typical diabetic complications occurred at a rate similar to that observed in other diabetic patients proving that the microvascular complications did not follow a separate genetic course but were due to the abnormal metabolic status.

7. In large-scale studies in which thousands of patients were analyzed over several decades, there was statistical evidence of an association between good control and fewer diabetic complications.

8. Swedish diabetic patients treated with a free diet and one daily injection of long-acting insulin had a 6- to 7-fold higher prevalence of severe retinopathy and glomerulosclerosis (nephropathy) as compared to a Swedish group treated with a strict diet and multiple injection of short-acting insulin; (the latter group was presumably more tightly controlled).

9. Normal human kidneys developed vascular lesions when transplanted into diabetic patients.

10. Diabetic kidneys with vascular changes showed clearing of these lesions after transplantation into nondiabetic recipients.

11. Several prospective studies (one of which followed over 4000 patients) have shown less retinopathy, nephropathy, and neuropathy when patients were maintained in strict control as compared to a more poorly controlled group.

12. Early lesions of retinopathy, neuropathy, and nephropathy were reversible when strict control of diabetes was introduced; more advanced structural changes, however, were not helped.

Thus, the goals of therapy are to attain as near euglycemia as possible without inordinate severe hypoglycemia and in a setting as consonant with the patient's preferred life style as possible. The challenge is to motivate patients to achieve this during the many years in which diabetes causes little symptoms in order to prevent the microvascular and neuropathic complications. Once these systems deteriorate, it is usually too late.

At the turn of the century, Sir William Osler stated that to know syphilis was to know all of medicine. Because diabetes mellitus can also affect almost all the organ systems in the body, it is not too much of an exaggeration to state that to know this disease is to know most of internal medicine. Although many of the complications cannot be entirely prevented, their onset can be delayed and their impact ameliorated by proper medical care. Helping the diabetic patient live a nearly normal life can be both challenging and satisfying for the physician.

CLINICAL PROBLEMS

Patient 1. This patient was given an oral glucose tolerance test (OGTT) in which the following plasma glucose concentrations were measured: Fasting, 85 mg/100 ml; 1 hour, 130 mg/100 ml; 2 hours, 108 mg/100 ml; 3 hours, 65 mg/100 ml; 4 hours, 43 mg/100 ml; 5 hours, 68 mg/100 ml.

QUESTIONS
1. What would the results have been if whole blood glucose had been measured?
2. List the differential diagnosis of reactive hypoglycemia.
3. Construct an OGTT representing hyperalimentation.
4. Construct an OGTT representing impaired glucose tolerance.
5. Construct an OGTT representing idiopathic reactive hypoglycemia.
6. What additional information is necessary to make a diagnosis of idiopathic reactive hypoglycemia?
7. What is the most likely diagnosis in the person with the OGTT depicted in this problem?

Patient 2. A 34-year-old man was admitted to the emergency room in a combative, disoriented state. When his children woke him for breakfast, he was abusive and responded inappropriately. When examined in the emergency room, this modestly obese man was oriented to name only, had no focal neurologic signs, and had a regular pulse rate of 120 beats/minute. The rest of the examination was negative. The astute emergency room physician suspected hypoglycemia, drew a plasma glucose (which returned at 23 mg/100 ml) and injected 50 ml of 50% glucose intravenously. Within 5 minutes, the patient calmed down, became completely oriented, and gave the following history. He had been to a party the night before and consumed a moderate amount of alcohol; he then drove home and went to sleep. The next thing he remembered was waking up in the emergency room. His wife recalled that he had often been difficult to arouse the morning following a party. On questioning, the patient reported that he ate frequently during the day to avoid intense hunger pains and occasional feelings of weakness. This practice had been going on for at least 3 years and had been associated with a 50-pound weight gain. His only exercise was mowing his lawn; this often caused palpitations, profuse sweating, and profound weakness, which was relieved by eating. He could not remember the last time he had missed a meal. He denied taking any drugs except aspirin for an occasional headache. His review of systems was negative except for nocturia thrice nightly. His physical examination revealed only mild hypertension (150/100) and obesity.

QUESTIONS
1. What kind of hypoglycemia does this man have?
2. His hypoglycemia is potentiated by two factors mentioned in the history. What are they, and what are their mechanisms?
3. What is the differential diagnosis of fasting hypoglycemia? Based on what you know so far, what are the possible causes for this patient's problem?
4. The following endocrinologic data were obtained: Twenty-four-hour urine for 17-hydroxysteroids-10.8 mg/24 hours (normal = 3 to 10). Symptoms of hypoglycemia appeared after 24 hours of fasting; at this time his plasma glucose concentration was 28 mg/100 ml and his insulin level, 35 μU/ml. Interpret these data.
5. In the routine work-up of this patient, a panel of blood chemistries revealed a serum calcium of 12 mg/100 ml (normal = 9.0 to 10.8). What is the probable diagnosis?

Patients 3 to 8. Match up the cause of hypoglycemia in each patient (numbers) with the appropriate signs or laboratory results (letters). Give reasons for your choices.
3. Adrenal insufficiency
4. Insulinoma
5. Factitious hypoglycemia
6. Hepatic failure
7. Fibrosarcoma
8. Ethanol ingestion
   a. glucose concentration—33 mg/100 ml; insulin concentration—30 μU/ml, C-peptide concentration—6.2 ng/ml (normal 1.0 to 4.2)
   b. abdominal mass on physical examination
   c. enlarged sella turcica

    d.   gluose concentration—18 mg/100 ml; insulin concentration—75 μU/ml; C-peptide concentration—0.4 ng/ml (normal 1.0 to 4.2).

    e.   dark urine, light stools

    f.   glucose concentration—21 mg/100 ml; insulin concentration—5 μU/ml; C-peptide concentration—0.5 ng/ml (normal 1.0 to 4.2).

    g.   peculiar odor on breath

    h.   serum thyroxine—15 μg/100 ml (normal 4 to 13).

Patients 9 to 14. Match up the correct diagnosis (letters) with the clinical description of each patient (numbers). Give reasons for your choices. (A diagnosis may be used more than once or not at all.)

    a.   Diabetes mellitus—type 1
    b.   Diabetes mellitus—type 2
    c.   Diabetes mellitus—other types
    d.   Impaired glucose tolerance
    e.   Gestational diabetes mellitus
    f.   Previous abnormality of glucose tolerance
    g.   Potential abnormality of glucose tolerance

9. A woman with no history of diabetes mellitus, whose 3 babies weighed 8 pounds, 9 pounds, and 10 pounds at birth.

10. A 12-year-old boy with a 1-week history of increased thirst, increased urination, a 6-pound weight loss, abdominal pain, nausea, vomiting, and difficulty catching his breath.

11. A 10-year-old girl with a fasting plasma glucose of 74 mg/100 ml, islet cell antibody positive, HLA genotype, DR3/DR5.

12. A 48-year-old man, who is 5'8" tall and weighs 189 lbs without any symptoms and a fasting plasma glucose concentration of 168 mg/100 ml.

13. A 24-year-old alcoholic with documented pancreatitis and a fasting plasma glucose concentration of 232 mg/100 ml.

14. A 52-year-old man who is 5'10" tall, now weighs 174 pounds after losing 15 pounds over the past month associated with polyuria and polydipsia and a urine test that is positive for glucose (½%), but negative for ketone bodies.

Patients 15 and 16. One patient has diabetic ketoacidosis and the other has hyperosmolar nonketotic coma.

QUESTIONS

Which of the following findings are similar in the two conditions and which are different? Give reasons for your choices.

    a.   polyuria
    b.   polydipsia
    c.   prodromal period
    d.   respiratory rate
    e.   neurologic examination
    f.   serum ketone levels
    g.   serum bicarbonate concentrations
    h.   total body sodium
    i.   total body potassium
    j.   plasma volume
    k.   arterial pH
    l.   arterial P_{CO_2}
    m.   prognosis
    n.   treatment after discharge

SUGGESTED READING

Metabolism

Cryer, P.E.: Glucose homeostasis and hypoglycemia. *In*: Williams Textbook of Endocrinology. 7th Ed. Edited by J.D. Wilson and D.W. Foster. Philadelphia, W.B. Saunders Co., 1985, pp. 989–1017.

Jefferson, L.S., and Neely, J.R.: Intermediary metabolism. *In*: Diabetes Mellitus and Obesity.

Edited by B.N. Brodoff, and S.J. Bleicher. Baltimore, Williams & Wilkins, 1982, pp. 3–26.

Rabin, D., and McKenna, T.J.: Clinical Endocrinology and Metabolism. New York, Grune and Stratton, 1982, pp. 111–131.

Seifter, S., and England, S.: Carbohydrate metabolism. *In*: Diabetes Mellitus: Theory and Practice. 3rd Ed. Edited by M. Ellenberg and H. Rifkin. New York, Medical Examination Publishing Co., 1983, pp 1–46.

Hypoglycemia

Burke, M.D.: Hypoglycemia: strategies for laboratory investigation. Postgrad Med, *66*:131, 1979.

Charles, M.A., Hofeldt, F., Schackelford, A., et al.: Comparison of oral glucose tolerance tests and mixed meals in patients with apparent idiopathic postabsorptive hypoglycemia. Absence of hypoglycemia after meals. Diabetes, *30*:465, 1981.

Davidson, M.B.: Hypoglycemia. *In*: Diabetes Mellitus: Diagnosis and Treatment. 2nd Ed, New York, John Wiley & Sons, 1986, pp. 511–565.

Ford, C.V., Bray, G.A., and Swerdloff, R.S.: A psychiatric study of patients referred with a diagnosis of hypoglycemia. Am J Psychiatry, *133*:920, 1975.

Lev-Ran, A., and Anderson, R.W.: The diagnosis of postprandial hypoglycemia. Diabetes, *30*:996, 1981.

Nelson, R.L.: Hypoglycemia: fact or fiction. Mayo Clin Proc, *60*:844,1985.

Selzer, H.S.: Severe drug-induced hypoglycemia: a review. Compr Ther, *5*:21, 1979.

Statement on hypoglycemia: Diabetes Care, *5*:72, 1982.

Yager, J., and Young, R.T.: Non-hypoglycemia is an epidemic condition. N Engl J Med, *291*:907, 1974.

Insulin Secretion (See Pathogenesis of Type 2 Diabetes Mellitus)

Cerasi, E.: Insulin secretion: mechanism of stimulation by glucose. Q Rev Biophys, *8*:1, 1975.

Howell, S.L.: The mechanism of insulin secretion. Diabetologia, *26*:319, 1984.

Kitabchi, A.E.: Proinsulin and C-peptide: a review. Metabolism, *26*:547, 1977.

Polonsky K.S., and Rubenstein A.H.: C-peptide as a measure of the secretion and hepatic extraction of insulin. Pitfalls and limitations. Diabetes *33*:486, 1984.

Diabetes Mellitus—Diagnosis and Classification

Davidson, M.B.: Diagnosis of diabetes mellitus. *In* Diabetes Mellitus: Diagnosis and Treatment. 2nd Ed. New York, John Wiley & Sons, 1986, pp.1–26.

Davidson, M.B.: Treatment—general principles. *In* Diabetes Mellitus: Diagnosis and Treatment. 2nd Ed. New York, John Wiley & Sons, 1986, pp. 27–52.

Harris, M.I., Wilbur, W.C., Hadden, M.A., et al.: International criteria for the diagnosis of diabetes and impaired glucose tolerance. Diabetes Care, *8*:562, 1985.

National Diabetes Data Group: Classification and diagnosis of diabetes mellitus and other categories of glucose intolerance. Diabetes, *28*:1039, 1979.

WHO Expert Committee on Diabetes Mellitus. WHO Tech Rep Ser, *727*, 1985.

Diabetes Mellitus—Pathogenesis of Type 1

Bennett, P.H.: Changing concepts of the epidemiology of insulin-dependent diabetes. Diabetes Care, *8* (Suppl 1):29, 1985.

Bottazzo, G.F.: Beta-cell damage in diabetic insulitis: are we approaching a solution? Diabetologia, *26*:241, 1984.

Bottazzo, G.H.: Death of a beta cell: homicide or suicide? Diabetic Medicine, *3*:119, 1986.

Cahill, G.F., and McDevitt, H.O.: Insulin-dependent diabetes mellitus: the initial lesion. N Engl J Med, *304*:1454, 1981.

Kromann, H.: Aspects of the aetiology and pathogenesis of insulin dependent diabetes mellitus: a critical review. Dan Med Bull, *29*:257, 1982.

Lernmark, A.: Molecular biology of type 1 (insulin-dependent) diabetes mellitus. Diabetologia, *28*:195, 1985.

Lernmark, A., and Baekkeskov, S.: Islet cell antibodies—theoretical and practical implications. Diabetologia, *21*:431, 1981.

Nerup, J., and Lernmark, A.: Autoimmunity in insulin-dependent diabetes. Am J Med, *70*:135, 1982.

Diabetes Mellitus—Pathogenesis of Type 2
Davidson, M.B.: Pathogenesis of impaired glucose tolerance and type 2 diabetes mellitus—
    current status. West J Med, *142*:219, 1985.
DeFronzo, R.A., Ferrannini, E., and Koivisto, V.: New concepts in the pathogenesis and treat-
    ment of noninsulin dependent diabetes mellitus. Am J Med, *74* (Suppl 1A):52, 1983.
Luft, R., Wajngot, A., and Efendic, S.: On the pathogenesis of maturity-onset diabetes. Diabetes
    Care, *41*:58, 1981.
Olefsky, J.M., Ciaraldi, T.P., and Kolterman, O.G.: Mechanisms of insulin resistance in non-
    insulin dependent (type 2) diabetes. Am J Med, *79* (Suppl 3B):12, 1985.
Pfeifer, M.A., Halter, J.B., and Porte, D. Jr.: Insulin secretion in diabetes mellitus. Am J Med,
    70:579, 1981.
Reaven, G.M., Bernstein, T., Davis, B., et al.: Nonketotic diabetes mellitus: insulin deficiency
    or insulin resistance? Am J Med, *60*:80, 1976.
Reaven, G.R., Chen, Y.I., Coulston, A., et al.: Insulin secretion and action in noninsulin-
    dependent diabetes mellitus. Is insulin resistance secondary to hypoinsulinemia? Am J Med,
    75 (Suppl 5B):85, 1984.
Savage, P.J., Dippe, S.E., Bennett, P.H., et al.: Hyperinsulinemia and hypoinsulinemia—insulin
    responses to oral carbohydrate over a wide spectrum of glucose tolerance. Diabetes, *24*:362,
    1975.

Diabetes Mellitus—Genetics
Christy, M., Mandrup-Poulson, T., and Nerup, J.: Genetic markers for insulin dependent diabetes
    mellitus. Ann Clin Res, *16*:53, 1984.
Galton, D.G., and Hitman, G.A.: DNA polymorphisms and the insulin gene: disease associations.
    Diabetic Medicine, 2:159, 1985.
Mandrup-Poulson, T., Owerbach, D., Nerup, J., et al.: Insulin-gene flanking sequences, diabetes
    mellitus and atherosclerosis: a review. Diabetologia, *28*:556, 1985.

Diabetes Mellitus—Abnormal insulin due to a point mutation
Tager, H.S.: Abnormal products of the human insulin gene. Diabetes, *33*:693, 1984.

Diabetes Mellitus—Malnutrition related
Rao, R.H.: The role of undernutrition in the pathogenesis of diabetes mellitus. Diabetes Care,
    7:595, 1984.

ANSWERS TO QUESTIONS

Patient 1
1. Each value would have been 15% lower (not 15 mg/100 ml).
2. Hyperalimentation (postgastric surgery), impaired glucose tolerance, idiopathic reactive
   hypoglycemia, adrenal insufficiency, beta-cell tumor (insulinoma), autoantibodies to the
   insulin molecule, and autoantibodies to the insulin receptor (the last 4 also cause fasting
   hypoglycemia).
3. The curve should be characterized by a normal fasting glucose concentration, high ½- to
   1-hour values, and hypoglycemia within 1 or 2 hours (early hypoglycemia).
4. The curve should be characterized by a normal to mildly elevated fasting glucose concentration, a 1-hour plasma glucose value of more than 200 mg/100 ml, a 2-hour value
   of between 140 and 200 mg/100 ml, and hypoglycemia between 3 and 5 hours during
   the OGTT (early hyperglycemia, late hypoglycemia).
5. The curve should be characterized by normal fasting, 1- and 2-hour glucose concentrations,
   and hypoglycemia between 3 and 5 hours during the OGTT (normal early part of curve,
   late hypoglycemia).
6. Do symptoms occur at time of low plasma glucose level? Are symptoms quickly (10 to
   20 minutes) relieved by carbohydrate snack? Does this pattern (i.e., symptoms consistent
   with hypoglycemia and quickly relieved by carbohydrate intake) occur on a regular basis?
7. Normal subject.

Patient 2
1. Fasting hypoglycemia, which is characterized by symptoms and signs occurring after not
   eating all night rather than after ingesting a (high carbohydrate) meal.
2. Ethanol and exercise.

Ethanol—(potentiation by alcohol can be inferred by the history of difficulty of arousal following a party)—interferes with hepatic gluconeogenesis probably because its catabolism uses nicotinamide-adenine dinucleotide (NAD), which is required for rate-limiting steps of gluconeogenesis.

Exercise–increases muscle utilization of glucose, which potentiates any tendency to hypoglycemia.

3. Drugs, ethanol ingestion, hepatic failure, adrenal insufficiency, extrapancreatic neoplasm, insulinoma, renal failure, autoantibodies to insulin, autoantibodies to the insulin receptor, and sepsis.

Drugs—especially insulin and sulfonylurea agents; propranolol, aspirin, and MAO inhibitors must also be considered. In view of negative drug history, this diagnosis is unlikely.

Ethanol ingestion—potentiates his basic problem but probably not the primary diagnosis.

Hepatic failure—no evidence.

Adrenal insufficiency—no historic or physical evidence for either primary or secondary adrenal insufficiency, but this diagnosis must be considered.

Extrapancreatic neoplasm—a 3-year-history, so this diagnosis is unlikely.

Insulinoma—must always be considered in patients with documented fasting hypoglycemia.

Sepsis and renal failure—no clinical evidence.

Autoantibodies to the insulin molecule and to the insulin receptor—rare syndromes usually occurring in females (like most autoimmune syndromes).

4. The normal value for urinary 17-OH steroids rules out both primary and secondary adrenal insufficiency. Although the insulin level of 35 μU/ml is not high considering this man's obesity (higher insulin concentrations are characteristic in obesity), it is inappropriately elevated for a plasma glucose of 23 mg/100 ml (insulin:glucose ratio = 1.5). Therefore, the patient probably has an insulinoma. (Factitious hypoglycemia secondary to either the surreptitious injection of insulin or oral ingestion of sulfonylurea agents is the only other possibility and is more likely to occur in patients connected with the medical profession.)

5. Multiple endocrine neoplasia type 1. This is a familial syndrome of multiple endocrine tumors of: (1) pancreas—insulin-producing (insulinoma) or gastrin-producing (Zollinger-Ellison syndrome), (2) parathyroid glands, or (3) pituitary gland (chromophobe adenomas some of which may secrete growth hormone causing acromegaly). Hyperplasia of the involved endocrine glands rather than discrete tumors is the pathologic change usually seen. Occasionally an adrenal tumor is associated with this syndrome. Multiple lipomas are often present. It is inherited as an autosomal dominant. The hypercalcemia in this patient is the probable cause of his nocturia since high blood calcium levels impair the concentrating ability of the distal tubules in the kidney.

Patients 3 to 8

3. c.—Pituitary mass causing ACTH deficiency and secondary adrenal insufficiency.
    f.—Appropriate low insulin and C-peptide concentrations in response to hypoglycemia.
4. a.—High insulin and C-peptide levels in association with hypoglycemia (insulin:glucose ratio = 0.91; normal = <0.30).
5. d—High insulin concentration in association with low C-peptide level indicates that the source of the insulin must be exogenous. (Endogenous secretion causes rises in both insulin and C-peptide concentrations.)
6. e.—Typical picture of bile duct obstruction (intrahepatic in this case).
    f.—Appropriate low insulin and C-peptide concentrations in response to hypoglycemia.
    g.—Odor of ammonia that accumulates in hepatic failure and can sometimes appear on the breath.
7. b.—Large retroperitoneal mesenchymal tumor.
    f.—Appropriate low insulin and C-peptide concentrations in response to hypoglycemia.

8.   f.—Appropriate low insulin and C-peptide concentrations in response to hypoglycemia.
     g.—Odor of alcohol.

Patients 9 to 14
9.   g.—Women who give birth to large babies have an increased risk to develop type 2 diabetes in the future.
10. a.—Typical clinical picture of patient in diabetic ketoacidosis.
11. g.—Individuals with a DR3 and/or DR4 in their genotype are at an increased risk to develop type 1 diabetes; presence of islet cell antibodies suggests autoimmune process of β-cell damage has already started to occur; normal fasting plasma glucose suggests that carbohydrate metabolism is still normal.
12. b.—Fasting hyperglycemia fulfills criteria for diabetes mellitus. Obesity and age strongly suggest that patient will be ketosis-resistant.
13. c.—Fasting hyperglycemia fulfills criterion for diabetes mellitus; cause is destruction of β-cells secondary to chronic alcoholic pancreatitis.
14. b.—Man with symptoms of uncontrolled diabetes mellitus (polyuria, polydipsia, weight loss) and glucosuria but no ketonuria.

Patients 15 and 16
Hyperglycemia is the common denominator in both diabetic ketoacidosis and hyperosmolar nonketotic coma. This condition causes an osmotic diuresis by the kidneys that can only lead to the symptom of *polyuria*. Because more water than solutes is lost, the urine osmolality is hypoosmolar to body fluids; this situation leaves a plasma osmolality that is hyperosmolar. The thirst center in the brain reacts to this hyperosmolar situation by signaling the person to drink more water; *polydipsia* then results. In the osmotic diuresis, tremendous amounts of sodium and potassium are lost causing *decreased total body sodium and potassium*. That loss combined with the fluid loss by the kidneys also causes a *decreased plasma volume*.

The following parameters are different in these 2 causes of coma for the following reasons:

Prodromal period—Acidosis supervenes quickly (1 or 2 days) when the effective insulin concentration becomes low; in hyperosmolar nonketotic coma, however, the chronic impairment of insulin action leads to a more gradual build-up of hyperglycemia over a much longer period of time. Since acidosis does not supervene, the patient can tolerate hyperglycemia for long periods of time, and it may be weeks before the patient seeks medical care.

Respiratory rate—Because acidosis drives the respiratory center in an attempt to compensate by a respiratory alkalosis, the respiratory rate in diabetic ketoacidosis is much higher than in hyperosmolar nonketotic coma, where it is usually normal.

Neurologic examination—Although the depth of coma may be similar in the two situations, it is common to have focal neurologic changes in hyperosomolar nonketotic coma; indeed, many of these patients are misdiagnosed initially as having cerebral vascular accidents.

Bicarbonate concentration—This level is low in diabetic ketoacidosis reflecting the metabolic acidosis.

pH—This level is low in diabetic ketoacidosis reflecting the metabolic acidosis; both pH and bicarbonate concentrations are normal in a "pure" case of hyperosmolar nonketotic coma.

Arterial PCO_2—In diabetic ketoacidosis, this level will be low reflecting the compensatory respiratory alkalosis; in hyperosmolar nonketotic coma there is no acidosis and thus no need for a compensatory respiratory alkalosis, so PCO_2 (as well as arterial pH and serum bicarbonate concentrations) is normal.

Serum ketones—These levels are elevated in diabetic ketoacidosis and should be either nondetectable or only minimally detectable in hyperosmolar nonketotic coma. One reason that any ketone bodies at all may be detectable in the latter condition is that patients who have been unable to eat or to use glucose may have "starvation ketosis." In this situation, ketone bodies are positive in the undiluted serum but negative when the serum is diluted because the concentration is so low; by contrast, in diabetic ketoacidosis, tests remain positive as the serum is diluted. Probably a more common reason for the presence of ketone bodies is that most often these patients have aspects of both diabetic ketoacidosis and hyperosmolar nonketotic coma (high glucose levels and ketosis with a compensated acidosis).

Prognosis—The prognosis in diabetic ketoacidosis is usually much more favorable than in hyperosmolar nonketotic coma. In the former, mortality rates range from 3 to 30% (but are usually around the lower level) and depend on the age of the patient and the depth of coma. In hyperosmolar nonketotic coma, mortality rates have been approximately 50% in the past, owing to failure to recognize the situation in some cases; moreover, the patients are usually older and have more complicating illnesses.

Treatment after discharge—In diabetic ketoacidosis, therapy after discharge always includes insulin. (There may be a "honeymoon phase" in which over the next several months insulin requirements drop and may even disappear; however, in over 95% of the cases insulin is required again, usually within 4 to 6 months, occasionally after a period as long as a year or two.) In hyperosmolar nonketotic coma, a large percentage of these patients can be treated by diet alone or by diet with the addition of oral hypoglycemic agents; this regimen indicates that these patients can still secrete some insulin.

These cases represent each end of a spectrum. Often patients have some aspects of both, that is, high glucose levels and mild acidosis.

9

Calcium, Phosphate, Magnesium, and Bone: Physiology and Disorders

Theodore J. Hahn

ABBREVIATIONS

ECF	extracellular fluid
FHH	familial hypocalciuric hypercalcemia
GFR	glomerular filtration rate
OAF	osteoclast activating factor
25(OH)D	25-hydroxy-vitamin D
1,25(OH)$_2$D	1,25-dihydroxy-vitamin D
PTH	parathyroid hormone
TmPO$_4$	tubular maximal reabsorption of phosphate
TRF	tubular reabsorption of phosphate

NORMAL MINERAL METABOLISM

Calcium

The concentration of calcium (Ca) in the extracellular fluid (ECF) plays a critical role in neuromuscular function, the clotting system, and various enzymatic and membrane transport systems. Ca balance is regulated by intestinal, skeletal, and renal factors which, under the influence of calcium-regulating hormones, act in concert to maintain the ECF and serum ionized Ca concentration constant within a remarkably narrow normal range. Approximately half of serum Ca is bound to protein, primarily albumin, and most of the remainder circulates as the free ion. It is the ionized portion of circulating Ca which is biologically important and subject to hormonal regulation. The normal range of serum total Ca concentration is 9.0 to 10.3 mg/dl (4.5 to 5.2 mEq/l).

The principal regulators of serum Ca concentration are (1) parathyroid hormone (PTH); (2) vitamin D, as its active metabolite, 1,25-dihydroxy-vitamin D (1,25(OH)$_2$D); and (3) the serum level of inorganic phosphate (PO$_4$). The rate of intestinal absorption of Ca is controlled primarily by 1,25(OH)$_2$D, which acts at the cellular level to stimulate Ca absorption. Large stores of both Ca and PO$_4$ are found in bone. The 8 kg of bone in the average adult contain approximately 1300 g of calcium. Approximately 90% of body Ca is in bone, 0.1% is in the ECF, and the remainder is intracellular. The interchange between bone and the ECF, which is regulated by PTH and serum PO$_4$ concentrations, appears to be the major factor that regulates serum Ca concentration. In addition, large amounts of Ca and PO$_4$ enter the glomerular filtrate and must be reclaimed by tubular reabsorption. Regulation of renal tubular Ca reabsorption by PTH and other hormones can be important in the control of blood Ca concentration, particularly when skeletal turnover is low. In addition, there is a reciprocal relationship between the blood levels of PO$_4$ and Ca, which is in large part a function of the solubility product of calcium phosphate; an increase in serum PO$_4$ concentration causes a fall in Ca due to deposition of Ca and PO$_4$ in bone and soft tissues.

Parathyroid Hormone. PTH is initially synthesized in the parathyroid glands as a 115 amino acid polypeptide, pre-pro-PTH. Rapid cleavage of 25 amino-terminal amino acids produces a 90 amino acid prohormone (pro-PTH) which is packaged into secretory vesicles. During transport to the cell surface, an additional 6 amino-terminal amino acids are removed, resulting in the secreted form of PTH which has 84 amino acids and a molecular weight (MW) of 9500 daltons. In response to a fall in blood ionized Ca, the 9500 MW form of PTH is secreted into the circulation where it has a half-life of about 20 minutes. PTH is rapidly degraded in the kidney and liver, generating carboxyl-terminal (C-terminal) fragments of 5000 to 7000 MW. These biologically inactive carboxyl terminal fragments are more slowly degraded than intact PTH, are eliminated from the body primarily by renal clearance, and are detected by many assays for PTH. The biologic activity of the PTH molecule resides in the amino (N) terminal portion (amino acids 1 to 34) which is degraded rapidly. PTH binds to cell-surface receptors in target tissues, including kidney and bone, where it activates adenylate cyclase, an enzyme that converts adenosine triphosphate (ATP) to cyclic adenosine-3',5'-monophosphate (cAMP). The cAMP then acts as a "second messenger" by activating a protein kinase (A-kinase), which mediates many of the intracellular effects of PTH. Additional PTH second messenger systems include stimulation of Ca flux into cells and activation of phosphoinositide turnover.

The combined effects of PTH on bone, kidney, and intestine increase the blood level of Ca and reduce the level of PO_4. When the serum ionized Ca concentration falls, PTH secretion is increased. In bone, PTH increases mineral resorption by stimulating osteoclast activity. This action releases both Ca and PO_4 into the circulation. In the kidney, PTH reduces the tubular reabsorption of PO_4, and augments tubular reabsorption of Ca. The fall in serum PO_4, which results from the increased phosphaturia, facilitates the increase in serum Ca by reducing the Ca $\times$ PO_4 product, thereby shifting the Ca-PO_4 equilibrium toward the ECF and away from Ca deposition in bone. In the kidney, PTH also stimulates the conversion of 25-hydroxy-vitamin D (25(OH)D) to $1,25(OH)_2D$ which stimulates the intestinal absorption of Ca and, to a lesser extent, PO_4. The net result of these various actions is an increase in serum Ca concentration, a decrease in serum PO_4, and a subsequent decrease in PTH secretion due to Ca feedback inhibition.

Vitamin D. It is now clear that vitamin D is a prohormone. The scheme of vitamin D metabolism is shown in Figure 9–1. Vitamin D_3 (cholecalciferol) is produced in the skin by solar irradiation of 7-dehydrocholesterol, and is ingested in the diet in animal fats and fish oils. Vitamin D_2 (ergocalciferol) is a synthetic form derived from irradiation of ergosterol. The D_2 and D_3 forms, and their metabolites, are equipotent in man and share identical metabolic pathways. Vitamin D ($D_2 + D_3$) is stored in body tissues, primarily fat and muscle. A small proportion is constantly released into the circulation and converted in the liver to 25(OH)D. The latter, which undergoes enterohepatic circulation, is the major circulating form of vitamin D. Its serum half-life is approximately 21 days. 25(OH)D is converted in the kidney to the most potent vitamin D metabolite, $1,25(OH)_2D$, by a mitochondrial enzyme system in the cells of the proximal convoluted tubule. $1,25(OH)_2D$ has a rapid serum half-life, on the order of 1 to 2 hours. Another vitamin D metabolite, $24,25(OH)_2D$, is also produced in the kidney; its biologic effects are unknown.

The actions of vitamin D appear to be mediated largely through $1,25(OH)_2D$. $1,25(OH)_2D$ acts on the intestine to increase the absorption of Ca and PO_4, and on bone, where it appears to facilitate bone resorption. This latter effect is probably mediated in part by stimulation of the synthesis of osteocalcin (also called bone Gla protein), a 5800 MW vitamin D-dependent, osteoblast-specific protein that binds to the Ca atoms in the hydroxyapatite crystal, and may function to facilitate Ca release from bone. Despite its ability to increase bone resorption, $1,25(OH)_2D$ in moderate doses can promote bone

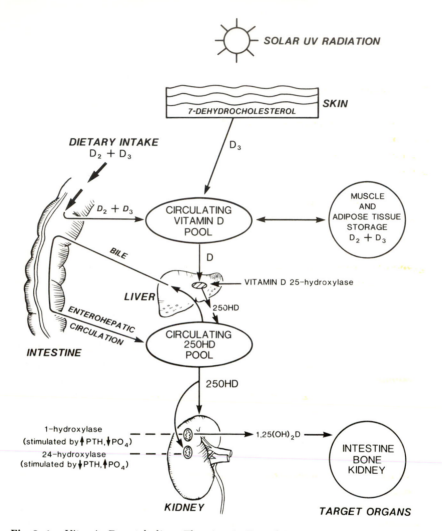

Fig. 9–1. Vitamin D metabolism. The vitamin D pool (vitamin D_2 + vitamin D_3) is derived either from dietary ingestion or from the conversion of 7-dehydrocholesterol to vitamin D_3 in the skin, in a process stimulated by solar UV radiation. Vitamin D is converted in the liver to 25(OH)D, the major circulating metabolite. 25(OH)D is subject to enterohepatic recirculation. The most biologically potent metabolite, $1,25(OH)_2D$, is produced from 25(OH)D by a mitochondrial enzyme system in the kidney that is regulated by PTH and PO_4 levels. $1,25(OH)_2D$ then acts on target organs including intestine, bone, and kidney.

mineralization in rickets, probably by elevating the serum levels of Ca and PO_4 and thereby favoring mineral deposition. $1,25(OH)_2D$ may also act on the kidneys and parathyroid glands, but effects on these two organs are not well defined. $1,25(OH)_2D$ acts on cells through the classic steroid hormone mechanism, being bound first to a cytosolic receptor protein, then transported to the nucleus where the receptor-sterol complex activates the synthesis of specific mRNA species.

The conversion of vitamin D to 25(OH)D is subject to only a minor degree of feedback regulation by both (25(OH)D and 1,25(OH)$_2$D. Thus, serum levels of 25(OH)D closely reflect vitamin D nutritional status, and increase substantially after vitamin D treatment or sunlight exposure. In contrast, the conversion of 25(OH)D to 1,25(OH)$_2$D in the kidney is under tight feedback control, and serum 1,25(OH)$_2$D levels therefore remain relatively constant. 1,25(OH)$_2$D production is stimulated by increased PTH activity and reduced PO$_4$ levels.

Calcitonin. Calcitonin is a peptide hormone of 3500 MW that is secreted by the parafollicular cells of the thyroid gland. It acts directly on osteoclasts to decrease their bone resorbing activity. This action produces a fall in serum Ca levels since bone formation is not affected. The hypocalcemic effect of calcitonin is more marked when bone turnover is high. Calcitonin may also act on the kidney to increase urinary excretion of Na, Ca, PO$_4$, and Mg.

The secretion of calcitonin is stimulated by a rise in serum Ca, and by administration of gastrin or pentagastrin. The normal physiologic role of calcitonin in man is unclear, and is almost certainly a minor one. It has been suggested that calcitonin may prevent an inordinate rise in serum Ca following the ingestion of a Ca-containing meal. In addition, calcitonin levels are higher in the fetus and in infants than in adults, suggesting a role during growth. Although calcitonin does not appear to play a significant role in normal human mineral metabolism, calcitonin in pharmacologic doses is useful in the treatment of Paget's disease, a high-turnover bone disorder associated with increased levels of osteoclastic activity, and is often used in the management of hypercalcemic disorders associated with increased osteoclastic resorption of bone.

Dietary Calcium and Calcium Balance. The average daily intake of calcium ranges from 400 to 1000 mg under normal circumstances; however, less than half of this amount is absorbed (Fig. 9–2). Daily losses of Ca from the body are nearly constant in normal individuals. Renal excretion of Ca is normally 100 to 300 mg/day (1.5 to 4 mg/kg ideal body weight), and this rate falls only slightly with restricted Ca intake. The endogenous fecal loss of Ca, from Ca that is excreted into the bile and intestinal fluids and not reabsorbed, is constant at approximately 200 mg/day. Another 10 to 20 mg/day is lost from the skin.

The efficiency of absorption of dietary Ca varies inversely with the amount ingested. With a low Ca diet, on the order of 200 mg/day, the efficiency of Ca absorption increases to about 60%. As dietary Ca is increased, absorption efficiency falls rapidly. Thus, at a dietary Ca intake of 800 mg/day, the minimum daily requirement recommended by the National Research Council, net Ca absorption averages approximately 25% of the amount ingested. There is considerable evidence that the efficiency of Ca absorption is regulated through feedback control of PTH secretion and 1,25(OH)$_2$D synthesis.

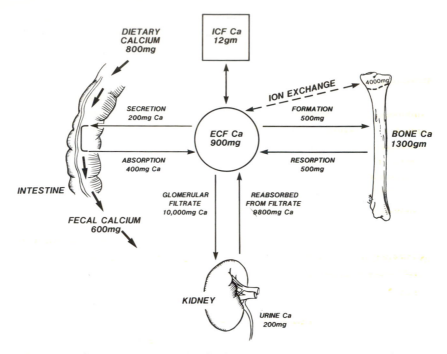

Fig. 9–2. Schematic representation of calcium metabolism in a normal individual ingesting an 800 mg calcium diet. Calcium concentration in the extracellular fluid (ECF) is controlled by absorption from the intestine, renal filtration and reabsorption, the balance of cell-mediated bone formation and resorption, rapid ionic exchange with a portion of bone calcium, and equilibrium with calcium in the intracellular fluid (ICF).

Calculations of total body Ca balance based on average losses in the urine, feces, and sweat suggest that the average adult rarely achieves a neutral or positive Ca balance at the recommended dietary Ca intake. Moreover, a significant fraction of the population may have an intake below the recommended daily allowance, resulting in a slightly negative Ca balance during most of adult life. Thus, low dietary Ca intake may contribute to the osteoporosis that occurs with aging.

Bone Metabolism and Serum Mineral Regulation. Since 99% of body Ca and 85% of body PO_4 are contained in bone, it is apparent that bone has an important regulatory role in Ca and PO_4 metabolism. The major cell types involved in normal bone turnover are the osteoblast, which is the primary bone-forming cell, and the osteoclast, the primary bone-resorbing cell. Although the activity of osteoblasts and osteoclasts is normally closely coupled, hormonal and local regulatory factors can rapidly change the formation/resorption balance. Normally approximately 500 mg/day of Ca is involved in hormonally-regulated bone turnover controlled by osteoblasts and osteoclasts, and another 4000 mg or so is available for ionic exchange controlled by various factors such as extracellular fluid (ECF) pH and concentrations of Ca and PO$_4$. These amounts are quite large in relation to the total ECF calcium pool of about 900 mg. Thus, changes in the ECF-bone equilibrium for Ca and PO$_4$ in response to hormonal, ionic, and other factors can rapidly alter ECF Ca and PO$_4$ concentrations.

Phosphate

Phosphorus plays a major regulatory role in body metabolism. It is present in the ECF as inorganic phosphate (PO$_4$) and exists within cells primarily as various phosphorylated organic compounds. A number of these compounds, such as ATP, are critical to energy metabolism. In addition, the phosphorylation and dephosphorylation of various enzymes play a major role in the regulation of their activity. In bone, phosphorus represents a significant portion of the mineral phase as calcium phosphate or as hydroxyapatite [Ca$_{10}$(PO$_4$)$_6$(OH)$_2$]. Approximately 85% of total body PO$_4$ is contained in bone, 1% is in the ECF and the remainder is intracellular. In contrast to Ca, serum PO$_4$ levels are not precisely controlled, and may fluctuate by 1 to 2 mg/dl throughout the day under the influence of dietary intake and hormonal changes.

Phosphate is usually abundant in the diet, and normal intake ranges from 800 to 1500 mg/day. Approximately 60 to 80% of dietary PO$_4$ is absorbed, and there are only minor changes in absorption rate in response to differing body needs. Only about 12% of serum PO$_4$ is bound to proteins, and PO$_4$ is freely filtered at the glomerulus, with 80 to 90% of the filtered PO$_4$ resorbed by the renal tubule. Thus, the kidney plays a primary role in regulating body PO$_4$ content. When dietary PO$_4$ intake increases, the rise in serum PO$_4$ tends to cause a reciprocal lowering of serum Ca, and PTH secretion is stimulated. This causes a decrease in renal tubular reabsorption of PO$_4$ (TRP), which increases renal excretion of PO$_4$ and restores the serum PO$_4$ toward normal. When PO$_4$ intake is reduced, TRP increases so that urinary PO$_4$ losses approach zero. Renal tubular PO$_4$ handling is assessed clinically by determining the renal threshold for phosphate concentration (Tm$_{PO_4}$/GFR). First, the TRP is calculated as $1 - (C_{PO_4}/C_{creat})$, and Tm$_{PO_4}$/GFR is then derived from a nomogram relating serum TRP to serum PO$_4$ (Fig. 9–3). PO$_4$ excretion is increased by PTH, expansion of ECF volume, and to a lesser extent by alkalosis, growth hormone, calcitonin, and glucocorticoids.

Magnesium

Magnesium (Mg) is a significant extracellular cation, and it is second only to potassium as the major intracellular cation. Approximately 65% of body magnesium is contained in bone, 1% is in the ECF, and the remainder is intracellular. Intracellular Mg levels are maintained constant, largely independent of serum Mg. The intracellular functions of Mg include serving as a cofactor for various enzymes and participating in the binding of enzymes to subcellular structures. In bone, approximately one-third of the Mg is freely exchanged with serum Mg, while the remainder is deep within bone crystals.

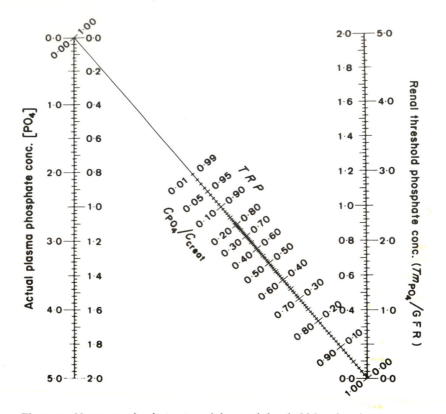

Fig. 9–3. Nomogram for derivation of the renal threshold for phosphate concentration (Tm_{PO_4}/GFR) from the serum phosphate level and the tubular resorption of phosphate (TRP). The TRP is calculated as $1 - (C_{PO_4}/C_{creat})$. There are two scales: an outer scale (0.0 to 5.0) in mass units and an inner scale (0.0 to 2.0) in SI units (mMol/L). The normal value for Tm_{PO_4}/GFR is 2.5 to 4.2 mg/dl. A low value indicates decreased renal tubular phosphate reabsorption, such as occurs in hyperparathyroidism. A value above 4.2 mg/dl indicates increased phosphate reabsorption, as in hypoparathyroid states. (From Walton, R.J., and Bijvoet, O.L.M.: Lancet, *2*:309, 1975.)

Normal dietary Mg intake is in the range of 175 to 300 mg (20 to 35 mEq)/day, of which about one-third is absorbed. Intestinal absorption of Mg is only minimally regulated by factors similar to those that regulate Ca absorption. Hence, Mg is absorbed largely independent of bodily needs. Fecal losses of Mg are increased in diarrheal and malabsorptive disorders. The kidney plays the major role in regulating body Mg content. Thus, when dietary Mg intake is reduced, there is a rapid reduction in urinary Mg excretion. When Mg intake is high, the maximal rate of renal tubular reabsorption of Mg is exceeded, and the excess Mg is excreted in the urine. Renal tubular reabsorption of Mg is reduced by several factors that decrease the reabsorption of sodium and water, including ECF volume expansion, hypercalcemia, alcohol, osmotic diuresis, and the use of loop diuretics (e.g., furosemide). PTH may increase the tubular reabsorption of Mg slightly.

DISORDERS OF SERUM MINERAL METABOLISM

Hypercalcemia

The serum Ca concentration is normally maintained within narrow and constant limits, and in most laboratories the normal range for serum total Ca is 9.0 to 10.3 mg/dl. Even slight persistent deviations from this normal range indicate a significant abnormality of Ca metabolism.

Clinical Presentation. Hypercalcemia is commonly encountered in clinical practice. It can vary in severity from an asymptomatic, long-standing condition, detected accidentally by routine screening blood tests, to an acute, life-threatening illness. The manifestations of hypercalcemia reflect both the degree of elevation of blood Ca and its duration. A serum Ca in excess of 15 mg/dl represents a serious medical emergency.

Several organ systems are affected by hypercalcemia, especially the kidneys and the central nervous system. The renal manifestations of hypercalcemia are largely due to hypercalciuria caused by the increased filtered load of Ca, and can vary from kidney stones to reversible, or even irreversible, renal failure. Among the earliest renal manifestations of hypercalcemia are polyuria and nocturia, which are caused by both the increased osmotic load of Ca and a loss of ability to concentrate the urine. The decreased concentrating ability and polyuria can predispose to dehydration. Kidney stones are usually a consequence of chronic hypercalciuria; thus, they are most common when the hypercalcemia is long-standing. With chronic, marked hypercalcemia, progressive renal failure can occur.

Calcium has a depressive effect on the nervous system, and impaired nerve conduction, hypotonia, hyporeflexia, and even paresis can occur as hypercalcemia progresses. Reduced intestinal motility can cause constipation, a frequent presenting symptom, and anorexia and nausea are common. With severe hypercalcemia, the patient's CNS functioning is usually impaired producing lethargy, confusion, and even coma. Hypercalcemia has a positive inotropic effect on the heart, and can alter the cardiac conduction system, resulting in a shortened Q-T interval and a tendency to arrhythmias. Hypercalcemia may also be associated with hypertension. Possible mechanisms include alterations in the renin-angiotensin system and direct effects on peripheral vascular resistance. Moreover, there is an increased incidence of peptic ulcer disease and pancreatitis. The tendency to peptic ulcer formation may be due to increased gastrin release as a consequence of increased serum Ca levels. Hypercalcemia may also be associated with increased deposition of Ca salts in soft tissues, with the lungs, kidneys, blood vessels, and joints being most susceptible. Soft tissue deposition occurs most commonly when there is an associated elevation in serum PO_4 concentration, as occurs in renal failure and vitamin D intoxication. A syndrome of "pseudogout" can be caused by increased deposition of calcium phosphate in joint tissues.

Hypercalcemia can be caused by a number of disorders (Table 9-1), and is the result of either increased bone resorption or increased intestinal ab-

Table 9–1.   Biochemical Findings in Patients with Various Hypercalcemic Disorders

	Serum						Urine	
	Ca	PO$_4$	Alk P'ase	iPTH	25(OH)D	1,25(OH)$_2$D	Ca	Tm$_{PO_4}$/GFR
Primary Hyperparathyroidism	I	D	N or I	I	N	I	I	D
Familial Hypocalciuric Hypercalcemia	I	D	N	N or I	N	N or I	D	D
Malignancy: Ectopic PTH-like Factor	I	D	N	D	N	N	I	D
Malignancy: Osteolytic Metastases	I	I	N	D	N	D	I	I
Vitamin D Intoxication	I	I	N	D	I	N or D	I	I
Sarcoidosis	I	I	N	D	N	I	I	I
Thyrotoxicosis	I	I	N	D	N	D	I	I
Immobilization	I	I	N	D	N	D	I	I

D, decreased; I, increased; N, normal.

sorption of Ca, or both. The severity of the hypercalcemia is frequently aggravated by a relative decrease in renal excretion of Ca due to decreased renal filtration rate as a result of dehydration. Of the disorders discussed in the following sections, primary hyperparathyroidism and neoplastic diseases are the most common causes of hypercalcemia.

Primary Hyperparathyroidism. Primary hyperparathyroidism is the cause of hypercalcemia in 10 to 30% of cases. It is a relatively common disorder, with an incidence of about 1:800 in adults. A parathyroid adenoma, usually single, is the cause in 80 to 85% of cases and parathyroid hyperplasia occurs in 15 to 25%. Parathyroid carcinoma is rare. A patient with primary hyperparathyroidism may have other endocrine disorders associated with the syndrome of multiple endocrine neoplasia (MEN), type 1 or type 2. Although PTH secretion is partially regulated by serum Ca concentration, in both parathyroid adenomas and in primary hyperplasia PTH secretion is greater than would normally be expected for the level of serum Ca. Also, urinary Ca excretion is almost always significantly increased due to the marked increase in filtered Ca load, despite the Ca-retaining effects of PTH on the kidney tubule.

The presentation of primary hyperparathyroidism is frequently asymptomatic, and the disorder is often detected incidentally on the basis of hypercalcemia observed on a routine blood chemistry profile. Common early symptoms include rather nonspecific weakness and fatigability. However, patients may have any or all of the symptoms of hypercalcemia. Hypertension is present in about 50% of patients, and a history of kidney stones in 10 to 30%. The diagnosis of primary hyperparathyroidism is established by the demonstration of: (1) increased serum Ca and decreased serum PO_4 in the fasting state, (2) increased serum immunoreactive PTH (iPTH) levels, and (3) increased 24-hour urinary Ca excretion (greater than 4 mg/kg ideal body weight). Renal phosphate wasting, as determined by a reduced Tm_{PO_4}/GFR, is universally present. Associated biochemical findings may include a mild hyperchloremic acidosis (increased serum chloride and decreased serum bicarbonate) due to enhancement of bicarbonate excretion by PTH. Serum uric acid levels may be mildly elevated due to PTH inhibition of urate excretion. In those relatively rare cases where clinically significant PTH-induced bone disease (osteitis fibrosa) is observed, the serum alkaline phosphatase, a marker of osteoblastic activity, may be increased, and radiologic findings of osteitis fibrosa may be observed (see Osteitis Fibrosa).

Care must be taken to distinguish primary hyperparathyroidism from *familial hypocalciuric hypercalcemia* (FHH), a familial autosomal dominant disorder that is also characterized by increased serum Ca and decreased serum PO_4 levels. Distinguishing features include the fact that in FHH the serum iPTH levels are generally not increased above the upper limits of normal, and urinary calcium excretion is universally decreased. The importance of making this distinction is that, in contrast to primary hyperparathyroidism, partial parathyroidectomy in patients with FHH does not cure the hypercalcemia. The hypercalcemia in FHH is currently thought to be the result of a "resetting" of parathyroid and kidney cell sensitivity to ECF Ca levels.

Primary hyperparathyroidism is best managed surgically in situations where there is marked elevation of the serum Ca, kidney stone formation, decreasing renal function, clinically significant bone loss, recurrent pancreatitis, or active ulcer disease. In the absence of these specific complications, selected patients with mild hyperparathyroidism can be managed medically with low calcium diet, enforced hydration, and careful follow-up.

Malignant Disease. Malignant disease is a common cause of hypercalcemia. The increase in serum Ca is most commonly due to metastases to bone (80% of cases), but can also occur in the absence of skeletal metastases. When hypercalcemia occurs in the presence of bone metastases, the destruction of bone and consequent hypercalcemia are due to release of local tumor factors that activate osteoclastic bone resorption. In the case of multiple myeloma and lymphomas, the responsible osteoclast-activating factor (OAF) has been identified as interleukin 1 or a closely-related peptide. As a result of osteoclast activation, Ca and PO_4 are released from bone, and the rise in serum Ca suppresses PTH secretion. Hence, serum Ca and PO_4 are elevated and serum iPTH is reduced. Malignancy-associated hypercalcemia that occurs in the absence of detectable metastatic disease is thought to be caused by various humoral factors, including a PTH-like substance produced by certain cancers, especially those of the lung and genitourinary system. This PTH-like tumor product mimics many of the effects of PTH on bone and kidney; thus, serum Ca is increased, serum PO_4 is decreased, and there is renal phosphate wasting. However, the substance is not detected by either N-terminal or C-terminal directed PTH immunoassays (iPTH), and serum iPTH levels are therefore low.

There is also evidence that parathyroid adenomas may occur with greater than expected frequency in patients with malignant disease. For this reason, one should not ignore the possibility of a coexistence of malignant disease and primary hyperparathyroidism.

Vitamin D Overdosage. Overdosage with vitamin D or one of its active metabolites [25(OH)D or 1,25(OH)$_2$D] can cause hypercalcemia due to stimulation of intestinal Ca absorption and increased bone resorption. Serum Ca and PO_4 are increased, and PTH is suppressed. This situation occurs primarily in patients with hypoparathyroidism, chronic renal failure, or various osteopenic bone disorders who are being treated with vitamin D metabolites. In patients treated with toxic doses of vitamin D, the serum 25(OH)D levels are markedly elevated, while 1,25(OH)$_2$D levels are normal or reduced. This observation suggests that 25(OH)D in high concentrations can mimic the effects of 1,25(OH)$_2$D. Toxicity due to severe vitamin D overdosage may last for months, since the sterol is sequestered in fat and muscle cells. Toxicity resulting from 25(OH)D or 1,25(OH)$_2$D overdosage lasts for a matter of a few weeks or 1 to 2 days, respectively, in accord with their relative circulating half-lives. Mild cases of vitamin D toxicity can be managed by discontinuing the sterol, restricting calcium intake, and enforcing hydration. In more severe cases, use of glucocorticoids to block the effects of vitamin D on intestinal calcium absorption produces a prompt lowering of serum Ca.

Sarcoidosis and Other Granulomatous Diseases. Hypercalcemia may occasionally occur in patients with sarcoidosis and other granulomatous diseases. Such individuals demonstrate increased intestinal Ca absorption, and the hypercalcemia can be aggravated by sunlight exposure or by the administration of small doses of vitamin D. The serum level of 25(OH)D is normal, but serum 1,25(OH)$_2$D is elevated, and the severity of the hypercalcemia correlates with the 1,25(OH)$_2$D level. Recent evidence indicates that the source of increased 1,25(OH)$_2$D production is the 1-hydroxylation of 25(OH)D in the granulomatous tissue, a process which may be mediated by activated lymphocytes. Receptors for 1,25(OH)$_2$D have been found in activated, but not resting, lymphocytes, and it has been suggested that 1,25(OH)$_2$D may play a role in regulating immune system function. The hypercalcemia of sarcoidosis responds rapidly to the administration of glucocorticoids, since steroid therapy both reduces the production of 1,25(OH)$_2$D by the granulomatous tissue and inhibits the action of 1,25(OH)$_2$D on the intestine.

Thyrotoxicosis. Severe hypercalcemia is unusual in patients with hyperthyroidism, but some will have mild transient elevations of serum and urine Ca, presumably due to increased thyroid hormone stimulation of osteoclastic bone resorbing activity. Occurrence of hypercalcemia is more common in children and young adults, due to their higher bone turnover rates. Moreover, the hypercalcemia may become severe if the patient is immobilized, thereby suppressing osteoblastic bone-forming activity. Serum Ca and PO$_4$ levels are elevated, and PTH is suppressed. The diagnosis is established by demonstrating increased serum levels of thyroid hormone. Management consists of hydration, mobilization, and treatment of the hyperthyroidism.

Immobilization. With total immobilization or prolonged bed rest, the balance between bone formation and bone resorption is disturbed. Immobilization eliminates the stress stimulus to osteoblastic activity; hence, bone formation is suppressed while resorption continues unabated. As a result, a net release of Ca and PO$_4$ from bone occurs. Prolonged immobilization can result in a marked loss of bone mass. Significant hypercalcemia may thus occur in totally immobilized children and young adults, and in older patients on bedrest who have disorders, such as Paget's disease and hyperthyroidism, that are associated with an increased bone turnover rate. Treatment consists of hydration and mobilization, where possible. In severe cases, calcitonin may be of benefit.

Recovery Phase of Acute Renal Failure. Hypercalcemia may develop during the diuretic phase of acute renal failure, particularly that caused by rhabdomyolysis. During the earlier oliguric phase, marked hypocalcemia is common in such patients, in part because marked elevations in serum PO$_4$ cause deposition of calcium phosphate salts in the damaged muscle and other soft tissues. With the appearance of decreased serum PO$_4$ levels during the diuretic phase, massive release of Ca from soft tissue deposits produces hypercalcemia. The hypercalcemia may be further aggravated by dehydration that leads to decreased renal Ca excretion. Treatment consists of hydration and maintenance of ECF fluid volume to promote renal Ca excretion.

Thiazide Diuretics. The administration of thiazide diuretics can occasionally cause a mild, transient elevation of serum Ca in apparently normal individuals. However, where thiazide-associated hypercalcemia persists for more than a day or so, an underlying disorder of Ca metabolism must be strongly suspected. Thiazide diuretics potentiate hypercalcemia by decreasing renal Ca excretion through two mechanisms: (1) decreasing the intravascular fluid volume due to sodium and water diuresis, and hence decreasing the renal filtration rate, and (2) directly enhancing renal tubular resorption of Ca. When thiazide-induced hypercalcemia occurs, the thiazide should be discontinued, rehydration promoted, and a search instituted for the underlying disorder of Ca or bone metabolism.

Other Causes of Hypercalcemia. Rarer causes of hypercalcemia include acute adrenal insufficiency, the milk-alkali syndrome, and factitious hypercalcemia due to increased protein binding of Ca. Serum total Ca concentration is frequently mildly elevated in patients with *adrenal crisis*. The hypercalcemia appears to be the result of increased serum protein concentration due to dehydration, enhanced tubular reabsorption of Ca, and increased complexing of Ca with citrate. Serum ionized Ca concentration is usually normal. The *milk-alkali* syndrome is a rare disorder in which patients with mild renal insufficiency who are treated with large amounts of calcium carbonate antiacids develop hypercalcemia, hyperphosphatemia, and progressive renal insufficiency. Increased Ca absorption may be facilitated by alkalinity in the intestinal lumen produced by the calcium carbonate. An underlying disorder of calcium metabolism such as mild hyperparathyroidism may play a predisposing role. *Increased protein binding* of Ca due to greatly increased amounts of abnormal globulin produced by certain hematologic malignancies such as multiple myeloma may rarely elevate the serum total Ca; however, the ionized Ca level remains normal.

Treatment of Hypercalcemia. A detailed discussion of the treatment of hypercalcemia is beyond the scope of this chapter. However, a general discussion of management techniques illustrates certain physiologic principles. The most important initial measure in the treatment of hypercalcemia is to restore normal intravascular fluid volume by replacing the sodium and water which have been lost as a result of the chronic Ca-induced osmotic diuresis. This approach will enhance renal Ca excretion by increasing renal blood flow and glomerular filtration rate. In addition, since sodium and Ca compete for reabsorption in the renal tubule, sodium loading further promotes Ca excretion. Sodium and water are given as alternating normal (0.9%) and half-normal (0.45%) saline solution until the central venous pressure is restored to normal levels. Fluid overload is prevented in the face of continuing saline administration by the periodic cautious administration of a loop diuretic such as furosemide. The resulting increased sodium delivery to the distal tubule further enhances Ca excretion. However, overzealous use of loop diuretics can lead to intravascular volume depletion and a worsening of the hypercalcemia. These general measures should significantly reduce the serum Ca level in virtually all hypercalcemic patients who have reasonably normal renal function. Additional general measures include restricting calcium intake, mobilizing the patient where possible to encourage calcium deposition in bone, and specific therapies aimed at the underlying disorder.

When these general measures do not produce a sufficient reduction in serum Ca concentration, a number of secondary measures can be employed. In hypercalcemic patients with reduced serum PO_4 levels (e.g., patients with primary or malignancy-associated hyperparathyroidism), oral PO_4 supplementation may reduce serum Ca levels both by binding dietary Ca and thereby reducing Ca absorption, and by raising serum PO_4 levels to normal, promoting Ca deposition in bone. Phosphate supplements should *not* be used in patients with normal or elevated serum PO_4 levels, since extensive soft tissue calcification may occur. Glucocorticoid therapy is a useful adjuvant in reducing intestinal hyperabsorption of Ca in states of increased vitamin D activity, and also blocks the stimulatory effect of OAF factors on bone resorption in the hypercalcemia associated with multiple myeloma and lymphomas. Calcitonin is often useful in malignancy-associated hypercalcemic states caused by increased osteoclastic activity. The concurrent administration of glucocorticoids with calcitonin delays the occurrence of osteoclast resistance to calcitonin. In more severe cases, the relatively toxic antitumor agent mithramycin can be used to inhibit osteoclast activity. When severely impaired renal function prohibits urinary excretion of the increased ECF Ca load, dialysis may be the only effective emergency treatment for hypercalcemia.

Hypocalcemia

Clinical Presentation. Hypocalcemia may be inadvertently detected by routine blood testing in an asymptomatic patient, or it may show significant symptomatology. It is a potentially dangerous disorder, and clinical manifestations are produced by disturbances in neuromuscular function. The symptoms of hypocalcemia include numbness and tingling sensations (paresthesias) of the hands, feet, tongue, or circumoral area. These are often most marked during periods of fatigue. Muscle spasms commonly occur in the forearm and hand, with the elbow, wrist, and metacarpal-phalangeal joints flexed and abducted across the palm; a similar pattern occurs in the ankle and foot (carpopedal spasm). Tetany is manifested first by muscle cramps and then by carpopedal spasm.

Latent tetany may be demonstrated by *Chvostek's sign*, a twitching of the ipsilateral facial muscles and upper lip following a sharp tap over the facial nerve in front of the ear. *Trousseau's sign* is a carpal spasm produced by obstruction of the blood flow in the forearm for 3 minutes with a blood pressure cuff inflated above the level of systolic pressure. The patient may also have mental instability, confusional episodes, or seizures. The ECG is usually normal, but may demonstrate a prolonged Q-T interval.

In the approach to a patient with hypocalcemia, it must first be determined whether there is a decrease in the serum ionized Ca. Since approximately 50% of serum Ca is protein-bound, mainly to albumin, measurement of total serum Ca includes both the metabolically active ionized Ca fraction and the protein-bound Ca. Consequently, if a patient has a low serum albumin, total serum Ca may be low, but ionized Ca can be normal. In this situation, ionized Ca can be measured, or a crude calculation can be applied to adjust the observed serum Ca for the degree of hypoalbuminemia; for example, add 0.8 mg/dl to the measured total Ca for each 1.0 g/dl decrease in the serum albumin below the normal value of 4.0 g/dl.

When it is determined that the serum ionized Ca is low, the factors that can produce hypocalcemia should be considered. A reduction in serum Ca often reflects a disturbance in the production, metabolism, or efficacy of either PTH or vitamin D. Hypocalcemia may also be caused by sudden removal of Ca from the serum as with acute hyperphosphatemia or increased deposition into bone. Enhanced urinary Ca loss may accentuate hypocalcemia in certain situations. The biochemical features of various disorders which produce hypocalcemia are shown in Table 9–2.

Disturbances of Parathyroid Hormone Production or Action. Disturbances in parathyroid hormone that produce hypocalcemia include impaired PTH secretion and inadequate end-organ response to PTH. PTH secretion is reduced in hypoparathyroidism, either post-surgical or idiopathic, and in Mg depletion. Conditions that are associated with inadequate end-organ response to PTH include pseudohypoparathyroidism, types I and II, acute or chronic renal failure, and Mg deficiency. Biochemical findings in hypoparathyroidism include hypocalcemia, increased serum PO_4, and undetectable iPTH.

Pseudohypoparathyroidism is a rare familial disorder manifested by hypocalcemia, hyperphosphatemia, and distinctive skeletal defects. The skeletal and developmental abnormalities, originally referred to as Albright's hereditary osteodystrophy, include short stature, a round face, obesity, and shortened third and fifth metacarpals and metatarsals. Pseudohypoparathyroidism is characterized by elevated levels of circulating iPTH and an apparent resistance in the bone and kidney to the actions of PTH. Pseudohypoparathyroidism type I is caused by the failure of PTH to activate adenylate cyclase due to a deficiency of the guanine nucleotide regulatory protein or G unit (also called N-protein), which provides functional coupling between the cell-surface PTH receptor and the intracellular adenylate cyclase catalytic unit. Pseudohypoparathyroidism type II is believed to be due to defective intracellular action of cyclic AMP. Renal insufficiency, either acute or chronic, may cause impaired end-organ action of PTH. The pathogenesis is complex, but may arise from altered metabolism of vitamin D and aluminum accumulation in bone. Severe Mg depletion, in addition to impairing PTH secretion, may also inhibit the response of bone to PTH.

Table 9–2. Biochemical Findings in Patients with Common Hypocalcemic Disorders

	Serum						Urine	
	Ca	PO$_4$	Alk P'ase	iPTH	25(OH)D	1,25(OH)$_2$D	Ca	Tm$_{PO_4}$/GFR
Hypoparathyroidism	D	I	N	D	N	D	D	I
Pseudohypoparathyroidism	D	I	N or I	I	N	D	D	I
Magnesium Deficiency	D	I	N	N or D	N	N	D	N or I
Vitamin D Deficiency	D	D	I	I	D	N	D	D
Renal Failure	D	I	N	I	N	N or D	D	D

D, decreased; I, increased; N, normal.

Disturbances of Vitamin D Metabolism or Action. A deficiency in, or reduced action of, the active metabolites of vitamin D can cause hypocalcemia. Due to the secondary hyperparathyroidism that results from decreased stimulation of intestinal Ca absorption, serum PO_4 is reduced and iPTH levels are elevated. Vitamin D deficiency can arise from defects in vitamin D metabolism at any step from intestinal absorption or synthesis in the skin to the final action of $1,25(OH)_2D$ at target organs. It is convenient to classify vitamin D deficiency in terms of the step in vitamin D metabolism affected: decreased availability of vitamin D, increased 25(OH)D loss, and decreased availability or action of $1,25(OH)_2D$. These disorders are managed by supplementation with vitamin D or its appropriate metabolite.

DECREASED AVAILABILITY OF VITAMIN D. Sufficient vitamin D may not be available to meet Ca homeostatic demands if there is markedly reduced vitamin D intake or decreased intestinal absorption, in combination with a minimal exposure to ultraviolet radiation from sunlight. Due to the widespread fortification of foods, such as milk, bread, and cereals with vitamin D, nutritional vitamin D deficiency is rare in the United States. Consequently, the most frequent cause of vitamin D deficiency is impaired absorption due to intestinal disorders that cause fat malabsorption such as chronic pancreatitis, celiac disease, Crohn's disease, and hepatobiliary disorders.

INCREASED 25-HYDROXY-VITAMIN D LOSS. In the face of normal availability and absorption of vitamin D, decreased levels of 25(OH)D may develop if there is an increased rate of metabolism of 25(OH)D to inactive metabolites. This process may occur during treatment with phenobarbital, phenytoin, glutethimide, or rifampin, agents that induce increased hepatic microsomal mixed-function oxidase enzyme activity. Increased activity of this system results in a more rapid breakdown and biliary excretion of both vitamin D and 25(OH)D. In states of maximal stimulation of mixed function oxidase activity, vitamin D requirements may increase more than 10-fold from the basal level of 100 to 200 units/day. Severe liver disease, in particular advanced biliary cirrhosis, may be associated with decreased synthesis of 25(OH)D or may cause impaired reabsorption of enterohepatic recirculated 25(OH)D.

DECREASED AVAILABILITY OR ACTION OF $1,25(OH)_2$ VITAMIN D. Reduced serum levels of $1,25(OH)_2D$ occur in: (1) chronic renal insufficiency, due to a reduction in functioning renal parenchymal tissue; (2) vitamin D dependency rickets, a hereditary defect in renal 25(OH)D-1-hydroxylase activity; (3) osteomalacia associated with certain mesenchymal tumors, presumably due to tumor production of substances which suppress renal 25(OH)D-1-hydroxylase activity, and (4) Fanconi's syndrome. In addition, serum levels of $1,25(OH)_2D$ are lower than expected, relative to serum PO_4 levels, in familial hypophosphatemic rickets. With the exception of chronic renal insufficiency, these disorders are uncommon. Finally, there are children with features of vitamin D dependency rickets who have end-organ insensitivity to $1,25(OH)_2D$.

Renal Failure. Hypocalcemia is common in both acute and chronic renal insufficiency. The mechanisms responsible for hypocalcemia include (1) phosphate retention, (2) altered vitamin D metabolism, and (3) impaired skeletal action of PTH.

Phosphate retention due to declining renal function causes a tendency to increased serum PO_4 and a reciprocal tendency to decreased serum Ca concentration. The resultant increased secretion of PTH then causes phosphaturia, which lowers serum PO_4. This results in the return of serum Ca to normal at the expense of increased PTH secretion. This process continues during progressive renal insufficiency until renal failure reaches such a degree of severity that the hyperphosphatemia is persistent. This series of events is postulated as a major cause of the secondary hyperparathyroidism of renal insufficiency.

Another cause of hypocalcemia in renal failure is impaired vitamin D metabolism. Since the kidney is the only significant source of $1,25(OH)_2D$, the production of this sterol declines during the course of progressive renal failure. Decreased $1,25(OH)_2D$ synthesis impairs Ca absorption, leading to a decrease in serum Ca; PTH secretion is thereby further stimulated. Increments in PTH secretion may maintain renal $1,25(OH)_2D$ generation at near-normal levels until more advanced renal failure prevents this compensatory mechanism. The PO_4 retention and altered vitamin D metabolism may be related, since hyperphosphatemia can decrease the generation of $1,25(OH)_2D$. Finally, there is evidence that the skeleton fails to release Ca normally in response to PTH in renal insufficiency. Although the mechanism is unclear, deficient bone responsiveness may be a consequence of decreased $1,25(OH)_2D$ effect.

Hypocalcemia is not invariably observed in uremic patients, particularly those undergoing long-term dialysis treatment. Indeed, hypercalcemia may occasionally be encountered following treatment with low doses of vitamin D metabolites. The probable mechanism is decreased bone assimilation of calcium due to aluminum toxicity (see Renal Osteodystrophy).

Removal of Calcium From Serum

HYPERPHOSPHATEMIA. Hypocalcemia may be caused by severe hyperphosphatemia. Although the mechanism responsible for this effect is not well defined, the most common explanation is that the solubility product of calcium phosphate is exceeded, leading to the deposition of Ca in soft tissues and bone. In addition, increased serum PO_4 can lead to decreased $1,25(OH)_2D$ production. Hyperphosphatemia is a principal factor in the hypocalcemia of acute or chronic renal insufficiency (see Renal Failure), occasionally develops after excessive intake of PO_4, and can occur after massive soft tissue breakdown as in acute rhabdomyolysis. Hypocalcemia is more likely to develop when serum PO_4 increases rapidly. Severe hyperphosphatemia is rare unless there is impaired renal function resulting in reduced PO_4 excretion.

CALCIUM DEPOSITION IN BONE. A tendency to hypocalcemia may be aggravated by processes causing rapid deposition of Ca into bone. This phenomenon is seen in osteoblastic metastases, particularly with tumors of the prostate, breast, and lung. In certain instances, the hypocalcemia is further aggravated by reduced renal production of $1,25(OH)_2D$ due to the effects of tumor-related inhibitors. Marked and protracted hypocalcemia can appear following the removal of a parathyroid adenoma, due to partial suppression of the remaining parathyroid glands in combination with a rapid bone uptake of Ca caused by accelerated bone formation. This situation can be anticipated preoperatively by the finding of increased serum alkaline phosphatase levels and radiologic evidence of parathyroid-related bone disease.

INCREASED RENAL EXCRETION OF CALCIUM. The kidney plays a role in the regulation of serum Ca concentration, and increased urinary losses of Ca can contribute to hypocalcemia. However, increased urinary loss is rarely the only factor causing hypocalcemia. An example of this situation is hypoparathyroidism, where the absence of circulating PTH leads to decreased Ca reabsorption in the kidney, thereby aggravating the hypocalcemia.

Miscellaneous Causes of Hypocalcemia. Hypocalcemia occurs frequently in severe *acute pancreatitis.* The pathogenesis of the hypocalcemia is probably multifactorial and is contributed to by local precipitation of Ca salts in the peritoneum, reduced PTH secretion due to coexistent hypomagnesemia, and vitamin D deficiency due to chronic fat malabsorption. Transient *neonatal hypocalcemia* is a relatively common disorder. Serum Ca levels normally decline in the neonate during the first 3 days of life. When the Ca level falls below 8.0 mg/dl at term or below 7.0 mg/dl in the premature infant, the hypocalcemia is pathologic. A number of mechanisms have been suggested including vitamin D deficiency, parathyroid immaturity, fetal parathyroid suppression caused by physiologic maternal hyperparathyroidism, Mg deficiency, and hyperphosphatemia due to the high content of PO_4 in cow's milk. *Citrate* present in transfused blood can bind ionized Ca, and a fall in Ca is occasionally seen after multiple transfusions with citrated blood.

Disorders of Serum Phosphate

In normal adults, the fasting serum PO_4 concentration ranges from 2.8 to 4.5 mg/dl. Higher values occur in growing children and in women after menopause. To accurately assess serum PO_4 status, fasting blood samples must be obtained, since increases of 1 to 2 mg/dl may occur after meals. The serum PO_4 level is not tightly regulated.

Hyperphosphatemia is often an asymptomatic condition, with the clinical symptoms being those of the underlying disorder. In severe cases, reciprocal reductions in serum Ca concentration can produce the typical symptoms of hypocalcemia. Prolonged elevations of serum PO_4 combined with normal or elevated serum Ca levels can produce ectopic calcifications, and pseudogout can result from calcium phosphate deposition in joint cartilage. Common causes of hyperphosphatemia include renal failure, hypoparathyroidism, states of increased bone resorption with suppressed PTH activity (cancer metastatic to bone, acute immobilization, thyrotoxicosis), and vitamin D intoxication. Increased serum PO_4 can also occur early in diabetic ketoacidosis due to decreased insulin stimulation of the cellular uptake of glucose and PO_4. The management of hyperphosphatemia includes hydration, PO_4 restriction, and treatment of the underlying disorder.

Hypophosphatemia, when severe, can produce various CNS symptoms including irritability, confusion, obtundation, seizures, and coma. There can be severe muscle weakness, and rhabdomyolysis may occur. Decreased oxygen delivery to tissues due to reduced erythrocyte 2,3-diphosphoglycerate levels may account for some of these symptoms, and myopathic symptoms may be further aggravated by reduced muscle ATP stores. Insulin resistance may occur due to decreased intracellular trapping of glucose as glucose-6-phosphate. Hypercalciuria may be present due to the shift of the $Ca-PO_4$ equilibrium away from bone, as well as to the effects of increased $1,25(OH)_2D$ synthesis due to reduced serum PO_4 levels. Severe hypophosphatemia (serum $PO_4 < 1$ mg/dl) may be caused by prolonged parenteral feeding without phosphate supplementation, chronic alcoholism, and prolonged severe diabetic ketoacidosis. Moderate hypophosphatemia (serum PO_4 1 to 2.5 mg/dl) may be caused by starvation, alcoholism, primary hyperparathyroidism, or severe secondary hyperparathyroidism, renal tubular PO_4 reabsorption defects, severe respiratory alkalosis, or prolonged use of phosphate-binding antiacids. Treatment consists of oral or parenteral phosphate replacement.

Disorders of Serum Magnesium

The normal range of serum Mg concentration is 1.4 to 2.2 mEq/l (1.7 to 2.6 mg/dl). Serum Mg concentration is not tightly controlled; hence, disorders of Mg intake, absorption, or renal excretion can markedly alter serum Mg levels. Disorders in serum Mg concentration produce symptoms both directly by altering cell membrane potentials and indirectly by altering the serum Ca concentration.

Hypermagnesemia of severe degree occurs almost exclusively in patients with severe renal insufficiency who have been treated with magnesium-containing antiacids, since in this situation the increased intestinal absorption of Mg cannot be compensated for by increased urinary excretion. When the serum Mg rises to 3 to 5 mEq/l, nausea, vomiting, and hypotension usually occur. Further elevation to 7 to 10 mEq/l produces drowsiness, muscle weakness, and loss of deep tendon reflexes. When the serum Mg level reaches 12 to 15 mEq/l, coma occurs and paralysis of the respiratory center is common. Various cardiac abnormalities may occur including prolonged Q-T interval, AV block, and cardiac arrest. Intravenous administration of Ca will temporarily reverse symptoms due to severe Mg elevation. In severe cases, dialysis may be required.

Hypomagnesemia occurs commonly in chronic intestinal malabsorption syndromes, chronic severe alcoholism, following correction of diabetic ketoacidosis, and after prolonged intravenous feeding combined with gastric suctioning. Decreased renal tubular reabsorption of Mg due to diuretic use, alcohol, hyperaldosteronism, or primary tubular defects can aggravate hypomagnesemia. Symptoms of hypomagnesemia usually occur only when the serum Mg falls below 1 mEq/l, and include weakness, muscle fasciculations, tremors, personality changes, and seizures. Many of these symptoms are attributable to the hypocalcemia that often accompanies chronic hypomagnesemia. The decline in serum Ca concentration is the result of a paradoxical decrease in PTH secretion, combined with intracellular shifts of Ca to replace Mg. The bone response to PTH may also be diminished. Administration of Mg will rapidly restore serum Mg and Ca concentrations to normal, and reverse the symptom complex.

METABOLIC BONE DISEASES

Bone Physiology

Bone has a dual function in man. First, it provides a physical basis for locomotion and affords protection to the internal organs. Secondly, the mineral phase of bone serves as a reservoir for essential ions and buffers. In the normal process of turnover and remodeling, bone is usually able to serve both functions. However, the critical role of maintaining a normal ECF Ca concentration always takes precedence over the mechanical supportive role, occasionally to the detriment of the latter.

Bone is composed of three major elements: a protein matrix, a mineral phase, and bone cells (Fig. 9–4). The matrix occupies about 50% of total

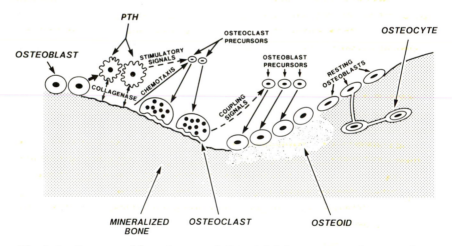

Fig. 9–4. Sequence of bone turnover (left to right): In response to bone-resorbing stimuli such as PTH, osteoblasts retract from the bone surface and secrete collagenase that initiates bone breakdown. Mononuclear osteoclast precursors are activated by chemotactic factors and stimulatory signals from the osteoblasts. Multinucleated osteoclasts then develop and begin to resorb bone. Coupling signals resulting from osteoclast activity stimulate the formation of osteoblasts from precursors. These new osteoblasts deposit bone protein matrix (osteoid) along lines of stress. The osteoid then mineralizes to become mature bone. "Retired" osteoblasts remain either as resting osteoblasts (lining cells) on the bone surface or as osteocytes embedded within lacunae. Osteoblasts and osteocytes are interconnected by an extensive network of cytoplasmic extensions.

bone volume and consists largely of the fibrous protein, collagen. The cross-linked collagen bundles serve as the structural core on which the mineral phase is deposited. Mineral accounts for most of the remaining half of bone volume, and for about two-thirds of the weight. It is comprised largely of hydroxyapatite, a crystalline material with the formula $Ca_{10}(PO_4)_6(OH)_2$. The bone cells occupy only about 3% of bone volume and are of three types: osteoblasts, osteocytes, and osteoclasts. The osteoblasts are the bone-forming cells and are derived from adjacent mesenchymal progenitors. Osteoblasts are found on the surfaces of newly forming bone, are rich in alkaline phosphatase, and produce the protein matrix. When the osteoblast completes a cycle of matrix synthesis, it either becomes buried in the lacunae of newly formed bone as an osteocyte or remains quiescent on the bone surface as a resting osteoblast or lining cell. The osteoblasts and osteocytes are interconnected by cellular processes that form a continuous layer over the bone surface, thus creating a local "bone ECF" that is separate from the remaining ECF. Osteoclasts are large multinucleated cells that are responsible for bone resorption. Their origin is a matter of controversy, but it has been hypothesized that they are recruited from mononuclear cells in the bone marrow. The recruitment and activation of osteoclasts appear to be dependent upon signals from the osteoblast. Osteoblast and osteoclast activity in adults is normally "coupled," presumably by local feedback signals.

The major factors regulating bone metabolism in adults are mechanical stress; ECF concentrations of Ca and PO_4; and hormones, the most important of which are PTH, glucocorticoids, the gonadal steroids, and the biologically active metabolites of vitamin D. In general terms, the metabolic bone diseases are caused by disordered bone cell function due to abnormal hormonal, physical, or ionic stimuli.

Osteopenia is a purely clinical and radiologic diagnosis that denotes that an individual has decreased bone mass relative to normal values for age, sex, and race. The bone histologic changes seen in patients with osteopenia are of three main types; (1) *osteoporosis*, in which there is a parallel loss of bone mineral and matrix; (2) *osteomalacia*, in which there is deficient mineralization of bone, resulting in an accumulation of unmineralized matrix (osteoid) and a decreased mineral/matrix ratio; and (3) *osteitis fibrosa*, in which there is increased PTH-stimulated osteoclastic resorption of bone, with replacement by fibrous tissue. Although these histologic classifications are often discussed as separate entities, many patients with osteopenia exhibit a mixture of pathologic changes with one form predominating.

Osteopenic Bone Disorders

Osteoporosis

PRIMARY (INVOLUTIONAL, POSTMENOPAUSAL) OSTEOPOROSIS. Primary osteoporosis is a common disease of late-middle and old age, which affects women 5 times more frequently than men. One-third of women over age 65 will have vertebral fractures due to osteoporosis, and the incidence increases with age. The lower incidence of osteoporosis in males appears to be at least partially a consequence of their greater initial bone mass, and to a degree reflects the anabolic effects of androgens. Racial differences in bone mass also exist; the incidence of osteoporosis in blacks is less than in Caucasians and Orientals. Bone mass declines with age after about the third decade, and the rate of loss is more rapid in trabecular bone (vertebrae, ribs, pelvis, ends of long bones) than in cortical bone (midshafts of long bones). Hence, fractures in patients with osteoporosis are most common in the vertebrae, distal forearm (Colle's fracture), and femoral neck. Mean annual rates of bone loss in mid-life average 1 to 2%/year. In the 5 to 8-year period immediately following menopause, women experience an accelerated rate of decline in bone mass related to the loss of the inhibitory effects of estrogens on bone turnover. Replacement with estrogen at this time will eliminate the accelerated phase of bone loss and thereby reduce the severity of subsequent osteoporosis.

The typical patient with osteoporosis is a light-framed Caucasian female between 50 and 70 years of age whose female relatives also have osteoporosis. The presenting complaint is often severe lower thoracic back pain of acute onset, which on x-ray examination of the spine is shown to be caused by a new vertebral compression fracture or by the extension of a previous fracture. A loss of 2 to 6 inches in height is common in advanced cases with mutliple vertebral compressions. Since the vertebrae compress anteriorly, an upper thoracic kyphosis (dowager's hump) is common. Osteopenia detectable by standard x rays indicates that a minimum 30 to 50% loss of bone mass has occurred. Quantitative CT scan and dual beam photon absorptiometry techniques are more sensitive and are capable of detecting a 5 to 7% loss of bone mass. Establishing the diagnosis of osteopenia by routine x rays is best done by examining lateral views of the thoracic and lumbar vertebrae. The earliest detectable change is a loss of density in the mid-body of the vertebrae with accentuation of the upper and lower end plates. This is followed by progressive vertebral compression which may be more marked in the mid-portions of the vertebra, giving the appearance of a bow tie or "codfish". Finally, there is near-complete collapse of the vertebral body (Fig. 9–5). The major biochemical feature which separates osteoporosis from other metabolic bone diseases is the absence of abnormalities of serum Ca, PO_4, alkaline phosphatase, and iPTH (Table 9–3). Bone histology reveals only a decreased amount of bone and variably reduced cellular activity. The diagnosis of osteoporosis is established by the clinical situation and by the exclusion of other osteopenic disorders.

The etiology of primary osteoporosis is probably multifactorial, and management is currently a matter of controversy. Achieving an adequate Ca intake (at least 800 mg/day), especially in early life during the bone-forming years, and maintenance of a good level of weight-bearing physical activity are probably the most useful general prophylactic measures. After menopause, due to the decreased efficiency of intestinal Ca absorption, an intake of at least

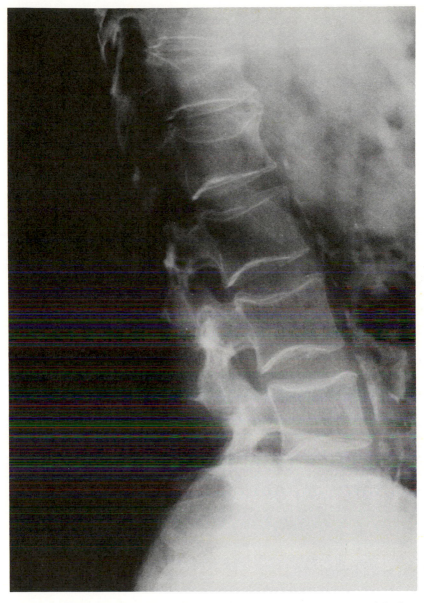

Fig. 9–5. Lateral x ray of the lumbar vertebrae demonstrating the typical findings of advanced osteoporosis. Note the distinct cortices on the upper and lower borders of the vertebrae, relative to the "washed out" appearance of the central portions of the vertebral bodies. Varying degrees of early compression of the midportions of the vertebral body are seen in the lower three vertebrae. The upper two vertebrae are partially collapsed.

Table 9–3.　Laboratory Findings in Common Metabolic Bone Disorders

	Serum				Urine	
Disorder	Ca	PO$_4$	Alk P'ase	iPTH	Ca	Tm$_{PO_4}$/GFR
Primary Osteoporosis	N	N	N	N	N	N
Primary Hyperparathyroidism (osteitis fibrosa)	I	D	N or I	I	I	D
Osteomalacia:						
Vitamin D Deficiency	D	D	I	I	D	D
Phosphate Depletion	N	D	I	N	I	N
Paget's Disease	N	N	I	N	N	N

D, decreased; I, increased; N, normal.

1500 mg of Ca per day is required to maintain Ca balance. High-risk patients should probably be maintained on estrogen supplements for 8 to 10 years following menopause, although the beneficial effects of estrogens on bone may be somewhat counterbalanced by the risks of undesirable complications such as uterine cancer and hypertension. Preliminary evidence suggests that sodium fluoride may be useful in stimulating osteoblastic bone-forming activity, and calcitonin may occasionally be of benefit in cases with increased osteoclastic activity.

SECONDARY OSTEOPOROSIS. A variety of systemic disorders can produce osteoporosis, particularly disorders of the endocrine system. *Premature ovarian failure* due to surgical procedure, ovarian disease, or radiation therapy almost invariably leads to severe osteoporosis unless estrogen replacement is initiated promptly. *Decreased testerone production,* due to primary testicular failure or pituitary disorders, is a common cause of osteopenia in adult males. The mechanism is undefined, but may be related to loss of the anabolic effects of androgens. *Glucocorticoid excess,* due either to steroid therapy for various disorders or to Cushing's disease, commonly produces severe osteoporosis. A major factor appears to be glucocorticoid suppression of osteoblast function. In addition, in long-standing cases glucocorticoid inhibition of intestinal calcium absorption may produce secondary hyperparathyroidism which further accelerates the bone loss. *Thyrotoxicosis* of long duration may occasionally produce significant loss of bone mass, due to a disproportionate enhancement of osteoclastic activity. *Juvenile-onset diabetes mellitus* is occasioanly associated with osteoporosis, which is apparently caused by deficient insulin stimulation of osteoblast function. Osteopenia is rare in adult-onset diabetes.

Immobilization frequently causes reduced bone mass due to absence of the weight-bearing stimulus for osteoblastic activity. Bone loss is most rapid with total immobilization, but even prolonged relative inactivity can produce significant osteoporosis. *Multiple myeloma* and certain other hematologic malignancies can occasionally appear as diffuse osteopenia, and must be excluded before assigning the diagnosis of osteoporosis. Severe chronic Ca and protein *malnutrition* have occasionally been reported to produce osteopenia. Rare congenital abnormalities of bone collagen formation, such as *osteogenesis imperfecta tarda,* may occasionally present as severe osteoporosis in children or adults.

Osteomalacia. Osteomalacia is caused by defective mineralization of bone due to either: (1) deficiency of biologically active vitamin D metabolites, or (2) chronic hypophosphatemia. Clinically, osteomalacia is characterized by bone pain and fractures, and is frequently accompanied by proximal muscle weakness. When the disorder occurs in children prior to the cessation of bone growth, bowing of the legs, and widening of the epiphyses produce the typical changes of rickets. There is x-ray evidence of generalized demineralization and occasionally pseudofractures (Looser's zone) are observed, appearing as painless lucent areas that extend partway through the bone.

VITAMIN D METABOLITE DEFICIENCY. Vitamin D deficiency osteomalacia is seen commonly in states of chronic intestinal fat malabsorption such as pancreatic insufficiency, celiac disease, diseases of the terminal ileum, and hepatobiliary disease. It can also result from chronic treatment with drugs such as phenobarbital, diphenylhydantoin, glutethimide, and rifampin that accelerate the hepatic degradation of vitamin D and 25(OH)D. Pure nutritional vitamin D deficiency is quite rare in the United States.

The disorder is characterized by reduced serum Ca, PO_4, and 25(OH)D levels, and increased levels of alkaline phosphatase and iPTH. Urinary calcium excretion is markedly reduced. These changes are caused by decreased vitamin D metabolite stimulation of intestinal Ca absorption that leads to secondary hyperparathyroidism. Bone histology demonstrates a decreased rate of bone formation and accumulation of unmineralized osteoid tissue. Osteoclast activity is somewhat increased. Treatment consists of vitamin D and Ca replacement.

Rarely, osteomalacia can be produced by mesenchymal tumors, apparently due to the elaboration of substances that inhibit renal $1,25(OH)_2D$ synthesis, and by rare congenital syndromes of cellular resistance to $1,25(OH)_2D$. Measurement of serum $1,25(OH)_2D$ levels is useful in establishing these diagnoses.

CHRONIC HYPOPHOSPHATEMIA (NORMAL VITAMIN D). Osteomalacia can be produced by chronic hypophosphatemia in the presence of normal levels of vitamin D metabolites. The reduced serum PO_4 levels can be caused either by renal tubular PO_4 wasting syndromes or by chronic PO_4 deficiency. The most common tubular PO_4 wasting syndrome is familial hypophosphatemic rickets (FHR), a sex-linked dominant disorder characterized by rickets, osteomalacia, and growth retardation. The basis of the disorder appears to be a defect in cellular transport of PO_4 in the intestine and kidney. Serum Ca concentration is normal, serum PO_4 is reduced, serum alkaline phosphatase is elevated, and iPTH levels are normal. Urinary Ca excretion is also normal, Serum 25(OH)D and $1,25(OH)_2D$ levels are within normal limits, although the latter might be considered inappropriately low in the face of chronic hypophosphatemia. Hypophosphatemic osteomalacia is also associated with a variety of other inherited and acquired renal tubular leak syndromes including distal renal tubular acidosis and the Fanconi syndrome. Bone histology demonstrates the typical changes of osteomalacia.

A chronic PO_4 depletion syndrome associated with osteomalacia, bone pain, muscle weakness, and increased urinary Ca excretion has been reported in patients who chronically take large amounts of aluminum hydroxide antiacids that interfere with intestinal PO_4 absorption. The increase in urinary Ca excretion is apparently due to increased $1,25(OH)_2D$ production associated with the chronic hypophosphatemia as well as to a rapid loss of Ca from bone.

Osteitis Fibrosa. This pathologic process occurs in hyperparathyroidism, either primary or secondary to chronic hypocalcemic stimuli such as occur in chronic renal insufficiency or severe Ca malabsorption. In severe, long-standing cases x rays may show subperiosteal resorption of bone, which is detected most readily in the hands, resorption of the distal ends of the clavicles, and cystic "brown tumor" accumulations of osteoclasts and fibrous tissue in the long bones. Histologically, osteitis fibrosa is characterized by a marked increase in osteoclastic activity, as demonstrated by increased numbers of osteoclasts and areas of osteoclastic resorption. The number and activity of osteoblasts is also somewhat increased; wide rows of osteoblasts overlie areas of collagen deposition and new bone formation. Bone turnover rate is accelerated. Moreover, a variable degree of peritrabecular fibrosis occurs in areas of bone resorption, a finding that led to the original descriptive term, osteitis fibrosa.

Renal Osteodystrophy. Renal osteodystrophy is an osteopenic bone disorder characterized by bone pain and increased fracture risk which occurs in patients with chronic renal insufficiency. Bone histology may demonstrate a mixture of any of four patterns: osteomalacia, osteitis fibrosa, osteoporosis, or osteosclerosis.

Osteomalacia is frequently the earliest skeletal lesion, and may in part reflect the effects of decreased renal $1,25(OH)_2D$ synthesis. Osteomalacia is more common in renal patients with low vitamin D intake. However, a large portion of the osteomalacia seen in chronic renal failure patients appears to be a result of the toxic effects of aluminum accumulation. The aluminum is derived either from dialysis fluids or from the aluminum-containing antiacids used in dialysis patients to reduce serum PO_4 levels. Due to renal insufficiency, the excess aluminum cannot be eliminated from the body and accumulates at the bone-forming surfaces where it both inhibits calcium phosphate deposition and suppresses osteoblast function. Patients with aluminum overload bone disease readily become hypercalcemic during treatment with even low doses of vitamin D and Ca, since their bones cannot readily assimilate additional Ca. Reversal of aluminum toxicity can be achieved through use of desferrioxamine, an aluminum-chelating agent. Osteitis is caused by markedly increased PTH secretion secondary to the chronic tendency to hypocalcemia that results from reduced renal $1,25(OH)_2D$ production and increased PO_4 retention. Osteoporosis usually occurs in association with other pathologic changes and appears to result in part from chronic acidosis and protein malnutrition. Osteosclerosis occurs in local areas of the skeleton and is usually seen late in the course of renal failure. It is often most prominent in the lower vertebrae and occurs as dense bands that alternate with less dense bone, producing a "rugger jersey spine" appearance on x ray. It usually occurs in patients with a high serum Ca $\times$ PO$_4$ product, and appears to be the result of locally increased production of matrix that then becomes calcified.

General measures in the management of the bone disease associated with renal insufficiency include reduction of PO$_4$ intake early in the course of renal failure to prevent hyperphosphatemia, later combined with the use of phosphate-binding antiacids to reduce PO$_4$ absorption. The tendency to development of secondary hyperparathyroidism is further circumvented by the use of vitamin D metabolite and Ca supplements. Limited use of aluminum-containing fluids and compounds reduces the severity of aluminum overload disorders.

Paget's Disease of Bone

Paget's disease of bone is a common chronic skeletal disorder of unknown etiology which affects about 4% of the population over 40. It is characterized by disordered, exuberantly increased bone turnover that leads eventually to localized bone enlargement, weakening, and deformity. The initial event appears to be a local increase in osteoclastic bone resorbing activity of unknown cause, followed by a chaotic increase in the formation of new bone that lacks normal patterns of trabecular organization.

The disorder is frequently asymptomatic. In symptomatic patients, bone pain, skeletal deformity, and problems caused by local bone overgrowth are the most frequent complaints. Commonly, there is only localized involvement of one or two bones; however, severe multifocal forms occur. The skull, lumbosacral spine, pelvis, femur, and tibia are the bones most frequently affected. The course of the disease is unpredictable; it may remain localized, wax and wane, or be rapidly progressive. Pain in Paget's disease may be due to: (1) direct involvement of bone, (2) impingement on nerves roots, especially in the lumbar spine, and (3) arthritic changes in the hip or knee due to leg bowing. The most common bone deformities are kyphosis, bowing of the extremities, and enlargement of the skull. When the disease involves the skull, there can be impingement on the long tracts of the spinal cord, and cranial nerve compression can lead to deafness or optic nerve atrophy.

Histologic examination of affected bone discloses a marked increase in bone resorption adjacent to areas of intense new bone formation. The collagen deposited in the new bone is abnormal and has a blotchy mosaic or woven pattern. The new bone is poor in tensile strength, and fractures are common. The pathogenesis of the disorder is unclear, although a viral etiology has been suggested.

The diagnosis is based on characteristic x-ray findings. Radionuclide bone scans provide the most sensitive radiologic means of evaluating the location and activity of Paget's disease. The characteristic laboratory finding is an increase in serum alkaline phosphatase concentration that may be quite marked and parallels the activity of the disease. Serum Ca and PO_4 are normal. Urinary excretion of hydroxyproline (a by-product of collagen formation and break-down) is increased.

Treatment of Paget's disease is directed toward suppressing the osteoclastic overactivity, which appears to be the primary event. Calcitonin therapy de-creases osteoclastic bone resorption, resulting in a coupled secondary reduc-tion in osteoblastic activity and a consequent decline in serum alkaline phos-phatase level. The resultant decrease in bone formation and turnover rate may lead to substantial symptomatic improvement. Diphosphonates, such as so-dium etidronate, act primarily by decreasing osteoclastic activity and are also useful in the management of this disorder.

CLINICAL PROBLEMS

Patient 1. A 48-year-old woman comes to your office complaining of fatiguability. Physical examination shows no obvious abnormalities.

LABORATORY DATA. Serum calcium 12.2 mg/dl (normal, 9.0 to 10.3 mg/dl), phosphate 2.6 mg/dl (normal 3.0 to 4.5 mg/dl), alkaline phosphatase 75 IU/L (normal, up to 80 IU/L), TmPO$_4$/GFR 2.1 mg/100 ml (normal, 2.5 to 4.2 mg/100 ml), 24-hour urine calcium 410 mg (normal 110 to 300 mg).

1. What is the most likely diagnosis, and what additional tests would be required?
2. What diagnosis is excluded by the urinary calcium value?
3. How would you manage this patient? Would you like any additional data to help you in this regard?

Patient 2. A 64-year-old man is brought to the emergency room because of confusion and incontinence. He was feeling well until approximately 6 months ago when he began to complain of back pain and fatiguability. Physical examination reveals a somewhat lethargic and disoriented man with pale conjunctivae and diffuse tenderness over the ribs and spine. X rays reveal diffuse osteopenia, and lytic lesions of the skull, ribs, and vertebrae.

LABORATORY DATA. Serum calcium 16.4 mg/dl, phosphate 4.9 mg/dl, alkaline phosphatase 78 IU/L, creatinine 1.6 mg/dl (normal, 0.7 to 1.3 mg/dl). Serum protein electrophoresis reveals an abnormal globulin, which proves to be gamma D, consistent with multiple myeloma.

1. What is the probable cause of the hypercalcemia and osteopenia in this patient?
2. What general measures should be used to control the hypercalcemia? Is there any urgency in treating this patient?
3. What specific agent would you recommend to treat this patient's hypercalcemia and why?
4. Would absolute bedrest be a good idea?

Patient 3. A 32-year-old man is referred to you for evaluation of hypocalcemia. At the age of 21, he was diagnosed as having Crohn's disease and subsequently required bowel resection, including removal of the terminal ileum. He complains of thigh and calf cramps, and intermittent circumoral paresthesias. On physical examination, he has positive Chvostek's and Trousseau's signs.

LABORATORY DATA. Serum calcium 6.0 mg/dl, albumin 4.1 mg/dl, phosphate 2.8 mg/dl, alkaline phosphatase 150 IU/L.

1. What is the likely diagnosis and what additional laboratory data are needed?
2. Would you expect a normal serum level of 25(OH)D? Would there be changes in serum 1,25(OH)$_2$D concentration?
3. What bone disease is associated with this disorder?
4. What physiologic and biochemical changes would be produced by vitamin D adminis-tration in this patient?

Patient 4. A 48-year-old woman is found to have hypocalcemia on a routine serum biochemical profile. Her only complaints are occasional tingling sensation in the lips and fingertips when she is tired. Fifteen years ago she underwent a near-total thyroidectomy for cancer of the thyroid.

LABORATORY DATA. Serum calcium 7.4 mg/dl, phosphate 4.8 mg/dl, alkaline phosphatase 67 IU/L.

1. What is the likely diagnosis and what additional data are needed?
2. She is started on estrogen therapy for menopausal symptoms, and her hypocalcemia worsens. Why?
3. How would you manage this patient?

Patient 5. A 54-year-old Causasian woman complains of the sudden onset of mid back pain with no history of trauma. At age 37 she underwent a hysterectomy with removal of both ovaries. No medical treatment was instituted at this time. For the past 5 years she has been treated with glucocorticoids for rheumatoid arthritis. Her physical activity has been limited due to her arthritis. Physical examination reveals tenderness over the mid thoracic spine. X rays of the spine demonstrate diffuse osteopenia and a vertebral compression fracture at T7.

LABORATORY DATA. Serum calcium 9.2 mg/dl, phosphate 4.1 mg/dl, alkaline phosphatase 78 IU/L, 24-hour urine calcium 138 mg.

1. What is the likely diagnosis and what are the contributing factors?
2. What other disorders need to be excluded?
3. What previous medical therapy would have been likely to reduce the severity of her current problem?
4. What treatment would you recommend at this point?

SUGGESTED READING

Bone Physiology

Avioli, L.V. and Krane, S.M. (eds.): Metabolic Bone Disease. 2 Vol. London, Academic Press, 1978.

Raisz, L.G., and Kream, B.E.: Regulation of bone formation, parts 1 and 2. N Engl J Med, *309*:29, 83, 1983.

Calcium, Magnesium, Phosphate, Parathyroid Hormone, Vitamin D

Agus, Z.S., Wasserstein, A., and Goldfarb, S.: Disorders of calcium and magnesium homeostasis. Am J Med, *72*:473, 1982.

Bell, N.H.: Vitamin D-endocrine system. J Clin Invest, *76*:1, 1985.

Coburn, J.W., Kurokawa, K., and Kleeman, C.R.: Divalent ion metabolism. *In* Contemporary Metabolism. Edited by N. Freinkel. New York, Plenum Publishing, 1979.

Habener, J.F., and Potts, J.T.: Parathyroid physiology and primary hyperparathyroidism. *In* Metabolic Bone Disease. Vol 2. Edited by L.V. Avioli and S.M. Krane. London, Academic Press, 1978.

Haussler, M.R., and McCain, T.A.: Basic and clinical concepts related to vitamin D metabolism and action. N Engl J Med, *297*:974, 1041, 1977.

Jaun, D.: The causes and consequences of hypophosphatemia. Surg Gynecol Obstet, *153*:589, 1981.

Rude, R.K., and Singer, F.R.: Magnesium deficiency and excess. Ann Rev Med, *32*:245, 1981.

Walton, R.J., and Bijovet, O.L.M.: Nomogram for derivation of renal threshold phosphate concentration. Lancet, 2:309, 1975.

Hypercalcemic Disorders

Mallette, L., et al: Primary hyperparathyroidism: Clinical and biochemical features. Medicine, *53*:127, 1974.

Marx, S.J., et al.: Divalent cation metabolism: familial hypocalciuric hypercalcemia versus typical primary hyperparathyroidism. Am J Med, *65*:235, 1978.

Mundy, G.R., Ibbotson, K.J., and D'Souza, S.M.: Tumor products and the hypercalcemia of malignancy. J Clin Invest, *76*:391, 1985.

Hypocalcemic Disorders

Breslau, N.A., and Pak, C.Y.C.: Hypoparathyroidism. Metabolism, *28*:1261, 1979.

Chase, L.R., and Slatopolsky, E.: Secretion and metabolic efficiency of parathyroid hormone in patients with severe hypomagnesemia. J Clin Endocrinol Metab, *38*:363, 1974.

Spiegel, A.M., et al.: Deficiency of hormone receptor-adenylate cyclase coupling protein: basis for hormone resistance in pseudohypoparathyroidism. Am J Physiol, *243*:E37, 1982.

Metabolic Bone Disease

Coburn, J.W.: Renal osteodystrophy. Adv Intern Med, *30*:384, 1984.

Ettinger, B., Genant, H.K., and Cann, C.E.: Long-term estrogen replacement therapy prevents bone loss and fractures. Ann Intern Med, *102*:319, 1985.

Frame, B., and Parfitt, A.M.: Osteomalacia: current concepts. Ann Intern Med, 89:966, 1978.

Hahn, T.J.: Drug-induced disorders of vitamin D and mineral metabolism. Clin Endocrinol Metab, *9*:107, 1980.

Ibbertson, H.K., et. al.: Paget's disease of bone: assessment and management. Drugs, *18*:33, 1979.

Riggs, B.L., and Melton, L.J.: Involutional osteoporosis. N Engl J Med, *314*:1676, 1986.

Seeman, E., et al.: Risk factors for spinal osteoporosis in men. Am J Med, *75*:977, 1983.

ANSWERS TO QUESTIONS

Patient 1

1. Primary hyperparathyroidism is the most likely diagnosis in this middle-aged, relatively asymptomatic, patient with hypercalcemia, hypophosphatemia, increased renal phosphate excretion (low Tm/GFR), and hypercalciuria. The diagnosis can be confirmed by demonstrating an elevated serum iPTH level.

2. Familial hypocalciuric hypercalcemia (FHH) should be excluded in all patients with a presumptive diagnosis of primary hyperparathyroidism based on serum biochemical values. This is especially important since parathyroid surgery is not indicated in patients with FHH. The elevated 24-hour urinary calcium excretion in this patient excludes FHH.

3. In view of the moderately elevated serum calcium and markedly increased urinary calcium excretion values, subtotal parathyroidectomy would be the most appropriate treatment of this patient. However, if the mean of repeated serum calcium and urinary calcium excretion values were only slightly above normal, if normal renal function was documented, and if there were no radiologic evidence of osteopenia or kidney stones, it would be reasonable to follow this patient on medical therapy. Medical management would include a reduced calcium intake, hydration, liberal salt diet, and a regular regimen of weight-bearing exercise.to stimulate bone formation. If these measures do not produce a satisfactory response, phosphate supplementation and estrogen therapy could be considered.

Patient 2

1. This patient's clinical picture is most compatible with multiple myeloma producing hypercalcemia through increased bone resorption. The causative agent in this process is an osteoclast activating factor (OAF) that is produced by the myeloma cells and stimulates osteoclasts to resorb bone.

2. The initial general measures that should be used in the management of this patient's hypercalcemia include: aggressive rehydration with saline (sodium chloride) solutions to restore intravascular volume and enhance renal calcium excretion, cautious intermittent use of furosemide (20 to 40 mg every 3 to 4 hours) to prevent volume overload, and restriction of calcium intake. The marked hypercalcemia and deteriorated mental status in this patient indicate that this is a medical emergency.

3. Glucocorticoid therapy is indicated in this patient to inhibit the stimulatory effects of OAF on osteoclast activity.

4. Absolute bedrest should be avoided if possible, since the loss of the weight-bearing stimulus for osteoblastic bone formation would further aggravate the hypercalcemia. This is also true in other hypercalcemic disorders where bone resorption greatly exceeds bone formation (primary hyperparathyroidism, hyperthyroidism). In addition, hypercalciuria and hypercalcemia can occasionally be produced by absolute bedrest in patients with a high bone turnover rate (children and young adults, patients with Paget's disease).

Patient 3

1. This patient has vitamin D deficiency caused by fat malabsorption due to absence of ileal function. The diagnosis could be confirmed by measuring the serum 25(OH)D level, and further substantiated by demonstrating an elevated iPTH concentration and markedly reduced 24-hour urinary calcium excretion (usually less than 40 mg). The patient's reduced serum phosphate level is the result of secondary hyperparathyroidism caused by the reduced serum calcium concentration: hence, Tm_{PO_4}/GFR would also be reduced.

2. The serum 25(OH)D level would be markedly reduced due to decreased vitamin D stores. In contrast, the serum $1,25(OH)_2D$ level is much more tightly controlled, and is usually normal to mildly elevated in mild to moderate vitamin D deficiency due to the stimulatory effects of increased PTH and reduced phosphate concentrations on renal $1,25(OH)_2D$ production. Only in severe vitamin D deficiency, when serum 25(OH)D levels are virtually undetectable, would the serum $1,25(OH)_2D$ decline. Therefore, the serum 25(OH)D level is the test of choice to document vitamin D deficiency.
3. Vitamin D deficiency produces osteomalacia. The patient's elevated serum alkaline phosphatase suggested that he has this disorder. Confirmation would require bone biopsy.
4. Vitamin D administration would stimulate intestinal calcium absorption, increasing serum calcium levels and restoring serum iPTH to normal. As a result, serum phosphate and renal Tm/GFR would also return to normal. Over a period of months, bone mineralization would improve, and the histologic changes of osteomalacia would resolve. Adequacy of vitamin D dose is best assessed by following the serum 25(OH)D level, and the adequacy of intestinal calcium absorption is followed by measurement of 24-hour urinary calcium excretion.

Patient 4
1. This patient appears to have hypoparathyroidism, probably the result of her previous thyroid surgery. Her symptoms are those of mild hypocalcemia. The low serum calcium and elevated serum phosphate fit with this diagnosis. The diagnosis would be confirmed by a low or undetectable serum iPTH level.
2. Estrogen therapy decreases the bone turnover rate and diminishes the response to PTH. In patients with impaired parathyroid function this can cause a worsening of hypocalcemia. The impaired bone and intestinal responsiveness produced by glucocorticoid therapy and the increased calcium demands associated with pregnancy can also worsen hypocalcemic symptoms in patients with hypoparathyroidism.
3. The patient should be treated with vitamin D (50,000 to 100,000 units/day) or $1,25(OH)_2D$ (0.5 to 1.5 µg/day) plus calcium supplementation (1000 to 2000 mg/day). Serum and 24-hour urinary calcium levels should be followed at 1- to 2-month intervals and doses adjusted to prevent overdosage. In resistant cases, reduction of dietary phosphate intake may be helpful. Doses of vitamin D and calcium can frequently be reduced if the patient is placed on hydrochlorothiazide (25 to 50 mg/day) to reduce urinary calcium loss.

Patient 5
1. This patient has osteoporosis due to premature menopause and glucocorticoid therapy, and aggravated by reduced physical activity.
2. The diagnosis is established by demonstrating normal serum and urinary mineral levels, and excluding all other disorders that could cause osteopenia, particularly endocrine disorders and multiple myeloma. When there is uncertainty regarding the diagnosis, bone biopsy may occasionally be necessary.
3. If the patient had been placed on estrogen replacement therapy starting at the time of her ovarian surgery, the severity of her osteoporosis would have been reduced.
4. At this point, general measures such as following a regular regimen of weight-bearing physical activity and maintaining good calcium intake (1500 mg/day) may slow her rate of bone loss. Estrogen therapy, even at this late date, may also retard the rate of further bone loss and reduce the risk of subsequent fractures. In a significant proportion of patients with osteoporosis, sodium fluoride therapy (50 to 75 mg/day for 2 to 3 years) can produce a measurable increase in bone mass.

10

Disorders of Water Metabolism

Myron Miller

ABBREVIATIONS

ADH	antidiuretic hormone
AVP	arginine vasopressin
LVP	lysine vasopressin
SIADH	syndrome of inappropriate ADH secretion

The ability to regulate volume and tonicity of extracellular body water within narrow limits is essential to the maintenance of health and preservation of maximal functional status of man. Involved in assuring the constancy of this important body compartment are the interactions of several hormonal systems, the integrity of thirst perception, and the function of the kidney as an excretory organ. Derangements of any of these elements can lead to marked alteration in extracellular fluid volume status and/or to clinically significant disturbance in tonicity of extracellular fluid, reflected as either hypernatremia or hyponatremia. The major hormonal regulator of water balance is the antidiuretic hormone (ADH, vasopressin), synthesized and released by the neurohypophysial system, and responsible for the ability of the kidney to reabsorb fluid in a precise fashion. It is through this hormone and effector system that large variations in fluid intake are modulated by the body to maintain constancy of water balance.

BIOCHEMISTRY AND PHYSIOLOGY

Biosynthesis of ADH

The neurohypophysial system is the site of ADH synthesis, storage, and release and is composed of the cell bodies of the supraoptic and paraventricular neurons of the hypothalamus, their axonal projections through the median eminence and pituitary stalk and the nerve terminals in the posterior lobe of the pituitary gland. In the nuclei of these cells, ADH is synthesized as part of a larger precursor molecule, prepropressophysin, which contains not only the hormone, but a specific carrier protein, neurophysin. The gene for vasopressin has been isolated and its structure determined. In the nuclei of the supraoptic and paraventricular neurons, the gene is transcribed into a precursor mRNA that is then converted to a mature mRNA, transported into the cell cytoplasm, and translated on ribosomes into the hormone precursor molecule, a protein composed of 166 amino acids. The precursor molecule is packaged by the Golgi complex into secretory granules and through a series of enzymatic cleavages is converted to a vasopressin-neurophysin complex. The secretory granules migrate down the axons and are stored in axon terminals in the posterior pituitary, a process estimated to take 12 to 14 hours. In response to stimuli reaching the neurosecretory neurons, an action potential is initiated that propagates to the axonal terminals and allows an influx of calcium from the extracellular space into the nerve terminal. Through the process of exocytosis, both ADH and its neurophysin are liberated into the bloodstream. While ADH is involved in regulation of body water, little is known of the biologic role of neurophysin.

In addition to the neural pathways originating in the supraoptic and paraventricular nuclei, there is evidence that ADH is also produced by cells of the suprachiasmatic nucleus. The axons of these cells do not project to the median eminence and posterior pituitary but instead to wide areas of the brain outside the hypothalamus. ADH liberated from these nerve terminals may act as a neuromodulator of neuronal activity in higher central nervous system centers, including those involved in learning and memory processes.

Structure

The released hormone is a nonapeptide made up of a three amino acid tail attached to six amino acids in a ring structure in which two cysteine molecules are linked by a disulfide bond. ADH occurs in two forms in mammalian species, with the difference being due to the amino acid in position 8 (Fig. 10–1). In most species the hormone contains an arginine residue (arginine vasopressin, AVP), while in the pig, hippopotamus and peccary, lysine occupies this position (lysine vasopressin, LVP). The neurophysins are larger polypeptides with a molecular weight of approximately 100,000 daltons. In man, there are two forms of neurophysin, one associated with vasopressin and the other with the neurohypophysial hormone oxytocin.

Circulation and Metabolism

In the bloodstream, vasopressin circulates as the free peptide with a half-life of 3 to 6 minutes. In normal man under conditions of ad libitum fluid intake, concentration of the hormone in blood ranges from 1 to 8 pg/ml. There is some evidence for a diurnal pattern to vasopressin secretion with maximum values being found late at night and early morning and with lowest values tending to occur in the early afternoon. Inactivation of vasopressin takes place in both the liver and kidney with the initial event being cleavage of the terminal glycinamide to produce a biologically inactive peptide fragment. Approximately 10% of secreted hormone is excreted in the urine as intact, biologically active vasopressin in amounts ranging from 27.5 to 140 ng/24 hours.

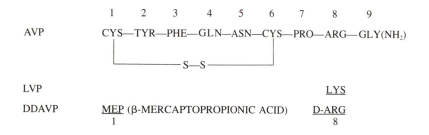

Fig. 10–1. Structural formula of arginine vasopressin (AVP) and the amino acid substitutions giving rise to lysine vasopressin (LVP) and desamino-D-arginine vasopressin (DDAVP).

Function

After release into the circulation, vasopressin has several functions and sites of action. Its most important physiologic action is on the distal and collecting tubule of the kidney, where it acts to conserve water and concentrate the urine by increasing cell permeability with resultant increase in hydro-osmotic flow of water from the luminal fluid to the medullary interstitium. In much higher concentrations, vasopressin can act on the smooth muscle of blood vessels to cause vasoconstriction.

Control Systems

Neural Regulation. A number of neurotransmitters and neuromodulators are capable of affecting ADH synthesis and secretion. There is much evidence to suggest that the final link connecting neural pathways to the magnocellular hypothalamic neurons is mediated by acetylcholine. Other neurotransmitter systems capable of affecting these neurons include dopamine, norepinephrine, glutamate, aspartate and gamma-aminobutyric acid. In addition, neuromodulators including prostaglandins, angiotensin II, and the endogenous opioids (enkephalin, beta-endorphin, and dynorphin) have been demonstrated to exert both stimulatory and inhibitory influences on vasopressin secretion. These actions appear to be due to a presynaptic modulation of neurotransmitter activity. In the case of the endogenous opioids, inhibition of ADH secretion has been associated with kappa receptor activity. Recent studies have demonstrated that a newly discovered hormone, atrial natriuretic peptide, is found in the hypothalamus and appears capable of inhibiting ADH release that occurs in response to the stimuli of dehydration and hemorrhage. Other neural factors capable of altering vasopressin secretion include pain and emotional stress, which can affect magnocellular function through direct afferent pathways from the limbic system to the hypothalamus. Emesis is also a potent stimulus for the release of vasopressin and most likely involves activation of neural pathways.

Tonicity. In the normal individual, the amount of hormone release is regulated by the tonicity of the blood through osmoreceptors located in the hypothalamus in or near the cell bodies of the magnocellular nuclei (Fig 10–2). Serum osmolality in normally hydrated individuals is usually maintained within a narrow range from 284 to 292 mosm/kg. Decrease of serum osmolality to less than 282 mosm/kg is usually accompanied by inhibition of ADH secretion with a resultant increase in urine volume and decrease in urine osmolality (Table 10–1). This hypotonic diuresis can produce urine flow rates as high as 1200 ml/hour and urine concentration to as low as 50 to 60 mosm/kg. In response to small increases in blood tonicity, usually due to change in serum sodium concentration, there is a progressive stimulation of ADH release with an accompanying progressive fall in urine volume and rise in urine osmolality (Fig. 10–3). Initiation of ADH release in normally hydrated subjects occurs when serum osmolality has risen to the range of 282 to 284

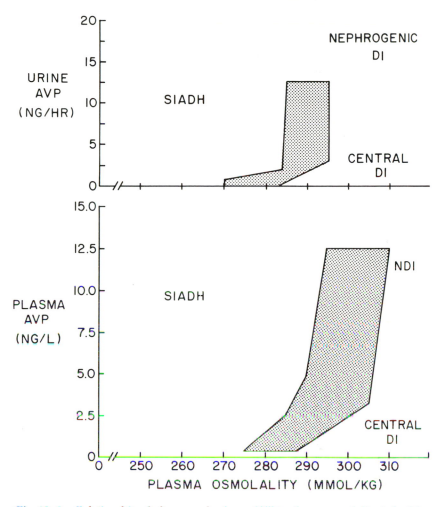

Fig. 10–2. Relationship of plasma and urinary AVP to plasma osmolality in healthy subjects. The shaded areas include values from the water load state, normal hydration, and dehydrated state. Regions shown are those in which values usually occur in patients with diabetes insipidus (DI), nephrogenic diabetes insipidus (NDI), and syndrome of inappropriate ADH secretion (SIADH). (From Miller, M.: Clin Lab Med, 4:729, 1984.)

mosm/kg. Maximum urine concentration, in the vicinity of 1200 mosm/kg, will usually occur when serum osmolality has reached 292 mosm/kg or greater.

Volume. Blood volume is an important determinant of the level of ADH discharge. Proportionally greater deviations from normality are required to affect hormone release than is needed for osmotic stimulation. Intrathoracic stretch receptors located in the left atrium are responsive to changes in blood volume and by means of alteration in vagal activity can modulate ADH release from the neurophypophysial system. This pathway involves relays in the nucleus of the tractus solitarius in the brain stem that project to the A1

Table 10–1. Alterations in the Physiologic Spectrum of States of Water Balance with Associated Typical Changes in Plasma Osmolality, Plasma AVP, Urine Osmolality, and Urine Flow Rate in Normal Subjects

Physiologic State	Plasma Osmolality (mosm/kg)	Plasma AVP (pg/ml)	Urine Osmolality (mosm/kg)	Urine Flow Rate (ml/hr)
Over-hydrated	<282	<1	50 to 100	600 to 1200
Initiation of ADH Release	282	1	100 to 200	400 to 800
Normal Hydration	284 to 292	1 to 8	500 to 1200	30 to 100
Thirst Perception	292	3 to 10	600 to 1200	15 to 25
Dehydrated (12–24 hr)	>290	5 to 15	600 to 1200	15 to 25

noradrenergic nucleus and in turn project to the cell bodies of the magnocellular hypothalamic nuclei. A decrease in blood volume of approximately 10% will provoke release of ADH, with progressively greater increases in hormone level occurring with further fall in blood volume. Plasma concentrations of AVP following reduction in blood volume far exceed those that can be achieved by osmotic stimulation. In a similar fashion, expansion of blood volume on the order of 10% results in inhibition of ADH secretion. There is an interaction between volume and osmotic stimuli for vasopressin release so that volume depletion results in an enhanced response to an osmotic stimulus while volume expansion necessitates a greater increase in blood osmolality in order to provoke ADH release.

Baroreceptor. Changes in blood pressure are capable of affecting vasopressin secretion. The receptors to change in systemic blood pressure (high-pressure baroreceptors) are located within the carotid body and arch of the aorta. Their afferent impulses are carried by the glossopharyngeal nerve to the brain stem and are subsequently relayed to the hypothalamus by the same pathways that carry information from vagal fibers in the atrium. A decrease in blood pressure of 5 mm Hg is usually sufficient to initiate an increase in vasopressin secretion. With larger falls in blood pressure, AVP levels in the circulation can reach concentrations 1000 times those seen in the basal state. These high concentrations may play a role in maintenance of blood pressure through the vasoconstrictive action of the hormone.

Aging Influences

Normal aging is associated with changes both in ADH secretion and in the renal responsiveness to the hormone. Plasma AVP concentration undergoes a gradual, progressive increase with advancing age. More significantly, the response of AVP to osmotic stimulation increases with age so that each increment in plasma osmolality in the older individual results in a greater increase in plasma AVP concentration. The basis for this enhanced osmotically induced AVP release with age is not clearly understood but may be related to the decline in baroreceptor function that also occurs with normal aging.

RELATION OF Posm TO Uosm IN VARIOUS STATES OF HYDRATION

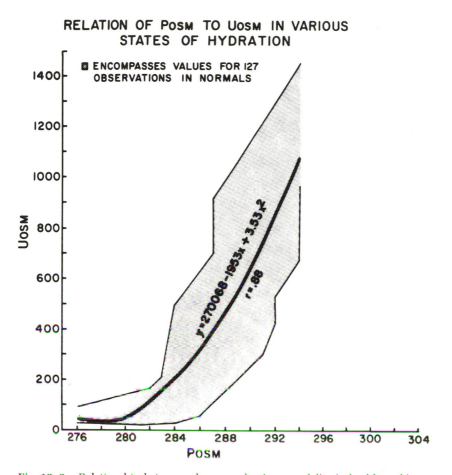

Fig. 10–3. Relationship between plasma and urine osmolality in healthy subjects. The solid line represents the curve of best fit determined from 127 values, while the shaded area encompasses the range of values actually observed. (From Miller, M., and Moses, A.M.: *In* Neurohypophysis. Edited by A.M. Moses and L. Share. Basel, Karger AG, 1977.)

Decreased baroreceptor activity would lead to a decline in inhibitory input into the hypothalamic magnocellular neurosecretory neurons.

In parallel with this change in ADH release is an age-related decline in renal concentrating response to the hormone. A decline in maximum achievable urine osmolality is usually present by age 60 years and undergoes progressive fall over the remainder of the life span. It is possible that this acquired impairment in renal responsiveness to ADH is a consequence of down regulation of renal AVP receptors, resulting from exposure to increased circulating levels of hormone. The degree of impaired concentrating ability is rarely of a magnitude sufficient to cause clinically significant disturbance of fluid balance.

Thirst perception also is affected by aging. Elderly healthy individuals exhibit a diminished sensation of thirst following exposure to water deprivation even though this stress raises plasma osmolality to higher levels than in young subjects. When access to water is resumed, the elderly consume less water in satisfying their thirst. These observations help explain the common clinical finding that older patients with a variety of illnesses often have features of dehydration, yet have poor fluid intake and need encouragement to drink sufficient fluid to correct their deficits.

MECHANISMS OF ACTION OF VASOPRESSIN

Numerous studies have established that vasopressin action involves binding of the hormone to specific cell membrane receptors. It appears that there are at least two classes of these receptors, designated V1 and V2, which differ in their biochemical mechanism of cellular action.

V1 Receptors

Vasopressin interaction with V1 receptors, found on myocytes of vascular smooth muscle, glomerular mesangial cells, and hepatocytes, is associated with increased Ca^{2+} cellular flux as mediator of response. This increase in Ca^{2+} movement into the cell leads to rapid hydrolysis of phosphatidylinositol, activation of phospholipase-A2, and release of arachidonic acid from membrane phospholipids. These events culminate in activation of an intracellular contractile system and/or increased synthesis of prostaglandins.

V2 Receptors

These receptors are associated with an adenylate cyclase within the contraluminal plasma membrane of cells of the renal collecting tubule. The interaction of vasopressin with the receptor leads to activation of the adenylate cyclase and generation of cAMP as a second messenger. In turn, this leads to activation of protein kinase and phosphorylation of protein substrates which results in enhanced movement of water across the luminal membrane of the cells of the collecting duct along an osmotic gradient. Figure 10–4 diagrams the regulation and actions of AVP.

Water Transport

The production of a concentrated urine requires the presence of an intact renal cortical-medullary concentration gradient for solutes. The main renal medullary solutes are sodium chloride and urea and it is their concentration in the medulla that determines the magnitude of the urine concentrating response to the passive flow of water across the tubular membrane that is induced by ADH. Blood flow in the vasa recti serves to maintain the gradient. Alteration of the blood supply to the medulla or administration of loop diuretics such as furosemide can lead to decline in the gradient with accompanying impaired ability to generate a concentrated urine.

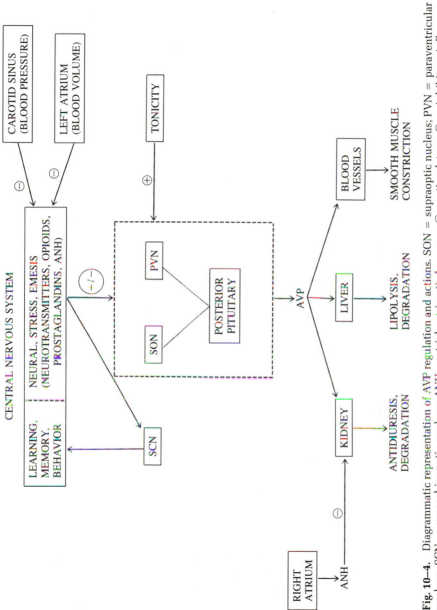

Fig. 10–4. Diagrammatic representation of AVP regulation and actions. SON = supraoptic nucleus; PVN = paraventricular nucleus; SCN = suprachiasmatic nucleus; ANH = atrial natriuretic hormone. ⊕ = stimulatory; ⊖ = inhibitory influence.

TESTS OF FUNCTION

Clinical Evaluation

When evaluating a patient suspected of having a disorder of water metabolism, initial assessment requires careful attention to the history and physical examination in an attempt to identify features suggestive of altered body water status. Thus, history is obtained of fluid intake, losses from such routes as urinary tract, gastrointestinal tract, or skin in association with fever, thirst perception, presence of known renal, cardiac, hepatic and endocrine diseases, and use of drugs that can affect water balance. Physical examination can reveal findings of water depletion such as decreased skin turgor, dry mucous membranes, orthostatic hypotension, and increased heart rate, or evidence of water overload such as edema, distended neck veins, and signs of congestive heart failure.

Basic laboratory determinations should include measurement of serum osmolality and the major serum components contributing to total serum solute concentration, including electrolytes, urea, and glucose. Determination of serum calcium and potassium may be of value since elevated calcium or low potassium can lead to reduced renal responsiveness to the action of ADH with resultant polyuria and volume depletion. Urinary measures such as osmolality and sodium concentration are valuable in evaluating the patient suspected of having water losing or retaining disorders. Estimation of osmotic excretion and clearance can be made. Free water clearance, which is inversely related to ADH action on the kidney, can be calculated from the formula $C_{H_2O} = V - C_{osm}$. It is often necessary to assess the function of components of the endocrine system by means of suitable tests of thyroid and adrenal function since disturbances of these systems can affect water handling capacity.

AVP Measurement

Diagnosis and treatment of patients with disorders of water metabolism rarely requires the direct measurement of AVP in the blood or urine. However, the ability to accurately measure AVP has greatly increased knowledge of the physiology of hormone regulation and has improved the understanding of mechanisms underlying pathologic states.

Early approaches to hormone measurement were based on bioassay procedures that reflected the action of AVP on arterial smooth muscle with resultant increase in blood pressure. These procedures were not sufficiently sensitive to quantitate the small amounts of hormone normally present in blood or urine. However, this assay is the basis for measuring the biologic activity of AVP extracted from animal posterior pituitary or manufactured synthetically and is used in estabishing reference standards of the hormone. Purified AVP has a potency of 400 pressor units per mg. Current assay systems often express AVP concentration in biologic unitage as well as in units of weight, with the accepted conversion factor relating biologic activity and weight being 1 μU = 2.5 pg of AVP.

In recent years, sensitive and specific radioimmunoassay (RIA) systems have been developed that are capable of accurately measuring AVP in small volumes of blood and urine. Because of the presence of substances in blood or urine that interfere with the assay technique, measurement of the hormone first requires extraction, partial purification and concentration before RIA can be carried out.

AVP in Blood. AVP can be measured by RIA in the serum or plasma of normal subjects (Fig. 10–2). The concentration is affected by both blood osmolality and the volume status of the individual. For normally hydrated individuals, whose plasma osmolality ranges from 284 and 292 mosm/kg, plasma AVP concentration has been found to range from 1 to 8 pg/ml. An increase in plasma osmolality in response to hypertonic saline infusion produces a progressive increase in plasma AVP but rarely exceeding 10 pg/ml. Modest dehydration, which provides both an osmotic and volume-mediated stimulus, can increase plasma AVP to approximately 15 pg/ml. A water load sufficient to reduce plasma osmolality to less than 282 mosm/kg will, in most normal subjects, suppress AVP secretion to levels at or below the detection limit of most assay systems.

AVP in Urine. Urinary AVP measurement has an advantage over measurement in blood by being an integrated value over a period of time and therefore is less subject to fluctuation from moment to moment in response to changes in physiologic state or environmental influences (Fig. 10–2). In the steady state, urinary AVP excretion represents approximately 15% of AVP secretion. A close relationship between plasma AVP concentration and urine AVP excretion rate has been demonstrated. In healthy normal male subjects, urinary AVP has been reported to range from 27.5 to 140 ng/24 hr. Healthy women have levels at the lower end of the range reported for men. Following water deprivation for 14 hours, urine AVP excretion can increase 2 to 3 fold over basal values. Water load suppresses AVP excretion, sometimes to undetectable levels.

FUNCTIONAL MEASURES OF AVP SECRETION AND ACTION

Dehydration Test

Comparison of renal concentrating capacity after dehydration to the subsequent urine concentration achieved following vasopressin administration provides a simple and reliable means of testing the capacity of the neurohypophysial system to release AVP (Table 10–2). The test is quantitative in that it allows for the detection of subnormal secretion of AVP. In addition, the test evaluates the capacity of the renal end organ to respond to the hormone. The procedure is based on withholding fluid until the maximal urine concentration due to endogenous vasopressin has been achieved and then administering exogenous vasopressin to determine the maximal capacity of the kidney to concentrate the urine. In normal individuals and in patients with mild degrees of polyuria, the period of fluid deprivation begins at approximately

Table 10–2.   Response to Water Deprivation Test*

Clinical Condition	Maximum Uosm at Plateau (mosm/kg)	Change in Uosm After Vasopressin (%)	Posm at Plateau (mosm/kg)
Normal	764±212†	<5	289±7
Partial DI	438±116	>9	294±4
Severe DI	168±59	>50	306±12
Nephrogenic DI	<150	<45	302 to 320
Primary Polydipsia	696±190	<5	>288
High-set Osmoreceptor	>600	<5	>295

*Adapted from Miller, et al., Ann Intern Med 73:721, 1970
†Mean ±S.D.

6 P.M. and is continued over the next 14 to 18 hours. In patients with severe polyuria who have urine volumes of 10 liters per day or greater, the period of fluid deprivation is begun at approximately 6 A.M. so that the patient can be carefully monitored and the test terminated if weight loss exceeds 2 kg or if untoward clinical symptoms occur. Hourly urine samples are obtained starting at 8 A.M. on the morning following initiation of water deprivation and urine osmolality is measured in each sample. Hourly collections are continued until two consecutive samples differ in urine osmolality by less than 30 mosm/kg. In normal individuals this occurs after 14 to 18 hours of water deprivation, while in patients with severe polyuria, a period of 6 to 8 hours is usually sufficient to reach a stable maximum urine osmolality. At this point, five units of aqueous vasopressin is given subcutaneously and urine osmolality is determined 1 hour later. Serum osmolality is measured prior to initiation of the fluid deprivation and again at the time of reaching the plateau in urine osmolality. In normal individuals, fluid deprivation for 18 to 24 hours rarely raises serum osmolality above 292 mosm/kg. To assure adequacy of dehydration, serum osmolality before injection of vasopressin should be above 288 mosm/kg. In subjects with normal neurohypophysial function, the maximum urine osmolality that can be reached after water deprivation varies considerably, depending on age, renal medullary solute concentration, and other intrarenal factors. Following injection of vasopressin, urine osmolality rises by less than 5% of the value obtained by fluid deprivation alone, whatever the absolute value of urine osmolality achieved by dehydration. This indicates that sufficient AVP release was induced by water deprivation to achieve a maximal effect on renal concentrating capacity as reflected by urine osmolality and therefore, the administration of exogenous vasopressin will fail to raise the urine osmolality to any significant degree.

Urine Osmolality to Serum Osmolality Relationship

In normal individuals there is a close relationship between urine osmolality and simultaneously measured serum osmolality (Fig. 10–3). This relationship can be defined for the normal population as a whole so that deviation due to disorders of ADH release or action can be recognized. Measurements of simultaneous serum and urine osmolality are obtained during periods of ad libitum fluid intake and during periods of water loading or water deprivation. In these circumstances, serum and urine osmolality should fall or rise in parallel and within the normal confidence limits.

Hypertonic Saline Infusion

Infusion of hypertonic saline intravenously, in the form of 5% saline solution, will cause a progressive rise in serum osmolality, which in healthy subjects will provoke the release of AVP from the neurohypophysial system. In water-loaded normal subjects, the serum osmolality at which ADH release is initiated is referred to as the osmotic threshold for ADH release. This point is recognized by the abrupt onset of a progressive decrease in urine volume and increase in urine osmolality in response to the released AVP. In a group of normal subjects, this value has been defined as a serum osmolality of 287.3 ± 3.3 mosm/kg. Elevation of the serum osmolality to higher levels leads to progressively greater decline in urine volume and increase in urine osmolality until maximum urine concentrating capacity has been reached, usually when serum osmolality exceeds 292 mosm/kg. The test is interpreted by calculating changes in free water clearance during the infusion in order to prevent masking of the antidiuretic response by an increase in urine volume that can occur in some patients due to large increase in urinary solute excretion following the saline infusion.

Water Load Test

The response to waterloading is a useful means of readily and quickly establishing the ability to normally suppress release of AVP (Table 10–3). Before the water load test is performed, conditions known to affect water handling must be excluded, including the presence of renal, cardiac, or hepatic disease, hypothyroidism, hypoadrenalism, and the use of drugs that may interfere with renal water excretion. In addition, the patient should not be exposed to stimuli that may provoke ADH release even in the presence of a fall in serum osmolality. Such stimuli include severe stress, pain, hypovolemia, and hypotension. The test is carried out by giving an oral water load

Table 10–3. Response to Oral Water Load Test, 20 ml/kg Body Weight

Clinical Condition	Minimum Uosm (mosm/kg)	% Water Load Excreted in 5 Hours	Posm Prior to Water Load (mosm/kg)
Normal	<100	>80	284 to 292
SIADH	>100	<80	<284*
Low Set Osmoreceptor	<100	>80	<284

*Posm may be normal if treated by fluid restriction prior to test

of 20 ml/kg body weight over a period of 15 to 20 minutes. Urine is then collected at hourly intervals for the next 5 hours for measurement of volume and osmolality in each specimen. The patient should remain in a recumbent position throughout the test except to void. Blood is obtained for measurement of serum osmolality prior to the administration of the water load. In normal individuals, more than 80% of the water load is excreted in 5 hours and urine osmolality will fall to less than 100 mosm/kg in at least one sample during the test, usually during the second hour. Such a response indicates normal suppressibility of ADH as well as normal capacity of the kidney to generate a dilute urine.

DIABETES INSIPIDUS

Diabetes insipidus is the polyuric state that results from impaired ability of the kidney to conserve water due to low blood levels of AVP following exposure to normal physiologic stimuli.

Table 10–4.   Causes of Hypotonic Polyuria

1. Hypothalamic Diabetes Insipidus
   Idiopathic and Familial
   Head Trauma
   Pituitary Surgery
   Tumor (Primary and Metastatic)
   Cerebral Anoxia
   Granulomatous Disease
      Histiocytosis
      Sarcoidosis

2. Nephrogenic Diabetes Insipidus
   Familial
   Spontaneous
   Acquired
      Renal Disease
      Potassium Deficiency
      Hypercalcemia
      Drug-Induced
         Lithium
         Demethylchlortetracycline

3. Primary Polydipsia
   Psychogenic
   Hypothalamic Disease
   Drug-Induced

4. Osmotic Diuresis
   Glucose (Diabetes Mellitus)
   Sodium
      Chronic Renal Disease
      Diuretic-Induced
      Excessive Intake
   Mannitol

Etiology

Many different disorders can lead to impaired ability to synthesize or release AVP and consequently to diabetes insipidus (Table 10–4). In a large series, approximately 25% of the cases were considered to be idiopathic in origin. In these individuals, diabetes insipidus frequently starts in childhood or in early adult life and appears to be slightly more common in males than in females. A small percentage of patients with idiopathic diabetes insipidus have the disorder as a result of familial disease inherited in an autosomal dominant fashion. More often, diabetes insipidus is a consequence of damage to the hypothalamus, pituitary stalk, or posterior pituitary gland as a result of tumor, head trauma, or surgical procedure in the area of the hypothalamus or pituitary. In these patients, there may be partial or complete loss of anterior pituitary function in addition to the diabetes insipidus. Diabetes insipidus occurring after head trauma or surgical procedures in the region of the hypothalamus and pituitary often is transient, occurring within several days after the trauma or surgical procedure and disappearing after several days.

Pathology

Examination of the hypothalamus of patients who have had long-standing diabetes insipidus reveals loss of most of the neurons in the supraoptic and paraventricular nuclei. The neural loss has been reported in patients with idiopathic diabetes insipidus as well as in patients whose disease was the result of trauma, surgery, or tumor. A loss of greater than 90% of the neurons is required before diabetes insipidus becomes clinically evident.

Symptoms and Signs

Because of deficiency of ADH, the major signs and symptoms are related to impaired ability of the kidney to conserve water. Thus, polyuria, severe thirst, and polydipsia are the most common presenting symptoms. Often these symptoms are sudden in onset whether due to idiopathic diabetes insipidus or to trauma or injury. The urine is pale in color and the volume increased to amounts as high as 25 liters per day. This massive polyuria is accompanied by urinary frequency as often as every 30 to 60 minutes throughout the day and night. In some patients, however, diabetes insipidus can be mild with urine volumes of 3 to 4 liters and with the patient being unaware of symptoms related to this mild polyuria. Classically, when thirst is present, cold drinks are sought out in an attempt to alleviate the thirst. Since the thirst center lies in close approximation to the nerve bodies responsible for ADH synthesis, some patients may have diabetes insipidus with impaired thirst perception as well. These individuals are at risk of severe dehydration with all of the accompanying features of severe volume depletion. Even when thirst perception is normal, fluid intake rarely is sufficient to compensate for urinary losses. Mild degrees of dehydration, however, are seldom clinically apparent. When access to water is interfered with, severe dehydration with accompanying symptoms of weakness, fever, dry mucous membranes, orthostatic hypotension, and tachycardia may occur.

Diagnostic Tests

Measurement of serum osmolality often reveals the presence of an increase in total solute concentration. This is usually accompanied by an increase in serum sodium concentration along with elevations of the serum BUN and creatinine, reflective of the fluid volume depleted state. At the same time, the urine is inappropriately dilute as indicated by urinary specific gravity and more accurately by the urine osmolality. The magnitude of the urine osmolality is dependent upon the severity of the ADH deficiency. In patients with severe diabetes insipidus and high urine volumes, urine osmolality may be in the range of 50 to 90 mosm/kg even though plasma osmolality or serum sodium are increased above the normal range. In milder degrees of diabetes insipidus in which there is a partial deficiency of ADH secretion, urine osmolality may be in the range of 200 to 500 mosm/kg.

The diagnosis and severity of the ADH deficiency can be established by means of the dehydration test (Table 10–2). Patients with deficiency of ADH will respond to the injection of vasopressin with an increase in urine osmolality achieved after water deprivation. In patients with severe diabetes insipidus and essentially complete loss of ADH secretory capacity, urine osmolality as a result of water deprivation will remain hypotonic to plasma. Patients with milder degrees of hormone deficiency may increase the urine osmolality to hypertonic levels but still less than the maximum achievable concentration that can be elicited by the injection of exogenous vasopressin. Serum osmolality measured at the time of the plateau in urine osmolality tends to be higher than in healthy subjects and is raised in proportion to the degree of severity of ADH deficiency. Thus, the dehydration test allows recognition not only of patients with complete hormonal loss and severe polyuria, but also of patients with mild degrees of AVP deficiency who often may not be clinically recognized because their polyuria is mild.

The hypertonic saline infusion test is also of value in establishing the diagnosis of diabetes insipidus. It is of particular importance in a small group of patients whose diabetes insipidus is not due to deficiency of ADH synthesis but rather to an inability to release ADH in response to an osmotic stimulus. In patients with complete ADH deficiency, saline infusion will not result in a fall of free water clearance even when plasma osmolality is raised well above the normal osmotic threshold to values of 300 mosm/kg or higher. There is a group of patients with polyuria who will respond to osmotic stimulation with hypertonic saline but only when plasma osmolality is raised far above normal values. These patients can be considered to have a high-set osmoreceptor as the reason for their disturbed water regulation.

Measurement of blood or urine AVP in response to water deprivation or hypertonic saline infusion has been used in establishing the diagnosis of diabetes insipidus (Fig. 10–2). Plasma AVP levels have been reported to remain below 0.9 pg/ml following water deprivation sufficient to increase serum osmolality from 288 to 312 mosm/kg. Patients with mild degrees of polyuria have had plasma AVP levels that were in the normal range but were low relative to the simultaneously determined serum osmolality. These patients are considered to have partial degrees of AVP deficiency as the basis for their polyuria. In a similar fashion, urinary AVP excretion has been found to be low or undetectable in many patients with severe polyuria with subnormal response to the stimulus of increase in serum osmolality. Most patients with diabetes insipidus demonstrate some AVP in the urine in response to water deprivation but these amounts are well below levels seen in normal individuals subjected to the same stimulus. These data further demonstrate that diabetes insipidus is often the result of varying degrees of partial ADH deficiency, rather than a result of complete failure to synthesize and release the hormone.

Therapy

The treatment of diabetes insipidus centers around hormone replacement therapy. AVP has a short duration of action and is destroyed in the gastrointestinal tract if taken orally. The hormone can be administered subcutaneously in an aqueous form that has a duration of action of 3 to 6 hours, or intramuscularly as a suspension in oil that has a duration of action of 24 to 72 hours. In recent years a potent AVP analog, DDAVP, has been synthesized that has markedly enhanced and prolonged antidiuretic activity and is almost completely devoid of pressor effects. This material can be taken intranasally once or twice a day and will control polyuria in most patients. Some patients can be successfully treated with the oral sulfonylurea chlorpropamide, which has the property of stimulating the release of AVP from the neurohypophysial system and also of enhancing the antidiuretic action of released AVP on the renal tubule. The hypolipidemic agent, clofibrate, is also capable of stimulating ADH release and may be used orally as a treatment for diabetes insipidus.

NEPHROGENIC DIABETES INSIPIDUS

Nephrogenic diabetes insipidus is a rare, usually inherited form of polyuria, most commonly affecting males, which results from inability of the kidney to respond to the antidiuretic action of ADH. The disease is usually evident shortly after birth and is recognized because of the severe polyuria and accompanying thirst and polydipsia. The signs and symptoms are the same as those in patients with severe forms of ADH deficiency. An acquired form of nephrogenic diabetes insipidus can occur in patients with chronic renal disease, after acute tubular necrosis, in patients with potassium deficiency or hypercalcemia, and after exposure to drugs such as lithium and demethylchlortetracycline (Table 10–4). Common to all of these situations is failure of the renal V2 receptor to respond to ADH. Vascular V1 receptors, however, show unimpaired responsiveness.

The diagnosis of nephrogenic diabetes insipidus is established by demonstrating failure to significantly concentrate the urine following injection of vasopressin or intranasal administration of DDAVP (Table 10–2). Measurement of plasma or urine AVP will show the hormone to be present in greater than normal amounts in response to the combined stimuli of volume depletion and hypertonicity (Fig. 10–2).

Hormone replacement therapy is not effective in managing the polyuria due to nephrogenic diabetes insipidus. Reduction in urine volume can be achieved by interfering with the ability of the kidney to generate a maximally dilute urine. This can be accomplished by chronic diuretic administration and a low salt diet to produce a sodium depleted state with consequent reduction in renal medullary gradient and decrease in intravascular volume and glomerular filtration rate.

PRIMARY POLYDIPSIA

Primary polydipsia is the condition resulting from chronic over ingestion of water that leads to suppression of ADH and production of hypotonic polyuria. The polydipsia and polyuria in this disorder are usually erratic in contrast to the sustained polydipsia and polyuria of diabetes insipidus. The patients often do not have nocturnal urinary frequency. The disorder is commonly seen in patients with emotional disturbances and occasionally can occur in individuals with central nervous system lesions that produce an increase in thirst perception.

Patients with chronic primary polydipsia may be difficult to distinguish from patients with true diabetes insipidus, but a correct diagnosis can be made following appropriate tests. The diagnosis should be suspected when, in addition to hypotonic polyuria, there is also low plasma osmolality or serum sodium concentration. The dehydration test can establish the diagnosis since a sufficiently long period of water deprivation will result eventually in maximal concentration of the urine (Table 10–2). Measurement of plasma or urine AVP may be low during the period of water ingestion but will reach normal values following prolonged water deprivation.

OTHER CAUSES OF POLYURIA

The excretion of increased amounts of solute in the urine can cause an obligatory water loss with resultant polyuria, increased thirst and polydipsia (Table 10–4). The most common circumstance is the osmotic diuresis secondary to glycosuria in patients with poorly controlled diabetes mellitus. Correction of the blood sugar abnormality will lead to resolution of the polyuric state. Polyuria can also occur as a result of increased sodium excretion such as may result from chronic renal disease, increased sodium intake or the use of diuretic agents. In all of these states, measurement of osmolal excretion and calculation of free water clearance will demonstrate that the increase in urine flow is attributable to the increase in solute excretion rather than to a primary free water diuresis.

SYNDROME OF INAPPROPRIATE ADH SECRETION

The syndrome of inappropriate ADH secretion (SIADH) is a disorder characterized by hyponatremia due to water retention caused by increased ADH. The excessive ADH in the circulation is due to inappropriate non-physiologic causes such as autonomous release from tumors or response to non-physiologic stimuli capable of overriding the inhibitory influence of hypoosmolality (Table 10–5).

Etiology

The most common cause of SIADH is the autonomous release of ADH from tumor tissue where it is synthesized, stored, and discharged in the absence of known stimuli. Of these tumors, small cell or oat cell carcinoma of the lung accounts for 80% of the patients. Prospective studies of patients with oat cell carcinoma of the lung have shown that more than 50% have impaired water excretion and elevated plasma ADH levels even in the absence of overt hyponatremia. Other malignancies that can be associated with SIADH

Table 10–5. Causes of SIADH

1. Malignancy with Ectopic Hormone Production
   Small Cell Carcinoma of Lung
   Pancreatic Carcinoma
   Thymoma
   Lymphosarcoma, Reticulum Cell Sarcoma, Hodgkin's Disease

2. Pulmonary Disease
   Pneumonia
   Lung Abscess
   Tuberculosis

3. Central Nervous System Disorders
   Trauma
   Tumor
   Infectious
   Vascular
   Acute Intermittent Porphyria
   Lupus Erythematosus

4. Drugs
   Chlorpropamide
   Vincristine
   Vinblastine
   Cyclophosphamide
   Carbamazepine
   Thiazide Diuretics
   Narcotics
   General Anesthetics
   Tricyclic Antidepressants
   Oxytocin

5. Other
   Hypothyroidism
   Positive Pressure Breathing

include pancreatic carcinoma, lymphosarcoma, reticulum cell sarcoma, Hodgkin's disease, and thymoma. In addition to tumor, non-tumorous lung tissue can acquire the capacity to synthesize and release ADH autonomously as a result of inflammatory diseases including tuberculosis and bacterial pneumonia. A third form of SIADH involves release of ADH from the patient's own neurohypophysial system as a result of a wide variety of central nervous system disorders or as a result of drug use. Virtually any disorder of the central nervous system including inflammatory, neoplastic, infectious, traumatic, or vascular diseases can result in SIADH. This may be transient as in the case of inflammatory or infectious diseases or chronic in the case of neoplastic diseases or head trauma. A number of drugs can stimulate the release of ADH. Chlorpropamide has been the most widely studied and has been shown to be capable not only of stimulating the release of ADH, but also of enhancing the antidiuretic action of submaximal concentrations of hormone at the level of the kidney. Other drugs capable of stimulating ADH release include: the antineoplastic agents, vincristine, vinblastine, and cyclophosphamide. Carbamazepine, used in the treatment of tic douloureux, can produce hyponatremia through stimulation of ADH release. A number of tricyclic antidepressant agents can also produce SIADH. Oxytocin given in large amounts to obstetrical patients can cause water intoxication due to its inherent antidiuretic activity. Exposure to general anesthetics or narcotics can stimulate release of ADH and cause water retention.

Pathophysiology

Because the release of ADH is not suppressible by volume expansion or hypo-osmolality, patients with the syndrome are unable to excrete a dilute urine and therefore retain ingested fluid. This results in expansion of the extracellular fluid volume. The expanded extracellular fluid volume is capable of suppressing the renin-angiotensin system with resultant suppression of aldosterone production by the adrenal gland. In addition, the increase in extracellular fluid volume activates the release of the atrial natriuretic hormone from the right atrium. These consequences of volume expansion lead to an increase in urinary sodium excretion and probably account for the observation that edema is rarely seen in patients with SIADH. As a result of the action of the increased ADH on the kidney, the urine is concentrated. Thus, the classical findings in SIADH are hyponatremia due to water retention with concomitant urine osmolality in excess of plasma osmolality. The ADH produced by tumors or by nontumorous lung tissue appears to be identical with native AVP and has the full biologic activity of the native hormone.

Symptoms and Signs

Patients with SIADH may have weight gain and symptoms due to the hyponatremia including weakness, lethargy, mental confusion, and ultimately, in patients with severe hyponatremia, convulsions and coma may ensue. Clinical signs of fluid overload such as edema or hypertension are rare.

Diagnostic Tests

Evidence of water overload may be manifest in routine laboratory measurements including low levels of serum BUN, creatinine, uric acid and albumin. The serum osmolality is reduced as is serum sodium concentration. At the same time, urine is inappropriately concentrated, generally being hypertonic to plasma. Urinary sodium concentration is usually increased to greater than 20 mEq/L and is often much higher.

The establishment of the diagnosis of SIADH requires exclusion of other causes of hyponatremia such as may occur from renal disease, congestive heart failure, or cirrhosis. Pseudohyponatremia can be seen in patients with high triglyceride levels because the lipids occupy significant volume and displace a similar volume of water. Hyperglycemia can result in lowering of serum sodium concentration due to an osmotic shift of fluid from the intracellular to the extracellular and intravascular spaces. Correction can be made using the assumption that each increase in blood glucose of 100 mg/dl above the normal will lower serum sodium concentration by 1.6 mEq/L. The presence of hypothyroidism and hypoadrenalism must be excluded since these disorders can result in impaired water excretion with dilutional hyponatremia. Careful history and physical examination must be performed to evaluate the patient for the possibility of tumor, inflammatory disease, central nervous system disorder, or drug use, which may be the cause of the SIADH.

The diagnosis may be established by means of the water load test (Table 10–3). Because the test may be dangerous in an already hyponatremic patient, it is not carried out until the serum sodium has been raised to a safe level, generally above 125 mEq/L and the patient is free of symptoms of hyponatremia. In patients with SIADH there will be impaired ability to excrete the water load in the following 5 hours, and this will be accompanied by impaired ability to dilute the urine to less than 100 mosm/kg. Patients who fail to excrete the water load in a normal fashion and who have no other apparent cause for impaired water excretion can be considered to have SIADH.

The test also allows for the recognition of patients with low-set osmoreceptor since these individuals have hyponatremia but are able to excrete the water load normally and dilute the urine when plasma osmolality is further lowered. When a water load has been given to a patient with SIADH, no further water intake should be permitted until the serum sodium concentration has returned to the pretest value.

Measurement of plasma and urinary AVP has been used in the evaluation of patients with hyponatremia (Fig. 10–2). Although levels of the hormone may be elevated in patients with SIADH, many such patients have hormone concentrations that fall within the normal range. However, these levels are excessive when related to the plasma osmolality. Some patients with SIADH will show partial suppression of plasma or urine AVP in response to water load, but even in these individuals, the levels remain inappropriately elevated. In response to stimulation, such as with hypertonic saline solution, some patients with SIADH show a progressive increase in plasma AVP that correlates with the induced rise in plasma osmolality, indicating that there is retention of osmotic control of AVP secretion in these patients. In other patients, raising plasma osmolality produces no clearcut relationship between the plasma AVP and corresponding plasma osmolality. In a small group of patients with SIADH, plasma AVP levels appear to be normally suppressed and the possibility is raised that the SIADH may be due to altered renal sensitivity to the hormone or to the production of some other antidiuretic substance.

Therapy

If the underlying problem responsible for the production of SIADH cannot be corrected, then treatment is directed at reduction of fluid intake and attempts to increase water excretion. In patients with mild features of water overload, fluid restriction to approximately 800 to 1000 ml daily should be sufficient to control the hyponatremia. Patients with severe water intoxication and associated central nervous system symptoms require more vigorous treatment. Intravenous administration of 200 to 300 ml of 3% saline solution over several hours is usually sufficient to raise the serum sodium to a level at which symptoms will improve. Occasionally, intravenous furosemide is given simultaneously to produce a natriuresis and diuresis. In this situation, careful attention must be paid to the correction of potassium and other electrolyte losses induced by the diuretic agent. Currently, there are no drugs that will effectively and reliably inhibit ADH release from either ectopic sources or from the neurohypophysial system in patients with SIADH. It is possible, however, to interfere with the action of ADH on the renal tubule through use of the tetracycline antibiotic, demethylchlortetracycline. Currently under development are vasopressin antagonists capable of blocking the activity of AVP on V2 renal receptors. These agents may be an important addition to the management of patients with SIADH as well as those with other forms of fluid retention secondary to increased ADH secretion or action.

CLINICAL PROBLEMS

Patient 1. A 22-year-old man without a significant prior medical history suffered a severe head injury in a motorcycle accident. Skull films revealed the presence of a basilar skull fracture. Approximately 48 hours after hospital admission, urine volume was noted to abruptly increase and urine specific gravity dropped to 1.001. Laboratory data obtained at that time revealed serum sodium 148 mEq/L, BUN 23 mg/dl, and urine osmolality 97 mosm/kg.

QUESTIONS
1. What is the most likely diagnosis?
2. How would you establish the diagnosis?
3. How would you manage the problem?

Six months later, he had recovered neurologic function, no longer had polyuria, and received no hormonal treatment. He complained of weight gain, fatigue, and loss of libido. Physical examination disclosed orthostatic hypotension, dry skin, and delayed relaxation phase of the deep tendon reflexes. Laboratory data revealed serum thyroxine 3.7 µg/dl, serum testosterone 124 ng/dl, and plasma cortisol 4.8 µg/dl at 8:00 A.M., serum sodium 141 mEq/L and urine osmolality 432 mosm/kg. He received hormone replacement therapy with 1-thyroxine, hydrocortisone, and testosterone injection. Over the next several days, he developed a progressive increase in urine volume and serum sodium was now 146 mEq/L with urine osmolality 138 mosm/kg.

QUESTIONS
4. What is the most likely diagnosis?
5. What is the explanation for the course of events?

Patient 2. A 73-year-old woman with a history of long-standing non-insulin dependent diabetes mellitus and congestive heart failure was admitted to the hospital because of symptoms of shortness of breath and edema that had not responded to diuretic treatment. She was taking digoxin 0.25 mg daily and had been started on treatment with an oral hypoglycemic agent 3 months previously because of poor control of blood sugar. Initial laboratory data disclosed serum sodium 127 mEq/L, serum potassium 2.8 mEq/L, BUN 8 mg/dl, urine osmolality 532 mosm/kg, and urine sodium concentration 89 mEq/L.

QUESTIONS
1. What is the likely cause of the hyponatremia?
2. How would you establish the diagnosis?
3. What role might the hypokalemia play in the hyponatremia?

Patient 3. An 83-year-old man was seen in the emergency room because of decreased ability to care for himself along with progressive confusion and disorientation. Past history was significant for hypertension and a fall 6 weeks previously during which he struck his head and lost consciousness for an undetermined length of time. On examination, blood pressure was 160/90 mm Hg, he was disoriented to time and place, and neurologic evaluation revealed weakness of the left arm and a positive left Babinski sign. Laboratory data were as follows: Serum sodium 118 mEq/L, BUN 6 mg/dl, urine osmolality 482 mosm/kg, urine sodium concentration 18 mEq/L.

QUESTIONS
1. What are likely causes of the change in mental status?
2. How would you manage the problem acutely?
3. How would you establish the diagnosis?
4. How would you manage the problem chronically?

SUGGESTED READING

Physiology
Dousa, T.P.: Renal actions of vasopressin. *In* The Posterior Pituitary. Edited by P.H. Baylis and P.L. Padfield. New York, Marcel Dekker, 1985.
Majzoub, J.A.: Vasopressin biosynthesis. *In* Vasopressin. Edited by R.W. Schrier. New York, Raven Press, 1985.
Miller, M.: Influence of aging on vasopressin secretion and water regulation. *In* Vasopressin. Edited by R.W. Schrier. New York, Raven Press, 1985.
Needleman, P., and Greenwald, J.E.: Atriopeptin: a cardiac hormone intimately involved in fluid, electrolyte, and blood-pressure homeostasis. N Engl J Med, *314*:828, 1986.
Robertson, G.L., and Athar, S.: The interaction of blood osmolality and blood volume in regulating plasma vasopressin in man. J Clin Endocrinol Metab, *42*:613, 1976.
Robertson, G.L.: Disorders of the posterior pituitary. *In* Internal Medicine. Edited by J.H. Stein and P.O. Kohler. Boston, Little Brown & Co., 1983.

Clinical Disorders
Bartter, F.C., and Schwartz, W.B.: The syndrome of inappropriate secretion of antidiuretic hormone. Am J Med, *42*:790, 1967.
Miller, M., et al: Recognition of partial defects in antidiuretic hormone secretion. Ann Intern Med, *73*:721, 1970.
Miller, M., and Moses, A.M.: Urinary antidiuretic hormone in polyuric disorders and in inappropriate ADH syndrome. Ann Intern Med, *77*:715, 1972.
Miller, M., and Moses, A.M.: Drug-induced states of impaired water excretion. Kidney Int, *10*:96, 1976.
Moses, A.M., and Streeten, D.H.P.: Differentiation of polyuric states by measurement of re-

sponses to changes in plasma osmolality induced by hypertonic saline infusions. Am J Med, 42:368, 1967.

Verbalis, J.G., Robinson, A.G., and Moses, A.M.: Postoperative and post-traumatic diabetes insipidus. Front Horm Res, 13:247, 1985.

Zerbe, R.L., and Robertson, G.L.: A comparison of plasma vasopressin measurements with a standard indirect test in the differential diagnosis of polyuria. N Engl J Med, 305:1539, 1981.

Zerbe, R.L.: The syndrome of inappropriate antidiuresis. In The Posterior Pituitary. Edited by P.H. Baylis and P.L. Padfield. New York, Marcel Dekker, 1985.

ANSWERS TO QUESTIONS

Patient 1

1. The abrupt onset of hypotonic polyuria following head trauma is characteristic of diabetes insipidus due to injury of the neurohypophysial system.
2. Hypotonic polyuria in the presence of elevated serum sodium and BUN is highly suggestive of diabetes insipidus. Restriction of fluid intake for 1 to 2 hours with consequent further increase in serum sodium and without effect on urine flow or osmolality will further support the diagnosis. Demonstration of responsiveness to injected aqueous vasopressin will confirm the diagnosis.
3. Initially, treatment is by hormone replacement using either injections of aqueous vasopressin or intranasal DDAVP. Each dose is given when "wearing off" of the previous dose is evident by abrupt onset of diuresis. If the diabetes insipidus persists for several days, treatment can either be continued with DDAVP or switched to longer acting injections of vasopressin tannate in oil.
4. Onset of hypotonic polyuria following initiation of treatment with hydrocortisone indicates unmasking of diabetes insipidus that had been obscured by the coexistence of hypopituitarism with associated hypoadrenalism and reduced excretion of free water.
5. The clinical and laboratory data are indicative of panhypopituitarism resulting from traumatic damage to the hypothalamus, pituitary stalk, or anterior pituitary gland. It is not unusual to find evidence of both anterior and posterior pituitary dysfunction after traumatic injury to the base of the brain.

Patient 2

1. The laboratory data suggest the presence of a dilutional hyponatremia, consistent with inappropriate secretion of ADH. The history of treatment with a diuretic and recent treatment with an oral hypoglycemic agent raised the question of drug-induced water retention.
2. Careful history and review of records will provide information regarding the specific drugs being taken. If the oral hypoglycemic agent is chlorpropamide, there is a strong likelihood of its being a causative agent in development of the hyponatremia. Discontinuation of the drug, followed by normalization of the serum sodium, will support this conclusion. When the serum sodium has risen to above 125 mEq/L and the congestive heart failure has improved, a water load test can be done to establish restoration of normal diluting capacity.
3. Severe hypokalemia may itself provoke release of ADH with resultant water retention. In this circumstance, correction of the hypokalemia by potassium replacement will lead to improvement in water handling capacity.

Patient 3

1. The progressive decline in mental status may be a consequence of head injury with chronic subdural hematoma. In addition, the changes could be due to hyponatremia, either by itself or additive to the brain injury. Brain trauma such as subdural hematoma can affect neurohypophysial function and result in increased ADH release with SIADH, as suggested by the laboratory data.
2. Acute management involves appropriate neurologic investigation and improvement of the hyponatremia. This can be accomplished by a combination of fluid restriction to 800 to 1000 ml/day and acute administration of 200 to 300 ml of 3% saline solution intravenously over a period of 4 to 6 hours. This should raise the serum sodium sufficiently to improve any symptoms that might be due to the hyponatremia.

3. After normalization of the serum sodium and improvement of mental status has been accomplished, an oral water load test can be performed.
4. If correction of any underlying brain injury fails to eliminate the SIADH, treatment will require long term fluid restriction to 800 to 1000 ml/day. If this is not adequate to maintain a serum sodium level sufficient to prevent recurrence of symptoms of hyponatremia, then oral demethylchlortetracycline can be given in a dose of 600 to 1200 mg daily to induce a state of moderate renal ADH resistance.

11

Lipoprotein Metabolism and Disorders

Robert A. Kreisberg

ABBREVIATIONS

C	cholesterol
FCHL	familial combined hyperlipidemia
FHC	familial hypercholesterolemia
FHTG	familial hypertriglyceridemia
HDL	high density lipoprotein
HMG CoA	hydroxymethylglutaryl coenzyme A
HTGL	hepatic triglyceride lipase
IDL	intermediate density lipoprotein
LCAT	lecithin cholesterol acyl transferase
LDL	low density lipoprotein
LPL	lipoprotein lipase
PHC	polygenic hypercholesterolemia
VLDL	very low density lipoprotein

LIPOPROTEIN STRUCTURE AND FUNCTION

Lipoproteins are complex macromolecules composed of carbohydrate, lipid, and protein. When viewed by electron-microscopy, they appear as particles with surface elements or "membranes" consisting of free cholesterol, phospholipid, and protein, and core elements consisting of cholesterol esters and triglyceride. The proteins are called apolipoproteins or apoproteins, and in addition to being structural components of lipoprotein, they serve a variety of other specific functions that will be discussed in detail later.

There are basically four major classes of lipoproteins:

1. Chylomicrons: derived from dietary fat; they deliver triglyceride to peripheral tissues to satisfy energy requirements or to be stored.

2. Very low density lipoproteins (VLDL): synthesized by the liver; they transport endogenously synthesized triglyceride to peripheral tissues to satisfy energy requirements or to be stored.

3. Low density lipoproteins (LDL): synthesized primarily from VLDL; they transport cholesterol to peripheral tissues to satisfy metabolic and structural requirements.

4. High density lipoprotein (HDL): synthesized from multiple sources: intestine, liver and as metabolic by-products of chylomicron and VLDL metabolism; they participate in the transport of cholesterol from peripheral tissues to the liver for excretion from the body (reverse cholesterol transport).

The lipid components of lipoproteins are distributed to varying degrees among all of the lipoprotein classes (Table 11–1). Chylomicrons are large particles consisting primarily of triglyceride with relatively small amounts of cholesterol, phospholipid, and protein, while VLDLs are smaller and have less triglyceride and more free and esterified cholesterol, phospholipid, and protein. The ratio of triglyceride to cholesterol in VLDL is 5:1. As the lipoproteins become heavier and more dense, the triglyceride content decreases, and the protein and phospholipid content increases. LDLs contain relatively little triglyceride and most of the circulating cholesterol (approxi-

Table 11–1.   Properties and Composition of Lipoproteins

	Chylomicrons	VLDL	LDL	HDL
Electrophoretic Mobility	Origin	Prebeta	β	α
Size (nm)	70–600	30–70	20	7–10
Density (g/ml)	<0.94	<1.006	1.019–1.063	1.063–1.21
Sf	>400	20–400	0–12	—
Composition (%)				
Unesterified Cholesterol	1–2	4–7	5–8	3–5
Esterified Cholesterol	1–2	15–22	45–50	15–20
Triglyceride	85–95	45–65	3–9	2–7
Phospholipid	4–6	15–22	16–25	26–32
Protein	1–2	6–10	18–22	45–55

mately 70%); a large percent of the molecule consists of protein and phospholipid. The ratio of triglyceride to cholesterol in LDL is approximately 1:5, the reverse of that of VLDL. The ratio of cholesterol to triglyceride in VLDL is used for calculation of the LDL cholesterol concentration. HDLs demonstrate a further increase in the phospholipid and protein components, and a reduction in the cholesterol and triglyceride content.

Apoproteins not only solubilize the lipid, so that otherwise insoluble substances can be transported in an aqueous medium, but they also have important structural and functional roles in lipoprotein metabolism and physiology (Table 11–2):

1. The amphipathic (solubilizing) properties of the apoproteins permit them to assume a 3-dimensional structure with a "nonpolar" or hydrophobic face that allows the interaction and binding of lipids on one side, away from the aqueous interface, while the "polar" regions interface with the aqueous media.

2. They serve as ligands or recognition proteins, thereby allowing lipoproteins to bind to specific cell receptors and be removed from the circulation.

3. They modify (activate and inhibit) the activity of two important enzyme

Table 11–2. Apolipoproteins

Apolipoprotein	Lipoprotein Class	Function
A–I	CM, HDL	LCAT Cofactor Structural role in HDL
A–II	CM, HDL	HL Cofactor Structural role in HDL
A–IV	CM	Unknown
ApoLp(a)	LDL, HDL	Unknown
B–48	CM	Structural role in CM
B–100	VLDL IDL LDL	Recognition protein (ligand) Structural role in VLDL and LDL
C–I	CM, VLDL, HDL	LCAT Cofactor
C–II	CM, VLDL, HDL	LPL Activator
C–III	CM, VLDL, HDL	LPL Inhibitor
D	HDL	Transfer CE to other lipoproteins
E	CM, VLDL, IDL, HDL	Recognition protein (ligand)
F	HDL	Unknown
G	HDL	Unknown
H	CM	LPL Cofactor

Abbreviations: CM, chylomicron; VLDL, very low density lipoprotein; IDL, intermediate density lipoprotein; LDL, low density lipoprotein; HDL, high density lipoprotein; LPL, lipoprotein lipase; HL, hepatic lipase; CE, cholesterol esters.

systems [lipoprotein lipase (LPL) and lecithin cholesterol acyl transferase (LCAT)] involved in lipoprotein metabolism.

4. They are responsible for the transfer of cholesterol esters from HDLs to other lipoproteins, as part of the process of reverse cholesterol transport.

Many of the apoproteins have been identified, isolated and characterized. Apoproteins are synthesized as propeptides and subsequently shortened proteolytically to become the active apoprotein, analogous in this regard to the synthesis of polypeptide hormones. Most of the apoprotein genes have been localized in the human genome, and human mutations have been identified (Table 11–3). Alterations in the structure of apoproteins can have profound effects on lipoprotein metabolism, and may predispose to the development of vascular disease, even in the absence of obvious lipid abnormalities. Specific apoprotein deficiencies have been temporarily corrected by the administration of normal plasma or the specific apoprotein.

Since apoproteins are under genetic control, gene abnormalities can produce a structurally and functionally abnormal apoprotein, leading to the development of a lipoprotein disorder characterized by hypercholesterolemia, hypertriglyceridemia, or both. In this manner, lipoprotein abnormalities may be analogous to other genetically determined diseases; an improperly substituted single amino acid may profoundly alter lipoprotein metabolism. In dysbetalipoproteinemia, also known as "broad beta disease" or Type III hyperlipoproteinemia, an improperly substituted amino acid at position 158 of apoprotein E interferes with the recognition and subsequent removal and metabolism of chylomicron remnants and intermediate density lipoproteins (IDLs). Apolipoprotein AI, the major structural apoprotein of HDLs and the activator of LCAT is another example. There are a number of mutations and genetic variants of apoprotein AI, which can be associated with a structural abnormality in HDLs or a reduction in HDL concentration.

Apoproteins belong to specific families, designated A, B, C, D, etc., and there may be several members within each family (CII, CIII, etc.). Apoproteins are commonly present in several lipoproteins where they can be minor or major constituents, and the lipoproteins usually contain several apoproteins. The exception is LDL where apoprotein B100 is the sole apoprotein.

Table 11–3.   Location of Apolipoprotein Genes

Chromosome			
1	2	11	19
AII	B	AI	CI
		AIV	CII
		CIII	E
			LDL-Receptor

Chylomicron Metabolism

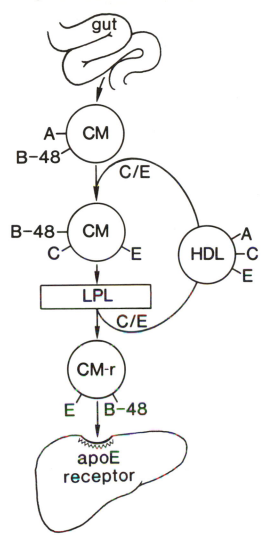

Fig. 11–1. Chylomicron Metabolism. Abbreviations as in Table 2.

LIPOPROTEIN METABOLISM

Chylomicrons (Fig. 11–1)

Chylomicrons are derived from dietary fat, and therefore reflect and constitute what is referred to as the "exogenous" pathway. Dietary fat is digested in the gastrointestinal tract. The free fatty acids and monoglycerides are absorbed by the gastrointestinal mucosa, where they are resynthesized into triglyceride, packaged with specific apoproteins, and released into the intestinal lymphatics. Apoproteins A and B48 are the major aproproteins of these nascent chylomicrons. When they enter the systemic circulation, there is an exchange of apoproteins with circulating HDLs. Apoproteins of the A family are transferred to HDLs, and those of the C family and E, transported by HDLs, are transferred to the chylomicrons. The apoprotein composition of the chylomicron now consists of B48, CII, CIII, and E. Apoprotein CII is required for activation of LPL, the enzyme system that is rate limiting for the hydrolysis of triglyceride. Apoprotein E is a recognition protein that permits the chylomicron remnant to be removed from the circulation by a specific liver receptor. Apoprotein C also prevents the chylomicron from being prematurely removed from the circulation (i.e., before optimum lipolysis has occurred). LPL, activated by apoprotein CII, hydrolyzes the triglyceride core of the chylomicron, releasing fatty acids to peripheral tissues to satisfy energy requirements, or to be stored for future use. As the triglyceride core is hydrolyzed, the apoprotein and phospholipid surface elements of the chylomicron become redundant, and spontaneously dissociate to form nascent HDLs. In this way, the apoproteins C and E are recycled to HDLs and reutilized. It is obvious that HDLs play a critical role in the regulation of triglyceride metabolism by providing both the chylomicrons and VLDLs with important apoprotein components. They accept and serve as a reservoir for the redundant apoproteins and phospholipids created during lipolysis. When the chylomicron remnant loses its complement of apoprotein C, it binds to a specific hepatic receptor, which recognizes apoprotein E, and it is removed from the circulation. During hydrolysis the remnant becomes progressively enriched with cholesterol and cholesterol esters that, by virtue of the receptor mechanism just described, returns dietary cholesterol to the liver for excretion from the body. In this manner, dietary cholesterol can influence hepatic cholesterol content and the activity of LDL receptor, which will be discussed in more detail later.

LPL is located in vascular endothelium, and hydrolysis of chylomicron triglyceride occurs at this interface. LPL is efficient and chylomicrons are removed with a half-life of 2 to 5 minutes.

Very Low Density Lipoproteins (VLDLs) (Fig. 11–2)

VLDLs are synthesized by the liver, and constitute the "endogenous" pathway for triglyceride transport. They resemble chylomicrons but contain less triglyceride and more cholesterol and protein. Although chylomicrons and VLDLs are separate lipoprotein families, there may be considerable overlap in size and composition between small chylomicrons and large VLDLs. Furthermore, while VLDLs are treated conceptually as a distinct lipoprotein it is, in fact, a heterogeneous family of lipoproteins with species of varying size and composition, within the limits displayed in Table 11–1. The smaller VLDLs may be intermediates in the lipolytic cascade, or may be directly secreted by the liver. The VLDLs released from the liver contain apoproteins B100, CII, CIII, and E. In the circulation, the VLDLs interact with HDLs

VLDL Metabolism

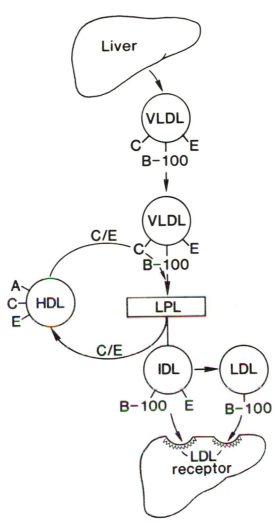

Fig. 11–2. VLDL Metabolism. Abbreviations as in Table 2.

in a manner analogous to that described for chylomicrons, and additional apoproteins C and E are transferred to them to optimize the content of these apoproteins. VLDLs are also metabolized by the LPL system, and apoprotein CII is required for activation of the enzyme. Nonetheless, the metabolism of VLDLs by LPL is less efficient than that of chylomicrons, and the half-life of the VLDL particle is considerably longer (hours vs minutes). This difference in the rate of metabolism of chylomicrons and VLDLs by LPL suggests that VLDLs do not serve as efficiently as substrate for the enzyme, perhaps related to their apoprotein composition. Again, apoprotein C also prevents premature hepatic removal of the VLDLs as lipolysis occurs.

HDLs play a critical role in the regulation of chylomicron and VLDL triglyceride metabolism, by serving as a reservoir of critical apoproteins, and by accepting the redundant apoproteins and phospholipids created during hydrolysis. In this manner, these components are preserved and used again.

An important intermediate of VLDL metabolism is the intermediate density lipoprotein (IDL). IDLs have lost significant amounts of triglyceride, and therefore, have become progressively enriched with cholesterol and cholesterol esters. The ratio of triglyceride/cholesterol in the IDLs is approximately 1:1, in contrast to VLDLs where the ratio is 5:1. Thus, in terms of their cholesterol and triglyceride content, IDLs are truly intermediate between VLDLs and LDLs. IDLs are created by the lipolytic cascade and retain only apoproteins B100 and E. Approximately 50% of the IDLs are removed from the circulation by the hepatic receptors for the chylomicron remnants and by the LDL receptors that recognize apoprotein E. The LDL receptor recognizes both IDLs and LDLs. The remaining 50% of the IDLs are converted to LDLs by incompletely defined mechanisms that involve another enzyme system, hepatic triglyceride lipase (HTGL), that hydrolyzes the remaining triglyceride. Factors that regulate the balance of these two competing routes of IDL metabolism are not well understood, but are of great importance. The number and affinity of the receptors for IDL, as well as the activity of HTGL, are obvious candidates for examination. HTGL, located in the vascular endothelium of the liver and the hepatocyte, is responsible for further hydrolysis of the triglyceride in the IDLs. As this occurs, there is additional loss of apoprotein E and the formation of LDLs, whose sole or predominant apoprotein is B100. HTGL may be genetically deficient and its activity is reduced in hypothyroidism. The hepatic uptake of IDL does not appear to be dependent upon HTGL activity.

Low Density Lipoproteins (LDLs)

LDLs are products of the lipolytic cascade and therefore of VLDL. The function of LDL is to deliver cholesterol to cells to support metabolic and structural requirements. Apoprotein B100 is the sole and critically important apoprotein, which is required for binding of LDLs to specific cell-surface receptors. After the LDLs bind to the receptor, they are internalized by endocytosis, and subsequently, degraded into their components. The LDL receptor is then recycled to the surface to function again.

The LDL receptor is under metabolic control and, in this way, differs from the hepatic receptor responsible for the removal of the chylomicron remnant. The properties of the LDL receptor are listed below:

1. It is present on all cells, but at least half of the receptors are in the liver.

2. It regulates or ''meters'' the entry of cholesterol into the cell, and may be protective for those cells that have LDL receptors.

3. It binds lipoproteins containing apoproteins B100 and E.

4. Its affinity for IDLs (apoprotein B100/E) is greater than for LDLs (apoprotein B100 alone).

5. Its molecular weight is approximately 160,000 daltons, and it consists of 1200 amino acids.

6. It is deficient (majority of patients) or abnormal in familial hypercholesterolemia.

7. It is under metabolic control and is primarily influenced by the hepatic content of cholesterol.

8. The number of LDL receptors may be also influenced by hormonal factors:

    a. Thyroid hormone (decreased in hypothyroidism, increased in hyperthyroidism).

    b. Estrogen (decreased with estrogen deficiency).

9. Age: In developed countries, receptor numbers may decrease with age.

The LDL receptor has a specific region that recognizes apoprotein B100, and allows it to bind to the surface of the cell (Fig. 11–3). After binding takes place, the receptor and the LDL particle are internalized, where they are disassembled and the receptor is recycled back to the surface of the cell. The LDL molecule is degraded into its amino acid and lipid components. The synthesis of cholesterol and the LDL receptor by the cell are controlled by the intracellular free cholesterol concentration. If the free cholesterol concentration is higher than normal, then receptor synthesis is decreased, and endogenous cholesterol synthesis is inhibited. Cholesterol inhibits the rate limiting enzyme of cholesterol synthesis, hydroxymethylglutaryl coenzyme

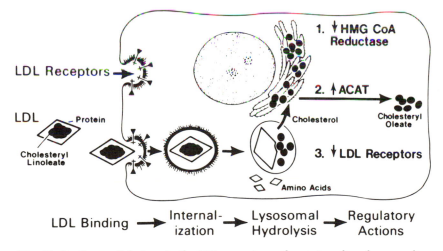

Fig. 11–3. Sequential steps in the LDL receptor pathway in cultured mammalian cells. Abbreviations: LDL, low density lipoprotein; HMG CoA reductase, 3-hydroxy-3-methyl-glutaryl CoA reductase; ACAT, acyl-coenzyme A: cholesterol acyltransferase. From Goldstein, J.L., and Brown, M.S. (Reproduced with permission Goldstein, J.L., Brown, M.S., and the Med Clin North Am.)

A reductase (HMG Co-A reductase). If the intracellular concentration of free cholesterol is low, then the synthesis of both the receptor and cholesterol is increased. By regulating both endogenous synthesis and the uptake of LDL cholesterol, intracellular cholesterol can be optimized and maintained within relatively narrow limits. Those cells that have LDL receptors are capable of carefully regulating the amount of cholesterol that enters the cell, and thereby can protect themselves from becoming overloaded with cholesterol. The LDL receptor is a high affinity, low capacity receptor, and therefore can easily maintain optimum intracellular cholesterol concentrations at relatively low LDL concentrations. All cells have a continuing structural requirement for cholesterol, and the adrenal glands and the gonads have an additional cholesterol requirement for steroid synthesis. Evidence suggests that some of the cholesterol required for steroid synthesis is supplied by LDL.

The amount of LDL cholesterol necessary to satisfy structural and metabolic needs, is relatively small. Newborn humans and experimental animals who do not develop atherosclerosis have relatively low serum concentrations of LDL cholesterol, 25 to 50 mg/dl. The LDL cholesterol concentrations that are characteristic of most Americans are greatly in excess of what is necessary to meet metabolic and structural demands. When the LDL cholesterol concentration has reached 120 mg/dl (equivalent to a plasma total cholesterol of 180 mg/dl), the median value for Americans, the LDL receptor number has decreased by approximately 35%. With regard to prevention of atherosclerosis, optimum LDL cholesterol concentrations should be less than this value. In patients with the heterozygous form of familial hypercholesterolemia, in whom LDL cholesterol concentrations are usually between 200 and 300 mg/dl, the LDL receptor number is reduced by 50%. In patients with the homozygous form of familial hypercholesterolemia, there are no functional LDL receptors. The progressive increase in LDL cholesterol concentration that occurs with age is associated with a reduction in the LDL cholesterol fractional catabolic rate, which indirectly reflects the number of LDL receptors. Not all societies display an age-related increase in LDL cholesterol concentrations, which suggests that modifiable environmental factors may be responsible for this increase.

High Density Lipoproteins (HDLs)

HDLs are a heterogeneous group of molecules of differing size and composition. They are the most dense of all of the circulating lipoproteins. Apoproteins AI and AII are the major apoproteins, but apoproteins C and E are also present. Apoprotein AI accounts for about 70% of the protein in the HDLs, apoprotein AII for 20%, and apoproteins C and E for approximately 10%. HDLs are synthesized in the liver and intestines, and are also derived from the metabolism of chylomicrons and VLDL as by-products. As previously discussed, HDLs serve as a reservoir for apoprotein C, and by virtue of the role of apoprotein C in activation of LPL, play an important role in triglyceride metabolism. Furthermore, HDLs are replenished as a ''spinoff'' of chylomicron and VLDL metabolism. An inverse relationship is frequently observed between the triglyceride and HDL-cholesterol concentrations. Nascent HDL particles, which contain little esterified cholesterol, have a disc-like structure and consist primarily of two layers of protein, phospholipid, and unesterified cholesterol (Fig. 11–4). As cholesterol esterification occurs under the influence of LCAT, the nonpolar cholesterol ester is transferred into the potential space between the bilayers and the particle becomes spherical in shape. As the cholesterol is esterified and moves from the surface to the interior, another free cholesterol molecule, derived from cells or other lipoproteins, replaces it. The phospholipid (lecithin) in the surface ''membranes'' provides the fatty acid required for esterification. All cholesterol esterification takes place in the HDL particle under the influence of LCAT, an enzyme synthesized and released into the circulation by the liver, and apoprotein AI, which activates LCAT. The process is dynamic. Cholesterol esters are continuously and simultaneously synthesized and transferred to other lipoproteins, principally VLDL and LDL. In this manner, cholesterol esters appear in all lipoproteins, but arise only in HDL. Most of the free cholesterol is derived from cells of the body. Following esterification in HDLs and transfer to other lipoproteins that are removed by the liver, the cholesterol is excreted from the body, hence the term ''reverse'' cholesterol transport. HDLs may also return cholesterol to the liver for excretion; hence they function both directly and indirectly in this process. Just as cells have LDL receptors, they also have specific HDL receptors. These HDL receptors also appear to be under metabolic control. Their role in the control of reverse cholesterol transport is reciprocal to that of the LDL receptor. Thus, if the intracellular concentration of cholesterol is too high, the synthesis of the LDL receptor is inhibited,

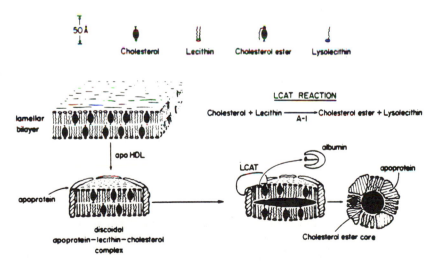

Fig. 11–4. HDL Structure and function. (Reproduced with permission of Tall, AR, Small, DM, and the N Engl J Med.)

while the synthesis of HDL receptor is stimulated. The inverse relationship between LDL and HDL receptor number provides another mechanism by which cellular cholesterol content can be finely regulated. The cell with high cholesterol content would "down-regulate" the LDL receptor to prevent further influx, and "up-regulate" the HDL receptor to promote cholesterol efflux. Alternatively, when intracellular cholesterol levels are low, LDL receptor synthesis will be "up-regulated" to promote cholesterol entry into the cell, and HDL receptor synthesis will be "down-regulated" to reduce the efflux of cholesterol from the cell. Relatively little is known about the factors and the biochemical events that regulate synthesis of HDL receptors.

The inverse relationship between HDLs and atherosclerotic disease is attributed to their role in reverse cholesterol transport. HDL concentrations are regulated by a number of factors that are shown in Table 11–4.

Lipoproteins As Risk Factors For Atherosclerosis

Lipoproteins are only one of a number of important risk factors for the development of atherosclerotic disease. These factors interact in an additive, or sometimes, synergistic way to accelerate the process. In addition, individuals without any of the identifiable risk factors may develop the disorder, indicating that there are other, as of yet, unidentified factors and that our "markers" for known risk factors are relatively unsophisticated. The latter is certainly true, as demonstrated now by numerous studies, in which apoprotein A and B measurements provide greater sensitivity than measurements of LDL- or HDL-cholesterol for identifying individuals at risk. Thus, the usual measurements of cholesterol and triglyceride represent a superficial approach to identifying and understanding lipoprotein disorders. The future

Table 11–4.   Factors Regulating HDL Concentrations

Increase	*Decrease*

1. Heredity
   a. Hyperalphalipoproteinemia
	1. Heredity
	   a. Hypoalphalipoproteinemia

2. Female Gender	2. Male Gender
3. Physical Activity	3. Poverty

4. Ethanol	4. Diet
	   a. High carbohydrate
	   b. Low fat

5. Drugs (lipid-active)
   a. Resins
   b. Nicotinic acid
   c. Fibric acid derivatives
	5. Obesity

	6. Hypertriglyceridemia

6. Drugs (nonlipid-active)
   a. β-adrenergic agonists
   b. Diphenylhydantoin
	7. Diseases
	   a. Diabetes mellitus
	   b. Renal failure

7. Chemicals
   a. Pesticides
	8. Drugs (lipid-active)
	   a. Probucol

	9. Drugs (nonlipid-active) a. β-adrenergic blockers

will emphasize measurement of apoproteins because most lipid problems are probably a result of apoprotein abnormalities.

A better understanding of the mechanisms by which lipoproteins may predispose to atherosclerosis may be gained by further discussion of processes, by which LDLs are removed from the circulation. As previously mentioned, LDL uptake is determined primarily by the LDL receptor. Under normal circumstances, the LDL receptor will remove 65 to 70% of the LDL particles, while 30 to 35% of the LDLs will be removed by another pathway, referred to as the scavenger pathway (Fig. 11–5). Monocytes and macrophages constitute the principal cells in this pathway. They are the ''foam''-filled cells demonstrated in early atherosclerotic lesions. In contrast to the receptor pathway where intracellular cholesterol synthesis and LDL receptor synthesis are

LIPOPROTEIN METABOLISM

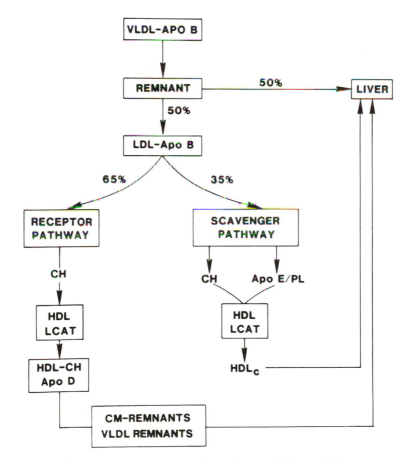

Fig. 11–5. Receptor and scavenger pathways for metabolism of LDL.

tightly controlled, such is not the case in the scavenger pathway. The scavenger cells possess receptors, thereby allowing lipoprotein removal, but intracellular free cholesterol neither inhibits cholesterol synthesis nor receptor synthesis, so that these cells can become progressively overfilled with cholesterol. Whether this occurs depends upon the amount of lipoprotein "traffic" through this pathway, as well as the capability for reverse cholesterol transport. An increasing concentration of LDL, either because of a reduction in LDL receptor number, such as might occur with age, or because of increased production diverts more LDL particles into the scavenger pathway. In fact, increased entry of LDL into the scavenger pathway could occur with a normal LDL level, if the number of LDL particles is increased, even though the LDL-cholesterol concentration is normal (i.e., a situation in which the amount of cholesterol per particle is reduced, but the number of particles is increased). Since entry into the receptor pathway is regulated not by cholesterol, but by apoprotein B100 content, an apoprotein abnormality could be solely responsible for down-regulating the LDL receptor and diverting LDLs into the scavenger pathway. While the scavenger receptor has high affinity for IDLs, it does not have a high affinity for LDLs, unless they are modified in some way. Recently, endothelial cells have been demonstrated to be capable of peroxidatively altering the lipid in LDL, via the generation of superoxide and free oxygen radicals, thereby converting LDL to a form readily removed by the scavenger cells. This observation is not only important for this hypothesis, but also emphasizes the importance of vascular factors, as well as non-vascular factors in the atherosclerotic process. It also suggests that a genetic predisposition to atherosclerosis could be represented at a vascular level and that hypertension, diabetes mellitus, and tobacco could predispose to vascular disease by alteration of this or other vascular processes.

Blood Lipid Measurements

Blood should be obtained after a 12- to 14-hour overnight fast for the measurement of the plasma cholesterol and triglyceride concentrations. Plasma cholesterol concentrations should always be interpreted on the basis of age. In an adult, plasma total cholesterol concentrations less than 200 mg/dl represent average or minimal risk for the development of atherosclerosis. As the plasma cholesterol concentration rises progressively above 200 mg/dl, there is a linear and continuously distributed increase in the risk for the development of ischemic heart disease. Since the total plasma cholesterol consists of cholesterol transported in VLDL, LDL, and HDL, it is often important to fractionate the cholesterol concentration in individuals with hypercholesterolemia, or in individuals with normal cholesterol concentrations, if they have co-existent atherosclerosis, or a strong family history of atherosclerosis. As they become available, apoprotein A and B measurements may be added to the testing procedure, or conceivably even replace the "tried and true" measurements of cholesterol and triglyceride. For now, however, fractionation of the cholesterol is the best that we can do to detect more subtle abnormalities in lipoproteins. The total plasma cholesterol and the HDL-cholesterol can be directly measured; the VLDL-cholesterol (VLDL-C) is derived from the triglyceride concentration, and the LDL-cholesterol (LDL-C) is calculated by subtraction of the HDL- and VLDL-cholesterol from the total, as shown below:

$$\text{LDL-C} = (\text{total cholesterol}) - (\text{HDL-C}) - (\text{VLDL-C})$$

The VLDL cholesterol represents 20% of the plasma triglyceride concentration, but this approximation is accurate only when the triglyceride is less than 400 mg/dl.

In general, an LDL-cholesterol concentration of 120 mg/dl would equate with a total plasma cholesterol concentration of about 180 mg/dl. Significant increments in the LDL-cholesterol concentration may exist in individuals whose plasma total cholesterol is normal or near normal, because there may also be a reduction in the HDL-cholesterol concentration. Alternatively, a low HDL-cholesterol (in a vegetarian, for example) might not infer high risk, if the corresponding LDL-cholesterol was also low. Therefore, risk is best assessed by developing an LDL/HDL-cholesterol ratio. A vegetarian has a low LDL-cholesterol, and under such circumstances, HDL-cholesterol is relatively unimportant. A woman may have mild to modest hypercholesterolemia due to a high HDL-cholesterol, and the LDL/HDL-cholesterol ratio may be normal. In some laboratories, the plasma total cholesterol to HDL-cholesterol ratio is used, which has certain obvious advantages, but considerable disadvantages in patients who have hypertriglyceridemia in whom the ratio would be increased, but the risk of atherosclerosis may not.

It is possible to classify hyperlipoproteinemias by measurement of plasma cholesterol and triglyceride concentrations and visual inspection of a plasma sample after it has been placed in a refrigerator overnight (Table 11–5). It should be obvious, however, that this is a relatively unsophisticated approach to understanding and treating lipoprotein disorders. While it has been helpful in the past, its utility is progressively diminishing as we learn that diverse genetic or molecular abnormalities can lead to phenotypically similar lipid and lipoprotein abnormalities. Identifying and understanding the specific defects leading to abnormalities should result eventually in the development of a classification system based upon pathophysiologic abnormalities. When this occurs, therapy can be developed in a more rational manner.

When the plasma cholesterol and/or triglyceride concentrations are elevated, secondary causes should be excluded. The secondary causes of hypercholesterolemia and hypertriglyceridemia are listed in Table 11–6.

The risk represented by hypercholesterolemia is best addressed by fractionation of the plasma total cholesterol into its LDL and HDL components. The significance of any given LDL cholesterol concentration must be based upon both the age and sex of the patient. Those individuals whose age and sex adjusted LDL-cholesterol is above the 90th percentile, and whose HDL-

Table 11–5.   Classification of Hyperlipoproteinemias

Type	Lipoprotein Abnormality				TG	CHOL	Appearance[1]
	CM	VLDL	LDL	IDL	Concentrations		
I	↑	N	N	N	↑	N	Cream Layer[2] with Clear Infranatant
IIa	N	N	↑	N	N	↑	Clear[3]
IIb	N	↑	↑	N	↑	↑	Lactescent[4]
III	N	N	N/↓	↑	↑	↑	Lactescent[4]
IV	N	↑	N	N	↑	N	Lactescent[4]
V	↑	↑	N	N	↑	↑	Lactescent[4] with Cream Layer

Abbreviations: CM, chylomicron; VLDL, very low density lipoproteins; LDL, low density lipoproteins; HDL, high density lipoprotein; N, normal; ↑, increased; ↓, decreased.
[1]Appearance of plasma placed in refrigerator overnight.
[2]Chylomicrons float to top of plasma.
[3]LDL particles do not alter light transmission.
[4]VLDL and IDL scatter light and cause lactescence; observed when the triglyceride is ≥350 mg/dl.

Table 11–6.   Secondary Causes of Hyperlipoproteinemia

Phenotype	Disorders
I	Diabetes mellitus Dysglobulinemia Lupus erythematosus
IIa	Hypothyroidism Nephrotic syndrome
IIb	Multiple myeloma Obstructive liver disease Porphyria
III	Dysglobulinemia Hypothyroidism
IV	Alcoholism Corticosteroids Diabetes mellitus Estrogens Glycogen storage disease Hypothyroidism Obesity Oral contraceptives
V	Alcoholism Corticosteroids Diabetes mellitus Estrogens Glycogen storage disease

cholesterol is less than the 10th percentile are at high risk of developing coronary heart disease (Table 11–7). The risk is moderate when the age and sex adjusted LDL- and HDL-cholesterol concentrations are greater than the 75th percentile, and less than the 25th percentile, respectively. Though uncommon, individuals may be encountered with moderate hypercholesterolemia, in whom the elevation is due to an increase in the HDL-cholesterol and not the LDL-cholesterol. Such individuals are not at increased risk of developing heart disease, and therefore, neither dietary nor drug therapy would be indicated. Without fractionation of the plasma cholesterol, inappropriate therapy could be undertaken.

PRIMARY DISORDERS ASSOCIATED WITH HYPERLIPOPROTEINEMIA

Lipoprotein Lipase Deficiency

Lipoprotein lipase (LPL) deficiency, Type I hyperlipoproteinemia, is a rare autosomal recessive abnormality that results in hyperchylomicronemia and a markedly increased plasma triglyceride concentration; the plasma cholesterol is normal or only slightly increased. Uninvolved family members may be heterozygotic for the abnormality, and demonstrate a reduction in LPL activity without hypertriglyceridemia. Clinical manifestations include lipemia retinalis, eruptive xanthomas, pancreatitis, and hepatosplenomegaly. The chylomicrons will form a cream layer when plasma is placed overnight in a refrigerator. There is no evidence that such patients are at increased risk for vascular disease, and therapy is directed at preventing pancreatitis and xanthomas. Therapy of this disorder depends primarily on elimination of fat from the

Table 11–7.

Age (years)	LDL Cholesterol				HDL Cholesterol				Triglyceride			
	Men		Women		Men		Women		Men		Women	
	Percentiles				Percentiles				Percentiles			
	75	90	75	90	10	25	10	25	75	95	75	95
20–24	118	138	118	141	32	38	37	44	146	165	135	168
25–29	138	157	126	148	32	27	39	47	171	204	137	159
30–34	144	166	128	177	38	38	40	46	214	253	140	163
35–39	154	176	139	161	39	36	38	44	250	316	170	205
40–44	157	173	146	165	37	36	39	48	232	318	161	191
45–49	163	186	150	173	33	38	41	47	218	279	180	223
50–54	162	185	160	186	31	36	41	50	244	313	190	223
55–59	168	191	168	199	31	38	41	50	210	261	229	279
60–64	165	188	168	191	34	44	44	51	193	240	210	256

(From The Lipid Research Clinics Population Studies Data Book, Volume 1, The Prevalence Study. U.S. Department of Health and Human Services: NIH Publ No. 80–1527, July, 1986.)

diet. There are no drugs that can reverse the abnormality in lipoprotein lipase activity.

Hypercholesterolemia.

Hypercholesterolemia can be monogenic or polygenic in origin:
I. Monogenic
    (a) Familial Hypercholesterolemia (FHC)
    (b) Familial Combined Hyperlipidemia (FCHL)
II. Polygenic (PHC)

Familial Hypercholesterolemia (FHC) is an autosomal dominant disease in which the LDL receptor is reduced in number or is defective. Patients with this disorder are unable to properly synthesize the LDL receptor. The prevalence of the heterozygotic form of FHC is 1/500 individuals, while that of the homozygous form is 1/1,000,000. In the heterozygotic form, the number of LDL receptors is reduced by approximately 50%, whereas homozygotes have no functional receptors (receptors are absent or defective). The presence of LDL receptors, even though reduced in number, has important therapeutic implications, and will be discussed in more detail later. The clinical manifestations include corneal arcus, xanthelasmas, tendon and tuberous xanthomas, and most importantly, premature coronary artery disease. Therapy of the disorder includes adherence to a diet that is low in animal fat and cholesterol, and when necessary, the use of lipid active drugs, which further reduce the LDL-cholesterol concentration. Many of these drugs accelerate the fractional catabolic removal of the LDL particle by decreasing intrahepatic cholesterol, thereby stimulating increased synthesis of the LDL receptor. In the homozygotic form of familial hypercholesterolemia, where receptors are absent or nonfunctional, such therapy is ineffective, because LDL receptor synthesis cannot be increased.

Familial Combined Hyperlipidemia (FCHL) is an autosomal dominant disease that may also be associated with hypercholesterolemia. It is relatively common with a prevalence of 1 to 2/100 individuals. It may present as hypercholesterolemia (Type IIa), hypertriglyceridemia (Type IV), or a combination of hypercholesterolemia and hypertriglyceridemia (Type IIb). In this disorder, there is increased synthesis of both VLDL and LDL, leading to a variable lipoprotein phenotype. FCHL accounts for 15 to 25% of patients with hypertriglyceridemia. The lipoprotein abnormality may not emerge until the 3rd or 4th decade. The risk of vascular and heart disease is clearly increased in such individuals, even if an increase in VLDL with attendant hypertriglyceridemia is the only manifestation of the disorder. Overproduction of apoprotein B-100 causes an increase in plasma apoprotein B levels, and identifies individuals at risk. Therapy should include the American Heart Association prudent diet (30% of calories as fat; less than 300 mg cholesterol daily) and use of drugs to reduce LDL-cholesterol concentrations (bile acid resins; nicotinic acid), to decrease VLDL synthesis (nicotinic acid), or to increase VLDL catabolism (fibric acid derivatives; clofibrate, gemfibrozil), depending upon the lipoprotein abnormalities present.

Polygenic Hypercholesterolemia (PHC) is the most common cause of hypercholesterolemia. By definition, it involves the upper 5% of the population, so that it is approximately 20 times more frequent than FHC among such patients, and it accounts for 95% of those individuals whose cholesterol concentrations are in the upper 5th percentile. The hypercholesterolemia is generally less severe than that observed in the heterozygotic form of FHC. Therapy of PHC is the same as that of FHC.

Dysbetalipoproteinemia or "Broad Beta" Disease

Dysbetalipoproteinemia is a relatively rare polygenic disorder that occurs in 1/10,000 individuals. It is most often due to a defect in the molecular structure of apoprotein E (apo E_2 isoform), an apoprotein necessary for hepatic recognition and removal of chylomicron remnants and IDL. A substituted amino acid near the binding portion of the apoprotein is responsible for the defective recognition of these particles by the hepatic receptors. The homozygous defect in apoprotein E (E_2/E_2; normal E_3/E_3) is actually quite common, occurring in 1/100 individuals, but, as stated, the phenotypic abnormality is much less common (1/10,000). The defect alone does not cause hyperlipoproteinemia, unless there is concomitant overproduction of VLDL (as in obesity or diabetes), or reduction in the LDL receptor (as in hypothyroidism or aging). The occurrence of the homozygous state for apo E_2 and familial hypertriglyceridemia (to be discussed) in the same individual would theoretically occur with a frequency of 1/10,000. These individuals have xanthelasmas, palmar and tuberoeruptive xanthomas and are predisposed to the development of premature coronary disease and peripheral atherosclerosis. The concentrations of cholesterol and triglyceride are both increased, often to the same magnitude. The plasma appears lactescent because of the accumulation of IDLs and may occasionally have a cream layer due to chylomicron remnants. Fibric acid derivatives are particularly useful in treating this disorder, but diet and the control of obesity and diabetes is also important.

Familial Hypertriglyceridemia (FHTG)

FHTG is a relatively common disorder occurring in 1 to 2/100 individuals and accounting for 10 to 20% of patients with hypertriglyceridemia. FCHL also accounts for an equal number of patients with hypertriglyceridemia. FHTG is an autosomal dominant trait, but the precise biochemical mechanism is not understood. The liver synthesizes normal numbers of compositionally abnormal VLDL particles; the ratio of triglyceride to protein in VLDL is increased. The plasma levels of apoprotein B in this disorder are normal, in contrast to FCHL where they are increased. When the plasma VLDL concentrations are high, clearance of chylomicrons may also be impaired, leading to the persistence of both lipoproteins in plasma and development of the Type V phenotype. These individuals are at no greater risk for the development of coronary heart disease than the normal population. This suggests that only those patients with hypertriglyceridemia and hyperapoproteinemia B are at increased risk of heart disease, and may explain why hypertriglyceridemia, per se, is not a risk factor.

THERAPY

Diet

The mainstay of treatment of lipoprotein disorders is diet. Although there were a variety of diets designed for each specific phenotypic abnormality, most physicians now rely primarily on the Prudent American Heart Association Diet, with limitation of intake of total fat and animal fat (30% of total calories), and cholesterol (less than 300 mg/day). When control of hypercholesterolemia is the object, the content of animal fat and cholesterol may be further reduced, until fat constitutes only 20% of calories and cholesterol intake is $\leq$ 100 mg/day. The maximum reduction in plasma cholesterol on such diets ranges from 10 to 20%, and often is inadequate as sole therapy. Since dietary cholesterol is incorporated into chylomicrons and is ultimately transported back to the liver in the chylomicron remnants, thereby increasing hepatic cholesterol content, a diet high in cholesterol leads to suppression of LDL receptor synthesis and decreased catabolic removal of LDL. By reducing dietary cholesterol, hepatic cholesterol content is reduced, LDL receptor synthesis is "up-regulated" and the LDL fractional catabolic rate is accelerated leading to a decrease in the LDL-cholesterol concentration. In this indirect manner, dietary cholesterol is an important determinant of LDL-cholesterol metabolism but not, as so many people believe, because dietary cholesterol is directly incorporated into LDL-cholesterol. In patients with carbohydrate-sensitive hypertriglyceridemia, the content of refined carbohydrate should be reduced and replaced with complex carbohydrate. In patients with hyperchylomicronemia (Type I or V), dietary fat should be severely restricted. Caloric restriction to promote weight loss in obese patients may be helpful, both for treatment of hypertriglyceridemia and diabetes mellitus.

Drugs

Cholestyramine and Colestipol. These drugs are anionic exchange resins that bind bile acids in the intestine, increase hepatic conversion of cholesterol to bile acids, and deplete hepatic cholesterol. The reduction in LDL-cholesterol is due to an increase in hepatic synthesis of LDL receptors and acceleration of LDL disposal. Cholestyramine and colestipol are particularly effective in the treatment of hypercholesterolemia, and because they are not absorbed, they are not associated with systemic side effects. They are, however, often accompanied by distressing gastrointestinal symptoms that include constipation, abdominal distention, flatulence, nausea, and vomiting. The side effects appear to be less troublesome if therapy is initiated with small doses, and increased gradually over several weeks. The maximum dose of cholestyramine is 32 g/day, and that of colestipol is 30 g/day. When used in satisfactory doses, they are capable of reducing the LDL cholesterol concentration by 20 to 25%, and reducing the risk of coronary heart disease. The HDL-cholesterol concentration is unchanged or increased slightly.

Nicotinic Acid. Nicotinic acid may be the most ideal of the lipid lowering drugs, since it reduces both VLDLs and LDLs and increases HDLs. Its precise mechanism of action is still poorly understood. In pharmacologic doses, it decreases the synthesis of VLDLs and LDLs. The increase in HDL concentration is due to a reduction in the fractional catabolic disposal of HDL and is not due to increased synthesis. In effective doses, nicotinic acid can reduce the plasma triglyceride and LDL-cholesterol levels by 20 to 40%, and increase the HDL-cholesterol by 20%. Therapy should be initiated with small doses taken 3 times per day, preferably with meals. The dose can be gradually increased to 1 g 3 times per day. The maximum tolerable dose of nicotinic acid is 9 g/day. The drug may be difficult for many patients to use, causing flushing of the skin, pruritus, skin dryness, and eye irritation. It may also produce abnormalities in liver enzymes, hyperuricemia, and hyperglycemia. The flushing can be diminished by taking one aspirin before each dose, and by avoiding foods that cause vasodilation and flushing, such as alcohol and hot liquids.

Fibric Acid Derivatives. The first generation drug in this class was clofibrate. It is capable of reducing plasma VLDL levels, and consequently, the triglyceride concentrations, while its effects on LDL-cholesterol are relatively inconsequential. Clofibrate also increases the HDL-cholesterol concentration. Although the mechanism of action is still incompletely understood, these drugs work primarily by enhancing VLDL clearance. They are most effective in patients in whom hypertriglyceridemia, alone or with hypercholesterolemia, is the major problem. They are particularly useful in patients with dysbetalipoproteinemia, and seldom useful in patients with isolated hypertriglyceridemia. The second generation drug, gemfibrozil, is similar to clofibrate, but may have fewer side effects. Its ability to increase the HDL-cholesterol appears to be somewhat greater than that of clofibrate. In many patients, these drugs are no more effective than diet.

Probucol. The mechanism of action of probucol is not completely understood. It appears to accelerate the fractional catabolic removal of LDL, but it inhibits apoprotein AI synthesis, and therefore reduces the HDL-cholesterol concentration. The HDL-cholesterol concentration is reduced to a greater extent than the LDL-cholesterol concentration, so that the net effect is an increase in the LDL:HDL ratio, which is undesirable. Consequently, it should now only be used as a ''second-line'' drug.

Inhibitors of Hydroxymethylglutaryl Co-A Reductase. A number of drugs are currently under investigation that reduce the LDL-cholesterol concentration by inhibiting the rate limiting enzyme of cholesterol synthesis (hydroxymethylglutaryl CoA reductase). As intracellular levels of cholesterol decrease, the synthesis of LDL receptors increases, leading to an increase in the fractional catabolic removal of LDL-cholesterol. LDL-cholesterol concentrations may be reduced by 20 to 40% with no appreciable changes in HDL-cholesterol.

Combined Therapy. The cholesterol lowering agents may be used in combination to take advantage of the specific actions of individual drugs. Thus, cholestyramine can be used in combination with nicotinic acid, probucol, and the inhibitors of cholesterol synthesis. Combined therapy may be capable of reducing the LDL-cholesterol concentration by 40 to 60% and normalizing it in some patients with heterozygous FHC.

CLINICAL PROBLEMS

Patient 1. A 42-year-old man developed eruptive xanthomas and recurrent bouts of abdominal pain. His plasma triglyceride concentration was 3275 mg/dl and his plasma cholesterol concentration was 860 mg/dl. Plasma placed in a refrigerator for 12 hours revealed generalized lactescence without a cream layer. He did not have diabetes mellitus, nor did he use alcohol. He weighed 235 pounds, and was 71 inches tall. His family history was noteworthy for several siblings with both hypercholesterolemia and hypertriglyceridemia, but not of the magnitude displayed by the patient. His two children also demonstrated hypercholesterolemia and hypertriglyceridemia, with cholesterol levels of 250 and 290 mg/dl, and triglyceride, levels of 325 and 300 mg/dl, respectively.

A weight reduction diet was instituted with a 65 pound weight loss over 6 months. His cholesterol decreased to 295 mg/dl (LDL-C, 195 mg/dl; HDL-C, 20 mg/dl), and his triglyceride decreased to 400 mg/dl. The addition of gemfibrozil reduced his cholesterol to 205 mg/dl, and his triglyceride to 250 mg/dl.

QUESTIONS
1. What is the lipoprotein phenotype?
2. What is the disorder that has produced this lipoprotein disturbance?
3. What is the role of obesity and how did weight loss benefit the patient?
4. What is the cause of his recurrent abdominal pain?
5. What is the risk of developing coronary heart disease in this family?

Patient 2. The patient is a 59-old-man referred for treatment of hypercholesterolemia. He underwent coronary artery bypass grafting at 50 years, and carotid endarterectomy at 56 years of age. He has had bilateral xanthelasmas most of his adult life, and has both achilles tendon xanthomas and xanthomas of the extensor tendons of his hands. He now exercises vigorously each day without chest pain, dizziness, or claudication. One of his two children, a daughter, has hypercholesterolemia and xanthelasmas, but is otherwise asymptomatic. His plasma is perfectly clear and his cholesterol is 300 mg/dl, and triglyceride, 110 mg/dl. On diet and full doses of cholestyramine, his cholesterol decreased to 235 mg/dl, but with a LDL-cholesterol of 180 mg/dl.

QUESTIONS
1. What is the lipid phenotype?
2. What is the disorder and is he a heterozygotic or homozygotic?
3. What is the mechanism of the disorder?
4. What are the secondary causes of hypercholesterolemia?
5. Should additional therapy be prescribed, and if so, which drug?

Patient 3. A 36-year-old successful businessman is referred because of obesity. A glucose tolerance test is normal, but the fasting plasma insulin and the insulin response to glucose is exaggerated. His plasma is slightly lactescent, and the cholesterol and triglyceride concentrations are 190 and 480 mg/dl, respectively. He is placed on a weight reduction diet, and advised to eliminate alcohol; his plasma triglyceride concentration decreases to 150 mg/dl. No other member of his family has a similar disorder.

QUESTIONS
1. What is the lipoprotein phenotype?
2. What are the secondary causes of hypertriglyceridemia?

3. What is the risk of coronary heart disease from the lipoprotein disturbance in this patient?
4. What is the effect of alcohol on HDL-C?

Patient 4. A 37-year-old sedentary man, is evaluated because of vague chest pains and a family history of heart disease. His physical examination was within normal limits. He developed chest pain and a markedly abnormal graded exercise ECG after 7½ minutes on the treadmill. Plasma lipid measurements disclosed a total cholesterol of 195 mg/dl, and a triglyceride of 110 mg/dl. Upon fractionation of the cholesterol, the LDL-C was 155 mg/dl, and the HDL-C was 19 mg/dl. His father and brother, both of whom had heart disease, also had low plasma HDL-cholesterol concentrations.

QUESTIONS
1. What is the role of HDLs in lipid physiology?
2. What are the risk factors for development of coronary heart disease in this patient?
3. What drug would be best for treatment of the lipoprotein disorder(s) in this patient? Why?
4. What drug would be theoretically contraindicated in this patient? Why?

SUGGESTED READING

Physiology and Pathophysiology
Eisenberg, S.: High density lipoprotein metabolism. J Lipid Res, *25*:1017, 1984.
Goldstein, JL, and Brown MS: The LDL receptor defect in familial hypertriglyceridemia: implications for pathogenesis and therapy. Med Clin North Am, *66*:335, 1982.
Goldstein, J.L., Kita, T., and Brown, MS: Detective lipoprotein receptors and atherosclerosis. Lessons from an animal counterpart of familial hypercholesterolemia. N Engl J Med, *309*:288, 1983.
Goldstein, J.L., Schrott, H.G., Hazzard, WR, et al: Hyperlipidemia in coronary heart disease. II. Genetic analysis of lipid levels in 176 families and delineation of a new inherited disorder, combined hyperlipidemia. J Clin Invest, *52*:1544, 1973.
Grundy, S.M.: Hyperlipoproteinemia: metabolic basis and rationale for therapy. Am J Cardiol, *54*:20C, 1984.
Grundy, S.M.: Hypertriglyceridemia: mechanism, clinical significance and treatment. Med Clin North Am, *66*:519, 1982.
Havel, R. (ed): Symposium on lipid disorders. Med Clin North Am, *66*:317, 1982.
Schaeffer, E.J., and Levy, R.I.: Pathogenesis and management of lipoprotein disorders. N Engl J Med, *312*:1300, 1985.
Sniderman, A.D., Wolfson, C., Teug, B., et al.: Association of hyperapobetalipoproteinemia with endogenous hypertriglyceridemia and atherosclerosis. Ann Intern Med, *97*:833, 1982.
Tall, A.R., and Small, D.M.: Current concepts: Plasma high density lipoproteins. N Engl J Med, *299*:1232, 1978.
Tolleshaag, I.T., Hobgood, K.K., Brown, M.S., et al.: The LDL receptor locus in familial hypercholesterolemia: multiple mutations disrupt transport and processing of a membrane receptor. Cell, *32*:941, 1983.

Lipoproteins and Coronary Heart Disease
Castelli, W.P.: Epidemiology of coronary heart disease: The Framingham Study. Am J Med, *76*(2A):4, 1984.
Gordon, T., Castelli, W.P., Hjortland, M.C., et al.: High density lipoprotein as a protective factor against coronary heart disease: the Framingham Study. Am J Med, *62*:707, 1977.
Kannel, W.B., Castelli, W.P., Gordon, T.: Cholesterol in the prediction of atherosclerotic disease. New perspectives based on the Framingham Study. Ann Intern Med, *90*:85, 1975.
Maciejko, J.J., Holmes, D.R., Kottke, B.A., et al.: Apoprotein AI as a marker of angiographically assessed coronary artery disease. N Engl J Med, *309*:387, 1983.
Reardon, M.F., Nestel, P.J., Craig, I.H., et al.: Lipoprotein predictors of the severity of coronary heart in men and women. Circulation, *71*:881, 1985.

Treatment
Brensike, J.F., Levy, R.I., Kelsey, S.F. et al.: Effects of therapy with cholestyramine on progression of coronary atherosclerosis: results of NHLBI Type II Coronary Intervention Study. Circulation, *69*:313, 1984.

Hoeg, J.M., Gregg, R.E., and Brewer, H.B.: An approach to the management of hyperlipo-proteinemia. JAMA, *255*:512, 1986.

Kane, J.P., and Havel, R.F.: Treatment of hypercholesterolemia. Ann Rev Med, *37*:427, 1986.

Kane, J.P., Malloy, M.J., Tun, P., et al.: Normalization of low density lipoprotein levels in heterozygous familial hypercholesterolemia with a combined drug regimen. N Engl J Med, *304*:251, 1981.

Lipid Research Clinics Program: The Lipid Research Clinics Coronary Primary Prevention Trial results. I. Reduction in incidence of coronary heart disease. JAMA, *251*:351, 1984. II. The relationship of reduction in incidence of coronary heart disease to cholesterol lowering. JAMA, *251*:365, 1984.

Mabuchi, H., Hava, T., Tatami, R., et al.: Effects of an inhibitor of 3-hydroxy-3-methylglutaryl CoA reductase on serum lipoproteins and ubiguinone-10 levels in patients with familial hypercholesterolemia. N Engl J Med, *305*:478, 1981.

Mattson, F.H., Erickson, B.A., and Kligman, A.M.: Effect of dietary cholesterol on serum cholesterol in men. Am J Clin Nutr, *24*:589, 1972.

Mellies, M.J., Gartside, P.S., Glatfelter, L, et al.: Effects of probucol on plasma cholesterol, high and low density lipoprotein cholesterol, and apolipoproteins AI and AII in adults with primary hypercholesterolemia. Metabolism, *29*:956, 1980.

The Coronary Drug Project Research Group. Clofibrate and niacin in coronary heart disease. JAMA, *231*:360, 1975.

ANSWERS

Patient 1

1. Phenotype IIb.
2. Familial combined hyperlipidemia.
3. Obesity is associated with insulin resistance and the development of hyperinsulinemia. Insulin stimulates VLDL synthesis and is probably responsible for the hypertriglyceridemia observed in obesity.
4. The recurrent abdominal pain in patients with severe hypertriglyceridemia is due to pancreatitis. Amylase levels may not be increased in blood or urine because an inhibitor of the reaction used for measurement of amylase develops in patients with hypertriglyceridemia. Lipase measurements will be more useful.
5. The risk of coronary heart disease is significantly increased and would be increased, even if the patient had normal LDL-cholesterol levels, because of an increase in apoprotein B levels. Such individuals may have greater numbers of LDL particles with less cholesterol per particle.

Patient 2

1. Phenotype IIa.
2. Familial hypercholesterolemia; heterozygote; homozygotes have plasma total cholesterol concentrations of 600 to 800 mg/dl.
3. The most common mechanism is a reduction (heterozygote) or absence (homozygote) of LDL receptors. Careful study reveals that some patients and their families have receptors that are present but function abnormally; they are clinically indistinguishable from the majority whose receptors are reduced or absent. Thus, even FHC is heterogeneous.
4. Hypothyroidism, nephrotic syndrome, dysglobulinemia, liver disease, and acute intermittent porphyria.
5. The next drug to be used should be nicotinic acid, in fact, some recommend it as the drug of choice with the resins to be used as "second-line" therapy. Both nicotinic acid and probucol will further decrease the LDL-cholesterol; nicotinic acid is preferable because it increases HDL-cholesterol, while probucol decreases HDL cholesterol. Since nicotinic acid decreases LDL synthesis and the resins increase LDL degradation, their mechanisms of action are complementary.

Patient 3

1. Phenotype IV.
2. Diabetes mellitus, obesity, alcoholism, nephrotic syndrome, dysglobulinemia, and hepatocellular disease.
3. Probably the same as that of the general population. Measurement of apoproteins A and

B more accurately reflect risk than measurement of cholesterol and triglyceride. Curiously, patients with hypertriglyceridemia often have low HDL-cholesterol levels that may not correct with control of the hypertriglyceridemia.

4. Alcohol (2 ounces per day of whiskey or the equivalent of beer or wine) raises HDLs and may protect against coronary heart disease. A recent study demonstrated that alcohol increased the HDL_3 subfraction and not HDL_2, which is the species that best correlates with protection against heart disease.

Patient 4

1. HDLs function to transport cholesterol from the periphery to the liver for excretion.
2. Both high LDL and low HDL; his LDL-C is at the 75th percentile for his age and his HDL-C is severely reduced. His LDL-C/HDL-C ratio is 7.75 and his mortality risk ratio is 2.5 to 3.0.
3. Nicotinic acid would be best for this patient because it decreases LDL and increases HDL.
4. Probucol should be avoided because it decreases HDL synthesis.

Index

Page numbers in *italics* indicate figures; numbers followed by "t" indicate tables.